Asian Medical Industries

This book develops the concept of *Asian Medical Industries* as a novel perspective on traditional Asian medicines.

Complementing and updating existing work in this field, the book provides a critical and comparative analytic framework for understanding Chinese Medicine, Ayurveda, Sowa Rigpa, and Japanese Kampo in the 21st century. No longer subaltern health resources or conservative systems of traditional knowledge, these medicines have become an integral part of modern Asia as innovative, lucrative industries. Ten original case studies employ insights from anthropology, history, geography, pharmaceutical sciences, botany, and economics to trace the transformation of Asian medical traditions into rapidly growing and dynamic pharmaceutical industries. Collectively, these contributions identify this as a major phenomenon impacting Asian and global healthcare, economics, cultural politics, and environments. The book suggests that we can learn more about Asian medicines today by approaching them as industries rather than as cultural or epistemic systems.

Asian Medical Industries is a highly original resource for students and scholars across a range of academic fields such as anthropology, history, and Asian studies, as well as medical practitioners, health sector actors, and policymakers.

Stephan Kloos is Acting Director of the Institute for Social Anthropology at the Austrian Academy of Sciences. His research on the development of Sowa Rigpa has been published in numerous articles and the co-edited volume *Healing at the Periphery: Ethnographies of Tibetan Medicine in India* (Pordié & Kloos).

Calum Blaikie is a Senior Researcher at the Institute for Social Anthropology, the Austrian Academy of Sciences. Focusing on pharmaceutical, institutional, and economic dimensions of Sowa Rigpa in the Himalayas, his research has been published in numerous leading academic journals and edited volumes.

NEEDHAM RESEARCH INSTITUTE SERIES
Series Editor: Christopher Cullen

Joseph Needham's 'Science and Civilisation' series began publication in the 1950s. At first it was seen as a piece of brilliant but isolated pioneering. However, at the beginning of the twenty-first century, it became clear that Needham's work had succeeded in creating a vibrant new intellectual field in the West. The books in this series cover topics that broadly relate to the practice of science, technology and medicine in East Asia, including China, Japan, Korea and Vietnam. The emphasis is on traditional forms of knowledge and practice, but without excluding modern studies that connect their topics with their historical and cultural context.

Celestial Lancets
A history and rationale of acupuncture and moxa
Lu Gwei-Djen and Joseph Needham
With a new introduction by Vivienne Lo

A Chinese Physician
Wang Ji and the Stone Mountain medical case histories
Joanna Grant

Chinese Mathematical Astrology
Reaching out to the stars
Ho Peng Yoke

Medieval Chinese Medicine
The Dunhuang medical manuscripts
Edited by Vivienne Lo and Christopher Cullen

Chinese Medicine in Early Communist China, 1945–1963
Medicine of revolution
Kim Taylor

Explorations in Daoism
Medicine and alchemy in literature
Ho Peng Yoke

Tibetan Medicine in the Contemporary World
Global politics of medical knowledge and practice
Edited by Laurent Pordié

The Evolution of Chinese Medicine
Northern Song dynasty, 960–1127
Asaf Goldschmidt

Speaking of Epidemics in Chinese Medicine
Disease and the geographic imagination in Late Imperial China
Marta E. Hanson

Reviving Ancient Chinese Mathematics
Mathematics, history and politics in the work of Wu Wen-Tsun
Jiri Hudecek

Rice, Agriculture, and the Food Supply in Premodern Japan
Charlotte von Verschuer Translated and edited by Wendy Cobcroft

The Politics of Chinese Medicine under Mongol Rule
Reiko Shinno

Asian Medical Industries
Contemporary Perspectives on Traditional Pharmaceuticals
Edited by Stephan Kloos and Calum Blaikie

Asian Medical Industries
Contemporary Perspectives on Traditional Pharmaceuticals

**Edited by
Stephan Kloos and Calum Blaikie**

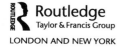

LONDON AND NEW YORK

First published 2022
by Routledge
2 Park Square, Milton Park, Abingdon, Oxon OX14 4RN

and by Routledge
605 Third Avenue, New York, NY 10158

*Routledge is an imprint of the Taylor & Francis Group,
an informa business*

© 2022 selection and editorial matter, Stephan Kloos and Calum Blaikie; individual chapters, the contributors

The right of Stephan Kloos and Calum Blaikie to be identified as the authors of the editorial material, and of the authors for their individual chapters, has been asserted in accordance with sections 77 and 78 of the Copyright, Designs and Patents Act 1988.

All rights reserved. No part of this book may be reprinted or reproduced or utilised in any form or by any electronic, mechanical, or other means, now known or hereafter invented, including photocopying and recording, or in any information storage or retrieval system, without permission in writing from the publishers.

Trademark notice: Product or corporate names may be trademarks or registered trademarks, and are used only for identification and explanation without intent to infringe.

British Library Cataloguing-in-Publication Data
A catalogue record for this book is available from the British Library

Library of Congress Cataloging-in-Publication Data
A catalog record has been requested for this book

ISBN: 978-1-032-11022-6 (hbk)
ISBN: 978-1-032-11025-7 (pbk)
ISBN: 978-1-003-21807-4 (ebk)

DOI: 10.4324/9781003218074

Typeset in Times NR MT Pro
by KnowledgeWorks Global Ltd.

Contents

List of illustrations ix
Notes on contributors x

Introduction: Asian medical industries 1
STEPHAN KLOOS

PART I
East Asian medical industries 29

1 Discovering new drugs in "Traditional" Chinese Medicine: Inside Guangzhou Huahai pharmaceuticals 31
LIZ P.Y. CHEE

2 Cultivation and paternalism in the service of the market: Medical industry and ethnicity in Southwest China 51
MANUEL CAMPINAS

3 The development of the Kampo medicines industry: "Good Practices" and health policy making in Japan 81
ICHIRO ARAI, JULIA S. YONGUE, AND KIICHIRO TSUTANI

4 The pharmaceutical industry of Toyama prefecture, Japan: *Haichi* household medicines, intersectoral collaboration, and industrial clustering 110
TOMOKO FUTAYA AND CALUM BLAIKIE

PART II
South Asian medical industries — 137

5 Globalising Ayurveda, branding India: Implications for the Ayurvedic pharmaceutical industry — 139
CHITHPRABHA KUDLU

6 Industry dynamics and clustering in Ayurvedic pharmaceutical production in South India: The case of CARe Keralam — 169
HARILAL MADHAVAN AND SAJITHA SOMAN

7 Untangling the web of raw material supply for Ayurvedic industry: The complex geography of plant circulations — 194
LUCIE DEJOUHANET AND SREELAKSHMY M.

PART III
Sowa Rigpa industries — 225

8 "Sourcery": Losing track of Tibetan medicinal plants between commerce and conservation in Northern India — 227
JAN M. A. VAN DER VALK

9 Making Tibetan medicine in Nepal: Industrial aspirations, cooperative relations, and precarious production — 253
CALUM BLAIKIE AND SIENNA R. CRAIG

10 The emergence of the Traditional Mongolian Medicine industry: Communism, continuity, and reassemblage — 280
STEPHAN KLOOS

Conclusion: Assembling Asian pharmaceuticals — 305
CALUM BLAIKIE

Index — 341

List of illustrations

Tables

6.1	Approved Ayurveda clusters in India in 2016	176
6.2	Initial costs of the CARe Keralam project	177
6.3	Constraints of the industry at various nodes	178

Figures

3.1	A comparison of prescription and OTC Kampo medicines sales in Japan (1976–2018). Source: Japan Kampo Medicines Manufacturers Association (2019).	90
7.1	The state channel for NTFPs used in Ayurveda (Dejouhanet 2014b).	200
7.2	Itineraries of NTFPs through hybrid networks.	204
7.3	The complex organisation of Ayurvedic raw material supply in central Kerala.	212

Notes on contributors

Ichiro Arai is a professor and dean of the graduate school of pharmaceutical sciences at Nihon Pharmaceutical University in Japan. His professional area of expertise is the regulatory sciences of traditional and complementary integrative medicine. He is also working to formulate health policies and standards in this area in international organisations.

Calum Blaikie is a senior researcher at the Institute for Social Anthropology, the Austrian Academy of Sciences. Focusing on pharmaceutical, institutional, and economic dimensions of Sowa Rigpa in the Himalayas, his research has been published in numerous leading academic journals and edited volumes. He currently leads an Austrian Science Fund project (P34010-G) investigating the integration of Sowa Rigpa into Indian governmental structures and healthcare systems (2021–2024).

Manuel Campinas is a pharmacist and a medical anthropologist specialising in the anthropology of pharmaceuticals. He completed his doctoral degree at the London School of Hygiene and Tropical Medicine. Having previously conducted fieldwork in Siberia on "folk medicine" and post-Soviet transformations, his recent ethnographic research focuses on the industrialisation of "ethnic minority medicine" in China. He is also a member of the Anthropology of Antimicrobial Resistance Research Group at LSHTM.

Liz P.Y. Chee is a research fellow in the S.T.S. Cluster of the Asia Research Institute (ARI) and a Fellow of Tembusu College, both at the National University of Singapore (NUS). She is the author of *Mao's Bestiary: Medicinal Animals and Modern China* (Durham: Duke University Press, 2021) and writes primarily about Chinese Medicine. She has previously published articles on shark-fin eating, Chinese proteomics, and the cultural boundaries between food and medicine.

Sienna R. Craig is a professor of anthropology at Dartmouth College in Hanover, NH, USA. As a cultural anthropologist and a writer, her work is centred on experiences of health and illness, cultures of medicine, and the dynamics of migration. Her publications include *The Ends of Kinship: Connecting Himalayan Lives between Nepal and New York* (University of Washington Press, 2020); *Healing Elements: Efficacy and the Social Ecologies of Tibetan Medicine* (University of California Press, 2012); and *Horses Like Lightning: A Story of Passage through the Himalaya* (Wisdom Publications, 2008).

Lucie Dejouhanet is an assistant professor in geography at the University of the French West Indies (AIHP-GEODE EA 929). Working on Ayurvedic raw material supply since 2004, she published *L'Inde, puissance en construction* (2016), and was appointed as Junior member of the Institut Universitaire de France in 2019.

Tomoko Futaya holds a PhD in economics from the University of Tokyo and is currently a professor of Japanese economic history at Aichi Gakuin University, Nagoya. Her current research concerns the economic history of consumption, healthcare, and the pharmaceutical industry in modern Japan. Her major recent publications include the book *Kindai Nihon no Shohi to Seikatsu Sekai* (with Satoru Nakanishi, Yoshikawakobunkan, 2018, in Japanese), and the chapter "Health and Medicine" in *Keizaishakai no Rekisi* (ed. Satoru Nakanishi, Nagoya University Press, 2017, in Japanese).

Stephan Kloos is acting director of the Institute for Social Anthropology at the Austrian Academy of Sciences. He has worked on Sowa Rigpa in India, China, Mongolia, and Russia since 2001 and led an ERC project (RATIMED) on the transnational Sowa Rigpa industry (2014–2019). He is coeditor (with Laurent Pordié) of *Healing at the Periphery: Ethnographies of Tibetan Medicine in India* (Duke University Press, 2022) and has published in numerous leading academic journals. His work can be accessed at stephankloos.org.

Chithprabha Kudlu received her PhD in psychology from the Indian Institute of Technology, Bombay (2000), and her PhD in cultural anthropology from Washington University in St. Louis (2013). She is currently an independent researcher based in India investigating the history and practice of Ayurveda in Kerala State.

Harilal Madhavan is a development economist and faculty member at the Indian Institute of Science Education and Research, Thiruvananthapuram (IISER TVM), India. His work specialises in the traditional pharmaceutical industry (especially Ayurvedic and Tibetan pharmaceuticals), global public health policy, and intellectual property rights.

Sajitha Soman is a columnist and an independent economist based in Thiruvananthapuram, India. Her research mainly focuses on trade in services and traditional health seeking practices of South Indians.

Sreelakshmy M. is an assistant professor at Nirmala College for Women in Coimbatore, Tamil Nadu, India, where she has taught geography for the last seven years to both undergraduate and postgraduate students. Her main research interests are water resources management and geomorphology.

Kiichiro Tsutani holds a PhD in clinical pharmacology and has worked as a medical officer for traditional medicines at the World Health Organization. His current research activities focus on health technology assessment, complementary medicine, and history of drug regulation.

Jan M.A. van der Valk is a scholar-practitioner trained in the fields of biology (University of Leuven), ethnobotany and anthropology (University of Kent), and Tibetan studies (Rangjung Yeshe Institute, Kathmandu University). For his PhD dissertation in anthropology (2017) and currently, as a postdoctoral researcher in the Austrian Science Fund project "Potent Substances in Sowa Rigpa and Buddhist Ritual" (University of Vienna), he has mainly focused on how natural substances are transformed into potent medicines by working with traders, manufacturers, and *materia medica* experts in Switzerland, India, and Nepal.

Julia S. Yongue is a professor in the Faculty of Economics at Hosei University in Japan. Her research intersects the history of business and medicine and focuses on how health policy has influenced the development of the Japanese pharmaceutical industry since the late nineteenth century.

Introduction

Asian medical industries

Stephan Kloos

Asian medicines are not what they used to be. No longer simply subaltern resources for the poor or struggling systems of traditional knowledge, they have become an integral part of modern Asia as official health care providers and innovative, lucrative pharmaceutical industries. While faith healers, village herbalists, and venerable scholar-practitioners remain important health resources in much of Asia and continue to shape popular images of "traditional" Asian medicine – not least as favourite subjects of anthropological studies and TV commercials marketing Asian medicines to urban audiences – their actual importance has declined throughout Asia. Conversely, mass-produced and professionally marketed "traditional" Asian health products and therapies have entered and altered mainstream healthcare not only in Asian countries but around the world. These developments constitute an industrial revolution of Asian medicines, the significance and magnitude of which cannot be underestimated. Long marginalised by biomedicine and government policies in the nineteenth and twentieth centuries, Asian medicines are today consumed by over half the world's population, command a market value far exceeding 100 billion USD,[1] have their own government ministries,[2] and even claim a Nobel Prize for medicine.[3] It is hardly surprising, therefore, that they play an increasingly important role in national and global health policies and, beyond the field of health, in Asia's economic and political ascendance. Yet while their remarkable trajectory of professionalisation, modernisation, and globalisation during the twentieth century

---

1 No reliable figures exist regarding the total economic value of Asian medicines, and especially data on the TCM industry – which dominates the field – vary dramatically (between 25 and over 130 billion USD).
2 For example, Ayurveda, Unani, Siddha, and Sowa Rigpa are administrated by the Indian Ministry of AYUSH since 2014.
3 In 2015, Tu Youyou won the Nobel Prize for extracting the antimalarial *artemisinin* from the Chinese herb *artemisia annua*, claiming to have drawn her inspiration from a fourth-century Chinese medical text (Chee, this volume; Hanson 2015; Hsu 2015). The TCM profession was quick to claim the Nobel Prize for itself, which led to a massive upgrading of state funded TCM research in China.

DOI: 10.4324/9781003218074-1

has been reasonably well studied, scholarship has by and large stopped short of explicitly focusing on and analysing the larger direction and outcome of this transformation: Asian medical industries.

The term Asian medical industries refers to the health industries that have emerged from the scholarly medical traditions of East, South, Inner, and Muslim Asia, including most notably Chinese medicine and related East Asian medicines like Japanese Kampo or Korean Hanbang, Ayurveda, Sowa Rigpa (Tibetan, Mongolian and Himalayan medicines), and Unani Tibb. While all these health industries have significant non-pharmaceutical aspects – think of acupuncture, different kinds of massage, and so on – this book only focuses on the pharmaceutical domain, which includes prescription drugs but also various categories of over-the-counter (OTC) medicines, nutritional supplements, and functional foods. Indeed, a key dimension of Asian medical industries is the fundamental *reformulation* (Pordié and Gaudillière 2014c) of Asian medicines, both in a literal, material sense concerning their ingredients and formulas, and in a figurative sense that encompasses their epistemologies, legal status, and regulatory aspects. Perhaps most significantly, this reformulation also entails a gradual, partial shift of focus from the clinical/medical sphere to the pharmaceutical/economic domain, where the main actors are no longer individual practitioners or local collectors (although, as this volume shows, they remain important), but companies and professional associations (cf. Gaudillière 2014b). While rooted in a general capitalisation of health (Gaudillière and Sunder Rajan 2021), the notion of "industry" itself exceeds the narrow economic domain of health products, corporations, and the market, encompassing the entire field of sociocultural, political, technological, scientific, and medical phenomena involved in the contemporary production, use, and transformation of Asian medicines in the widest sense. Consequently, Asian medical industries produce not only health commodities and economic profits but also political, social, cultural, and moral values.

Asian medical industries constitute a wider field than can be comprehensively covered within the space of one book. Thus, this volume does not contain chapters on the industries of Unani Tibb, Korean Hanbang, Siddha, Miao medicine, and Southeast Asian medicines (e.g. Thai, Khmer, Vietnamese, Indonesian, Myanmar), even if Unani has a significant presence in Muslim South and Central Asia (Attewell 2005; Schmidt Stiedenroth 2020), the Miao medicine industry in China is reportedly of similar value as the Ayurveda industry (Yang and Peng 2015), and the Korean herbal medicine industry is comparable to that of Kampo in Japan (Ma 2015, 2019). For the most part, these medical traditions – and particularly their emerging industries – remain under-researched, which is especially true for Southeast Asian medicines (see Coderey and Pordié 2019 for some notable exceptions). Yet even the industries of the classical and relatively well-studied medical traditions of East, South, and Inner Asia, which this volume focuses on, are only beginning to attract serious scholarship. Indeed, despite excellent initial forays, they remain largely uncharted territory for the social sciences, perhaps partly due to their enormous size, multiple dimensions, and rapid transformations. Building on existing work on the professionalisation, modernisation, commercialisation, pharmaceuticalisation, and globalisation of Chinese medicine, Kampo, Ayurveda, and Sowa Rigpa,[4] we thus seek to critically trace the ongoing industrial revolution of these Asian medicines and explore the characteristics of Asian medical industries as a larger phenomenon in the contemporary world.

Asian medical industries can also be understood to encompass the vast and dynamic Asian biomedical and biotech sector, where especially China and India act as major global players. Although this volume does not focus on Asian biomedicines per se, it centrally underscores the increasing obsolescence of a hard conceptual division between "traditional" and "modern" (i.e. biomedical) pharmaceuticals in the Asian industrial context. Kampo medicines, for example, need to comply with mainstream biomedical drug laws and regulations, while the Japanese biomedical pharmaceutical industry was significantly developed by herbal medicine producers; the research-and-development processes of many Ayurvedic products do not significantly differ from those of Western healthcare commodities; and "traditional Chinese medicines" (TCM itself being a modern invention) are produced in the same kind of high-tech factories – even, at times, by the same companies – as biomedicines. Conversely, Asian pharmacopeias are subjected to extensive biomedical research and bioprospecting, leading to successful biomedical drugs such as Novartis' antimalarial drug Coartem® or Roche's anti-viral Tamiflu®. Biomedical and consumer goods companies the world over increasingly respond to Asian medical competition by marketing their own herbal health products or even participate directly in the Asian medicines sector, such as Procter & Gamble's Ayurvedic Vicks® products. As Asian medicines can no longer be considered "traditional" and increasingly share the same scientific, regulatory, and market space as biomedicine, the modern-traditional dichotomy makes less sense than ever. Similar to the Asian biotech sector (e.g. Sunder Rajan 2006, 2017; Ong and Chen 2010) or the biomedically conceived "pharmaceutical nexus" (Petryna and Kleinman 2006), Asian medical industries constitute transnational and capitalist pharmaceutical assemblages (Kloos 2017a). Yet too often, they are still implicitly framed as marginal domains of tradition and culture, rather than as the important public health, economic and political – but also cultural – assets they have become.

---

4 For work on the professionalisation of Asian medicines, see Leslie (1968, 1973), Scheid (2002), Craig (2008). On modernisation, see Leslie (1974), Adams (2007), Adams and Li (2008). On commercialisation, see Banerjee (2002), Hsu (2008b), Madhavan (2009). On pharmaceuticalisation, see Banerjee (2008), Blaikie (2015), Kloos (2017a). On globalisation, see Alter (2005), Zhan (2009), Kloos (2020).

How did "traditional" Asian medical systems become "modern" industries? How do they operate today, and what is their role in ongoing transformations of health, medicine, and society in contemporary Asia? How can we study Asian medicines as industries rather than as "traditional culture," and what might this contribute to medical anthropology and other social studies of medicine and Asia? In addressing some of these questions, the present volume provides a comparative perspective on Asian medicines *as industries* in a larger regional and historical context. In doing so, it offers new insights into the emergence and evolution of Asian medical industries, their various paths of integration into official health care systems, and their sources of raw materials. Even more importantly, *Asian medical industries* outlines and applies a new analytic framework that transcends, like its subject, the conceptual domains of "tradition," "culture," or "medical systems." This opens Asian medicines to the kind of critical scholarly inquiry that has so far largely remained limited to biomedicine, while at the same time challenging the unnecessarily narrow biomedical focus of notions like pharmaceutical reason (Lakoff 2005), the pharmaceutical nexus (Petryna and Kleinman 2006), biocapital (Sunder Rajan 2006), pharmaceutical capitalism (Gaudillière and Sunder Rajan 2021), most work on global health (e.g. Biehl and Petryna 2013; Farmer et al. 2013), and the field of medical anthropology itself (cf. Scherz 2018).[5] There is no good reason why Asian medical industries should not be considered in critical explorations of contemporary health and healthcare, especially as they explicitly and strategically address public health issues like care and aging, mental health, and chronic illness (e.g. Lock 1980, 1993; Cohen 1998; Lang 2018).

Beyond medical systems

Both in its pan-Asian comparative approach and its insistence on a fundamental reframing of its subject, this book follows a similar agenda as Charles Leslie's seminal volume *Asian Medical Systems* (Leslie 1976b). Studying Asian medicines as *cultural and epistemic systems* yielded unprecedented insights into their histories, medical theories, healing modalities, the transmission of knowledge, and encounters with the "other" in the form of biomedicine, modernity, or the world – the very foundation that current scholarship on Asian medicines, including this volume, builds on. It was thanks to Leslie's intervention that Asian medicines began to be taken seriously as medical, scholarly, and indeed civilisational systems in Western academic circles, substantially contributing to the development of the nascent fields of medical

---

5 The strong biomedicalisation of medical anthropology over recent decades is well demonstrated by the otherwise comprehensive and wide-ranging Routledge Handbook of Medical Anthropology (Manderson et al. 2016), which remarkably does not cover "traditional and complementary medicine" at all.

anthropology and Asian medical history. Topics like medical pluralism, explanatory models, professionalisation, modernisation, and later also globalisation became central problems addressed by medical anthropological research up to this day, while medical historians began to challenge biomedically dominated historiographies by tracing previously invisible histories of Asian medicines. Leslie's work and legacy – including successor volumes to Asian Medical Systems (Leslie and Young 1992; Bates 1995; Connor and Samuel 2001; Alter 2005) and the large number of studies on each of these systems individually – both documented and participated in the gradual emergence of Asian medicines as markers of national identity (e.g. Langford 2002; Kloos 2011), intellectual history (e.g. Prakash 1999), and alternative modernities (e.g. Hsu 2009; Pordié and Gaudillière 2014a) in different parts of the continent. In order to contextualise the chapters that follow, a brief overview of the East, South, and Inner Asian "medical systems" is necessary.

Classical Chinese medicine can be traced back to the writing of its foundational texts between the third century BCE and the third century CE (Unschuld 1985; Scheid 2007), including the *Huangdi Neijing* (Yellow Emperor's Inner Canon), the *Shang Hanlun* (Treatise on Cold Damage Disorders and Miscellaneous Illnesses), and the *Huangdi Bashiyi Nanjing* (Yellow Emperor's Canon of Eighty-One Difficult Issues). Although these canons provided its core concepts and cosmology, it was not before unprecedented state involvement during the Song dynasty (960–1279 CE) that Chinese medicine emerged as a systematic scholarly medicine (Goldschmidt 2008), which also spread to neighboring Japan, Korea, and Vietnam (Otsuka 1976; Park et al. 2012). The impact of Western medicine and modernity from the nineteenth century onwards constituted a third major turning point in the history of Chinese medicine, leading to the creation of a new, modern "species" of Chinese medicine in the Republican Period from the 1920s onward, which – somewhat ironically – came to be called "Traditional Chinese Medicine" or simply TCM (Lei 2014). During the early years of the communist People's Republic of China, this still marginal "mongrel medicine" (ibid.) was reworked into a standardised theoretical system with a nationwide network of institutions (Taylor 2005) and was later successively integrated into national health care policy (Farquhar 1994; Park et al. 2012). China's transition to a market economy in the 1990s, the inclusion of TCM in China's national health insurance in 1999, and the country's WTO entry in 2001 created the conditions for the emergence of a fully fledged TCM industry. In 2017, China's first law on Chinese medicine came into effect, explicitly positioning Chinese medicine – the term now also including China's minority medicines – on an equal level to biomedicine. Meanwhile, TCM (including acupuncture) has spread around the globe (Hsu 2008a, 2008b) and moved out of Chinatowns into mainstream healthcare, fundamentally remaking itself in the process (Zhan 2009).

Despite the overwhelming size and importance of Chinese medicine and an outstanding body of scholarship concerning it, its *industry* remains among the least studied among major Asian medical traditions. To be sure, scholars have noted the emergence of a Chinese herbal industry and the concomitant pharmaceuticalisation of Chinese medicine from the 1950s and especially the 1990s onwards (Scheid 2002; Taylor 2005: 77–78), the onset of Chinese medicine entrepreneurship and its commercialisation during the 1980s (Farquhar 1996), and the entrance of Chinese proprietary medicines into global wellness markets in the 2000s (Hsu 2009). Nonetheless, most of these studies treat the Chinese medicine industry as peripheral to other concerns, with only a few scholars - most notably Liz Chee (2021) - addressing it more directly (Kuo 2015; Smith 2019; Wang 2019), including scholars of Ayurveda providing interesting comparative perspectives (Islam 2017; Kudlu and Nichter 2019). Similarly, Japanese Kampo and Korean Hanbang, which originated from Chinese medicine but were shaped by centuries of independent development (van Put 1995; Hanson 2016; Kang and Kim 2016), remain understudied as medical industries. A small number of articles on the Japanese Kampo medicines industry (Arai 2009; Umemura 2011) and a larger number on the Korean herbal medicines industry (Cho 2000; Kim 2006, 2009; Ma 2015, 2019; Lee 2016) are notable exceptions. Nonetheless, the comparative dearth of serious social science research on East Asian medical industries stands in sharp contrast to the large number of botanical, pharmacological, and clinical studies being published on these medicines in China, Japan, and South Korea, underscoring the importance of placing such industry-driven knowledge production in social, political, and historical context. The four chapters dedicated to East Asian medical industries in this volume thus break new ground in presenting hitherto non-existent historical and ethnographic insights into the Chinese medicine and Japanese Kampo industries.

The roots of Indian medicine are often traced back to the Vedic Period (ca. 1500–500 BCE), but Ayurveda (the "science of longevity") as a distinct medical tradition emerged only around the time of the Buddha (fifth to fourth century BCE) in the North Indian ascetic milieu (Zysk 1991). Its foundational compendia, the "great triad" consisting of the *Caraka Samhita*, *Sushruta Samhita*, and *Ashtangahridaya Samhita*, were compiled between the last centuries BCE and the seventh century CE (Wujastyk 1998; Meulenbeld 1999–2002), defining Ayurveda in its classical form. They were also widely translated and known far beyond India. Referring to a fifth-century description of public hospitals, Dominik Wujastyk (1998: 2) remarks that "India may have been the first part of the world to have evolved an organised cosmopolitan system of institutionally-based medical provision." Even after what is considered its golden age, Ayurveda continued to refine its knowledge and dynamically adapt to India's changing sociocultural, political, and religious context, including the decline of Buddhism after the seventh century, Muslim influx beginning in the eleventh century, and the period of Mughal dominance from the fourteenth to the eighteenth centuries (Smith and Wujastyk 2008). This was also true for the early colonial period from the sixteenth to the nineteenth century when Indian medical knowledge was treated with sympathetic interest and respect by the European traders and colonialists (Patterson 1987). However, the emergence of modern medicine in Europe and a radical change in British colonial policy in 1835 led to the invalidation and marginalisation of Indian medicines, while Western medicine was instituted as the only legitimate form of official healthcare. Faced with existential crisis and in resistance to such colonial policies, Ayurvedic practitioners began organising themselves to respond to the challenge of modern biomedicine. Subsequently, during the early and mid-twentieth century, they gradually transformed Ayurveda "from an eclectic set of healing practices to a quintessentially Indian medicine" (Langford 2002: 7), laying the foundations for its more recent revival.

Ayurveda's modernisation and professionalisation in the second half of the twentieth century have been extensively studied (e.g. Leslie 1968, 1974, 1976a; Brass 1972; Langford 2002; Wujastyk and Smith 2008), and its increasing commercialisation and pharmaceuticalisation have already been noted in the late 1980s and 1990s (Leslie 1989; Nichter 1996). A decade later, Maarten Bode and Madhulika Banerjee first considered Ayurveda and Unani as industries, analysing Ayurvedic pharmaceutical companies' combination of traditional and modern knowledge, practices, and identities (Bode 2008), and critically tracing Ayurveda's gradual industrialisation from colonial times up to the present (Banerjee 2009). Based on the notion of "reformulation regimes" (Pordié and Gaudillière 2014c), Laurent Pordié and Jean-Paul Gaudillière's special journal issue *The Herbal Pharmaceutical Industry in India* (2014a) explored innovation processes and intellectual property rights as central to the reinvention of Ayurveda as a pharmaceutical industry. Pointing to a merging of cultural and economic politics in Asian medicine, Nazrul Islam (2017) and others (Halliburton 2011; Meier zu Biesen 2018; Kudlu and Nichter 2019) identified the recent boom in Ayurvedic patent drugs, lifestyle health products, and cosmetics as an instance of nation branding. Other publications deal with the problem of drug regulation and quality control in the Ayurveda industry, often with an applied focus (e.g. Shankar et al. 2007; Sahoo et al. 2011). Such research has significantly advanced critical scholarship on contemporary Asian medicines, making Ayurveda the best-studied Asian medical industry so far. Based on this groundwork, this volume's chapters on the Ayurveda industry are able to pursue important new directions of research while highlighting the sheer scope of this field of inquiry.

The classical medical tradition of Highland and Inner Asia, Sowa Rigpa ("the science of healing") originates from Central Tibet, where it was assembled from elements of Tibetan, Indian, Chinese, Persian, and Central Asian medical knowledge from at least the seventh century CE onwards (Garrett 2008; Kilty 2010). Best known as "Tibetan medicine," it actually constitutes a family of regional medical traditions – also including Mongolian, Bhutanese, and Himalayan Buddhist medicine (Kloos et al. 2020) – that are all based on the *Gyushi* (Four Tantras), Sowa Rigpa's twelfth-century standard treatise (see Yang Ga 2014). Between the thirteenth and the seventeenth centuries, this medical tradition spread, together with Tibetan Buddhism, from Central Tibet throughout the Tibetan plateau (Wangdue 2016), Mongolia (Bold 2013), and the Himalayan range (e.g. Wangchuk 2008; Kloos and Pordié 2022). Particularly during and following the Fifth Dalai Lama's reign in the late seventeenth century, Sowa Rigpa was institutionalised as part of the Ganden Phodrang state's hegemonic power (Gyatso 2015), coming to serve much of Inner Asia as the sole professional health resource. In the early and mid-twentieth century, however, Sowa Rigpa's existing medical structures were largely destroyed following large-scale political upheavals (particularly the Stalinist purges in Mongolia and Mao's annexation of and violent reforms in Tibet) coupled with the forceful introduction of biomedicine. Decades of official repression in Tibet, Mongolia, and Siberia (e.g. Hofer 2018; Kloos, this volume), and governmental neglect in the Himalayan areas (e.g. Craig 2012; Pordié and Kloos 2022) ensued before Sowa Rigpa began to reemerge in the 1980s and 1990s as an increasingly popular primary health resource (Janes 1999; Craig and Adams 2008; Hofer 2018; Blaikie 2019), and a placeholder for various national and ethnic identities (e.g. Janes 1995; Janes and Hilliard 2008; Kloos 2017b).

Although translations of, and general introductions to, Tibetan medicine already began to appear in the 1970s (see Kloos 2015), critical scholarship on the topic was pioneered by Vincanne Adams (1988, 1998, 1999, 2001a, 2001b, 2005, 2007) and Craig Janes (1995, 1999, 2001, 2002). Tracing Tibetan medicine's transformations and changing sociocultural roles since the late twentieth century, they were soon joined by other scholars exploring its encounters with mainstream science, the market economy, and nationalist politics in different locations (e.g. Craig 2007, 2008, 2012; Schrempf 2007; Pordié 2008; Fjeld and Hofer 2010–2011; Adams et al. 2011; Hofer 2018; Pordié and Kloos 2022). While some of this work already considered aspects of Sowa Rigpa's industrialisation, such as the introduction of modern scientific standards (Adams 2002a, 2002b) and pharmaceutical quality control (Craig 2011; Saxer 2012), the development of a Tibetan medicine industry per se was first studied by Martin Saxer (2013). Since then, the scope of inquiry expanded beyond Central Tibet to the transnational Sowa Rigpa industry (Kloos 2017a), with new insights published on its size, shape, and dynamics (Kloos et al. 2020), its integration into intellectual property rights regimes (Madhavan 2017), and its role in public (Blaikie 2019) and global health (Kloos 2020). While Sowa Rigpa studies have become a vibrant field of scholarship, it remains disproportionately small compared to Sowa Rigpa's size, diversity, and regional importance, and mostly limited to a few key sites of Tibetan medicine in Tibet and India. This volume, therefore, strategically focuses on under-explored domains of the Sowa Rigpa industry, including Mongolia, Nepal, and the raw materials trade.

As this impressive body of scholarship on Asian medicines demonstrates, Leslie's notion of *Asian medical systems* was an extremely productive one. His intervention, furthermore, not only made Asian medicines legible to academics, but also to governments, administrators, and wider domestic and international publics (see e.g. Kloos 2013, 2016), leading to increasing levels of popularity, official recognition, commercial development, and eventually their reassemblage as Asian medical industries. In short, the reframing of Asian medicines as systems was a resounding success on multiple levels. In the contemporary context, however, almost half a century after Leslie established "medical systems" as a conceptual framework, these strengths increasingly become limitations. The coherent, rational, fixed, and ultimately closed character of the concept tends to direct the analytic focus to issues of identity and the geographic, cultural, and epistemic boundaries of these medicines-as-systems, often producing unresolvable binary oppositions, such as traditional-modern, local-global, East-West, Indian-Chinese, and so on. The resulting emphasis on purity, coherence, and (in)compatibility, as well as its cultural/epistemic analytic framework, seriously distorts our understanding of the theory, practice, and development of Asian medicines today (cf. Pordié and Gaudillière 2014b: 3).

As industries, Asian medicines have outgrown the framework and analytical capacity of the "medical system" – not despite but precisely because of the success of the concept. The "worlding" of Chinese medicine (Zhan 2009), contemporary reformulation regimes in Indian medicines (Pordié and Gaudillière 2014c), or the pharmaceutical assemblage of Sowa Rigpa (Kloos 2017a), for instance, are all rooted in and strategically utilise terms like "traditional medicine" or "medical systems," but also transcend them. In contrast to the stable classical core, internal epistemological coherence, clear outer contours, and historical continuity implied by medical systems, Asian medicines today are marked by fluid external boundaries and ongoing reformulations of core epistemologies. As becomes clear in the chapters that follow, their internal coherence and historical continuity are open-ended processes rather than established facts, with considerable efforts made to (re-)affirm them in radically new circumstances, be it through simple marketing strategies, official regulation and standardisation, or new historiographies. While there exists a small but growing body of cutting-edge literature on specific sites and aspects of Asian medical industries as outlined above, this volume is an attempt to articulate a larger comparative framework that informs and connects such scholarship. It thus builds on and broadens the scope of collective volumes such as *Asian Industrial Medicines* (Pordié and Hardon 2015) and *Circulation and Governance of Asian Medicines* (Coderey and Pordié 2019), which played a pioneering role in applying a comparative pan-Asian approach to the rapid industrialisation of Asian medicines, even without explicitly conceptualising the phenomenon as such. What all of this work makes clear, then, is that we need a new perspective and approach to account for the dramatically changed, and changing, world of Asian medicines. Asian medical industries, this volume suggests, offer such an approach.

Characteristics of Asian medical industries

Even the rudimentary overview above of Asian medicines and their industrial development suggests that, from a comparative perspective, their overall development is remarkably consistent (see also Meyer 1995). Indeed, their similar historical trajectories in the twentieth and early twenty-first centuries – some of which are explored in this volume – are striking, considering their vastly different contexts and generally weak relations of exchange. While the exact timelines, the degree of their transformation, and local details vary, what is today known as Chinese medicine, Kampo, Ayurveda, or Sowa Rigpa all underwent existential crises following political upheavals/reforms and the introduction and establishment of biomedicine as the sole legitimate form of healthcare. Forced to radically reinvent themselves in a context of rapid modernisation, they all began to align themselves with national political agendas and to (re-) organise, professionalise, and standardise their medical knowledge, clinical practice, training modalities, and professional institutions. Consequently, Asian medicines began to be recognised and developed as domains of significant economic and public health potential in the 1990s, which initiated a still-ongoing phase of unprecedented industrial growth driven by their increasing commercialisation, official regulation, and integration into national economies and health care systems. Of particular importance in this latest phase were state-enforced regulation and standardisation regimes: invariably, the compilation of pharmacopeias, the establishment of drug registration procedures, and the implementation of modern quality and safety standards have been the most essential feature of Asian medicines' transformation into industries (Kloos et al. 2020) and market commodities (Coderey and Pordié 2019), and thus also constitute a major focus of this book (see Chapters 1, 3, 5, and 10). Yet besides the commonality of similar historical trajectories and the centrality of regulation and standardisation regimes, it is also possible to identify a number of other features that characterise contemporary Asian medicines as industries, that enable comparison between them, and that make it possible to consider them as a larger phenomenon.

To begin with, Asian medical industries are *global in scope*: no longer merely local or regional phenomena, Asian medicines today are known and consumed all around the world, which is directly connected to their industrial development. Thus, stakeholders from individual practitioners to large corporations and governments actively seek to create und supply not only domestic demand but also export markets across the globe for Asian medical expertise and products (e.g. Hsu 2009; Zhan 2009). In order to succeed, pharmaceutical producers often need to shift to increasingly large-scale mass-production, as well as engage with "regulatory globalisation"

(Kuo 2015) by complying with international food and drug standards (see Kudlu, this volume), trade agreements, and intellectual property regimes (see Madhavan 2017). Similarly, producers are forced to increasingly diversify and globalise their sources of pharmaceutical raw materials, whose price and availability are subject to international market fluctuations and biodiversity protection regimes (see Campinas, Dejouhanet and Sreelakshmy, and van der Valk, this volume). A single Tibetan or Ayurvedic pill may contain herbs and minerals from several different regions, countries, and even continents, and Asian medical practitioners and their patients frequently traverse multiple national boundaries and legal contexts to offer or receive treatment. Asian medical industries are thus not only global in scope but also *transnational in constitution*: they are fundamentally made in and through translocal encounters and entanglements (Zhan 2009), assembling elements (actors, ingredients, knowledge, technologies, etc.) from many different places (see Blaikie and Craig, this volume). Recent efforts by Chinese and Indian representatives to open "Tibetan" medical centers in Siberia in order to secure medicinal plant supplies and cheap pharmaceutical labor to supply their own TCM and Ayurveda markets are only one illustrative case in point. As industries rather than epistemic systems, finally, Asian medicines are also increasingly being recognised and taken seriously for their potential role in global health (WHO 2008, 2013), further underscoring their recent shift in status and scope (Kloos 2020).

Secondly, Asian medical industries are *based on capitalist logic*, even as they remain partially rooted in non-capitalist – often religious – value systems. While this does not mean that economic profit-maximisation has become their sole logic and driving force – quite to the contrary, many practitioners and institutions strongly resist such commercialisation on ethical or religious grounds – their existence is nonetheless predicated upon capitalist forms of health care (Nichter 1996; Kloos 2021). Money may be considered as morally problematic but has at the same time become the prime index of ethical, social, and professional value. Whether profits are used for personal gain or reinvested in charity, public health, or the expansion of medical services is beside the point here: they need to be made for Asian medical industries to function. Facilities and labour for pharmaceutical mass production, compliance to quality control regulations, drug registration procedures, or national and international distribution networks are expensive and demand capital investment. As Asian medicines are increasingly integrated into official health care systems and policies, even non-industrial, individual practitioners or pharmaceutical producers find themselves with little choice but to participate in the money economy (Hofer 2018; Pordié and Kloos 2022). As the contributions by Chee, Futaya and Blaikie, Madhavan, van der Valk, and Kloos in this volume show, it is no longer possible to study Asian medicines as a cultural domain outside of, distinct from, or even antagonistic to a supposedly uniform, global, and non-cultural capitalism. Rather, as John and Jean Comaroff (2009) and Anna Tsing (2015) point out, it is the mutual incorporation of culture and capitalism (and, one might add, medicine) in the widest sense of the word – each transforming and becoming part of the other – that needs to be a central focus of any serious work on contemporary forms of capitalism. Critical explorations of Asian medical industries can thus offer a unique perspective on ongoing socioeconomic changes in Asia.

Third, Asian medical industries revolve around the object of the drug, which is to say that they *function through processes of pharmaceuticalisation*. While non-pharmaceutical interventions like acupuncture, cupping, massage, or dietary and behavioral counseling are important parts of these industries, especially in contexts where herbal drugs cannot legally be prescribed or sold, there is no doubt that the industrialisation of Asian medicines is closely related to a global trend of reducing health care to pharmaceutical interventions (Biehl 2007; Banerjee 2009; Kloos 2017a) and economic logics (Adams 2013; Gaudillière 2014a; Gaudillière and Sunder Rajan 2021). As a consequence, the development, production, distribution, sale, and regulation of drugs, as well as their safety, efficacy, and availability have become central concerns of contemporary healthcare industries, including Asian medicines. Numerous studies on Ayurvedic reformulation practices (e.g. in Pordié and Gaudillière 2014a) or Good Manufacturing Practices (GMP) in Tibetan medicine (Craig and Adams 2008; Craig 2011; Saxer 2012), not to mention a large body of clinical/pharmacological research on the safety and efficacy of individual Chinese, Ayurvedic, or Sowa Rigpa drugs (Zhang et al. 2009; Li et al. 2013; Reuter et al. 2013), serve to underscore this point. This trend of pharmaceuticalisation has been accompanied by a growing interest in an "anthropology of pharmaceuticals" (van der Geest et al. 1996), which has moved from an initial focus on the social lives of medicines (Whyte et al. 2002) to more serious considerations of their materiality (Blaikie et al. 2015). Virtually all chapters in this volume trace, directly or indirectly, such processes of pharmaceuticalisation and reveal them as foundational to the emergence and functioning of Asian medical industries.

Fourth and directly connected to this, Asian medical industries *rely existentially on natural ingredients* consisting mainly of plants but also animal substances, minerals, and metals. Indeed, such natural ingredients are commonly perceived and presented as their main distinguishing feature and advantage compared to synthetic biomedicines and constitute an important factor of Asian medicines' commercial success. Yet, at the same time, this reliance also exposes the industry to attacks regarding the real or alleged use of endangered animal species (Chee 2021) and to serious shortages of essential raw materials (Dejouhanet 2014). While a part of Asian medicines' materia medica consists of commercially cultivated (and therefore widely available) plants, a significant number of herbal ingredients continues to be wildcrafted and traded through complex and often informal networks. As Campinas, Dejouhanet and Sreelakshmy, and van der Valk describe in this volume, the availability of such raw materials is impacted not only by unsustainable harvesting practices, environmental degradation, and climate change but equally by international biodiversity protection regimes, national bureaucracies, and diverse socioeconomic factors on the local and regional level. At the core of Asian medical industries thus lies an unresolved tension between rapid industrial expansion on the one hand, and diminishing supplies of ingredients on the other, fuelling further attempts at regulation, experiments with cultivation, the globalisation of supply networks, widespread pharmaceutical reformulation, and even practices of counterfeiting and corruption. Yet despite their industrial expansion and the use of non-local ingredients, Asian medical industries remain embedded in, and shaped by, the social ecologies (Craig 2012) of particular places and their interdependent cultural and natural environments. Indeed, as uncultivated plants become valuable commodities through the application of cultural expertise, previously marginal places and communities are rendered central sites not, as is often the case, of primary sector resource extraction but of sophisticated knowledge industries.

Fifth, besides their economic dimension but closely related to it, Asian medical industries have high *symbolic and political value as key sites for the promotion of (postcolonial) nationalist interests*. While this was already the case for most Asian medicines well before their industrialisation, and indeed contributed to their modern development (Prakash 1999; Taylor 2005; Banerjee 2009; Kloos 2011; 2017b; Lei 2014), today it is precisely their economic success and increasing scientific legitimacy that translate back into the symbolic and political realm. More than ever, Asian medicines today symbolise, *as industries*, their nations' cultural identity, intellectual genius, and political/economic success. In contrast to earlier periods, however, they now do so from a position of economic strength rather than marginality. Imbued with real economic and political power, they have become more than just symbols: although still serving larger political purposes, they now also utilise national identities and politics for their own economic interests. The issue of *nation branding*, analysed by Kudlu in this volume, thus works in two directions: national identities are used to brand and market Asian medical products, while their industries are also involved in producing, branding, and marketing Asian ethnic and national identities (cf. Comaroff and Comaroff 2009). At times, this conjuncture of political and economic value and interests can lead to the creation of separate traditions and industries along national lines, such as "Tibetan," "Mongolian," or "Sowa Rigpa" medicine in China, Mongolia, and India, respectively, or even to competing UNESCO applications for "cultural heritage" status for the same medical tradition.

Sixth, such nation branding and market competition notwithstanding, Asian medical industries *cannot be demarcated by stable boundaries* in the same way as Asian medical systems. Indeed, the very attempt to delineate these industries as distinct "bodies" or "systems" is a futile exercise. The above-mentioned connections between herbal and biomedical pharmaceutical industries involving Asian medicine-derived ingredients like artemisinin or shikimic acid are a case in point. Other examples include Chinese medicine companies who produce Mongolian medicines, vitamins, or even biomedical drugs alongside Chinese proprietary formulations; Indian Ayurvedic firms who manufacture and market all kinds of non-classical Ayurvedic products, from toothpastes to beauty creams to plant fertilisers, under the label of "traditional Ayurveda" (Khalikova 2017, 2020); or the Japanese *haichi* medicine industry described by Futaya and Blaikie in this volume. The partial disappearance of dividing lines between what can or cannot be considered as Chinese medicine, Kampo, Ayurveda, or Sowa Rigpa is also reflected in the heterogeneity and unreliability of economic figures concerning the size of Asian medical industries. For example, the size of the Chinese medicine industry in China in 2016 was variously reported as 25 billion USD (ibisworld.com 2021), 68 billion USD (Frost and Sullivan 2016), or even over 130 billion USD (Dang et al. 2016), showing a variation of almost 100 billion USD. While there are a number of explanations for such inconsistencies, including the relatively poor regulation of the industry and widespread over- and underreporting of economic data, at their root lies the very fluidity of this industry's limits and the different statistical inclusion/exclusion criteria that result from it. Instead of defining Asian medical industries, against all evidence, as stable and coherent epistemological and territorial bodies, it makes more sense to understand them in terms of *partially overlapping pharmaceutical assemblages* (Kloos 2017a), which may share certain elements with biomedicine and each other.

To be sure, practitioners and patients usually do have clear ideas and concerns about the boundaries of their medical systems[6] – what qualifies as "real" Chinese medicine, Ayurveda or Tibetan medicine – and so does, implicitly, a large body of scholarly literature problematising issues like hybridity, syncretism, or an epistemic clash between tradition and modernity (Nandy 1988; Bhabha 1994; Ernst 2002). Yet Asian medical industries increasingly displace classical notions of purity and authenticity into techno-legal and economic registers, as when their purity is defined and measured in terms of pharmaceutical quality control, and their authenticity becomes a matter of marketing strategies. Rather than being problematised as a deviation from a norm, hybridity and syncretism are increasingly idealised as lucrative innovation strategies or transcended in the development of entirely new products. The internal coherence and historical continuity of Asian medicines have thus almost imperceptibly morphed from supposedly established facts into open-ended processes requiring constant attention and work. It is precisely the productive tension created by the partial disappearance of distinct boundaries between various Asian medicines on

---

6 The exact locations of these boundaries as delineated by practitioners change over time, despite frequent claims about their stable nature.

the one hand, and the increasing political and economic value of distinct ethnomedical identities on the other, that informs contemporary efforts of (re-)organising Asian medicines and revising their historiographies to ensure their intellectual/structural coherence and historical continuity in radically changed circumstances.

Asian pharmaceutical assemblages

Understanding and studying Asian medicines as industries constitutes not so much a change of terminology than a change in approach and perspective. It is not that terms like medical systems, tradition, modernity, authenticity, or purity have disappeared or become irrelevant, but they have shifted registers, lost their assumed stability, and acquired new and often provisional meanings and functions that are explicitly used by and within the industry. Having thus become part of the phenomenon in question, they can no longer serve well as analytic or descriptive concepts but rather need to be problematised – and taken seriously – as elements of ethnographic reality and historical change. This, and the sheer size, heterogeneity, and novelty of Asian medical industries, raises important methodological-conceptual questions: how can we understand, explore, and engage with contemporary industrial Asian medicines? What is the best way to analyse their emerging forms and larger role, trace their evolving development in real time, and contextualise them in the contemporary world? It is clear that any scholarly engagement with this topic must, first and foremost, rely on fine-grained, locally grounded empirical research. At the same time, it is crucial that such research also addresses and makes visible the larger shape and dynamics of Asian medicines today; analytically accounts for the multiple, at times conflicting, and frequently shifting parts and dimensions of Asian medical industries; and contextualises them within ongoing Asian and global socioeconomic, political, scientific, and health developments.

One methodological/analytic framework for combining empirical attention to local and historical specificity with a focus on the bigger picture is the *pharmaceutical assemblage* (Kloos 2017a), which provides a productive model for understanding the distinctive features of Asian medical industries. Defined as a contingent ensemble of different elements, which may include people, things, practices, knowledge, interests, or values that may not be reducible to a single logic (Collier and Ong 2005) and may even appear incommensurable, the assemblage is centrally marked by an ongoing process of deterritorialisation and reterritorialisation (Deleuze and Guattari 1980; Sassen 2008). More specifically, *pharmaceutical assemblages* refer to constellations that emerge through the de- and reterritorialising effects of pharmaceuticalisation where, for example, elements of Asian medical knowledge, modern technoscience, capitalist interests, cultural markers, religious discourses, nationalist politics, local ecologies, and global regulatory systems come together in new and evolving forms. Besides providing a coherent analytic frame for entities with heterogeneous elements and fluid identities/boundaries on a territorial axis, the pharmaceutical assemblage's temporality is emergent and open-ended. All of this applies directly to Asian medical industries, which – despite having acquired considerable size and force over the past twenty years – are still in a formative phase characterised by a continuous process of inclusion and exclusion of materials, knowledge, discourses, people, and institutions. Not yet stabilised into more permanent apparatuses, their medium- and long-term future remains indeterminate. While relying on fine-grained local data, using the concept of the pharmaceutical assemblage enables us to account for the heterogeneous parts and dimensions of Asian medical industries, grasp their larger shape and dynamics, and contextualise them as a distinct and powerful phenomenon in contemporary Asia and the world.

Due to these characteristics of emergence, indeterminacy, and fluidity, assemblages can be difficult to grasp, which may explain the dearth of research on Asian medical industries. Consequently, we need concrete empirical and analytical vantage points from which to approach and explore them. The pharmaceutical assemblage defines four such vantage points, which are also central domains of inquiry of this volume: raw materials, pharmaceutical production, the market, and intellectual property rights. Thus, one chapter in each of this volume's three sections (Campinas, Dejouhanet and Sreelakshmy, van der Valk) directly addresses the domain of raw materials, presenting not only original data but also critically innovative approaches to understand this existential foundation of Asian medical industries. More indirectly, this topic is also dealt with in the chapters by Madhavan and Soman, Blaikie and Craig, and Kloos. Similarly, a number of chapters in each section (Chee, Futaya and Blaikie, Madhavan and Soman, Blaikie and Craig) approaches Asian medical industries through the vantage point of pharmaceutical production, providing unique insights into how Asian medicines are – in a literal, material sense – assembled today. The central role of the market in shaping as well as regulating Asian medicines and their industries is explored by all chapters, but perhaps particularly so by Arai et al., Futaya and Blaikie, Madhavan, and Soman, and Kloos. The role of Intellectual Property Rights, finally, is less directly visible in the context of this volume, but nonetheless addressed as a significant presence by Chee, Arai et al., Kudlu, and Madhavan and Soman. As all chapters demonstrate clearly, these four domains are so interconnected that none of them can be considered in isolation from the others. Behind all of this looms the state as a dominant force determining the form and development of Asian medical industries (see especially Kloos), an observation further taken up by Blaikie in conclusion.

It is clear that the size, complexity, and dynamics of Asian medical industries cannot be adequately explored and understood by one discipline – or, indeed, one book – alone. Consequently, this volume consciously adopts a multi-disciplinary approach, assembling contributions and insights from medical anthropology, history, economics, geography, pharmaceutical science, and ethnobotany, not merely across but in many cases also within its chapters. Yet multidisciplinarity alone is not sufficient without a larger aim and purpose. The larger aim of *Asian Medical Industries* is to move toward an integrative approach to health and medicine, which does not rely on an outdated separation of modern and traditional. This volume thus carries forward the efforts of Sean Lei (2014), Volker Scheid (2002) and others to overcome this separation and the resulting divisions of intellectual labor – in Lei's case, referring to histories of biomedicine in China and histories of traditional Chinese medicine, each virtually independent from the other – that prevent us from understanding Asian medicines as constitutive parts of modern Asia. Indeed, when we begin to study Chinese medicine, Ayurveda, or Sowa Rigpa not as instances of "traditional culture," but as dynamic, transnational industries of significant public and global health relevance, social science explorations of contemporary healthcare, biotechnologies, pharmaceutical regimes, or global health acquire a new and as-yet unexplored dimension. By placing Asian medical industries on the same conceptual level as biomedical industries, we are able to expand the reach of analytic tools developed by scholars of biomedicine, biotechnology, or global health by applying them to Asian medicines and vice versa. Beyond enabling radically new questions and perspectives, this integrative approach is also informed by an underlying postcolonial agenda of decentering familiar tropes and concepts (by means of de- and reterritorialisation), something that is underscored by the diverse backgrounds of this volume's contributing authors. The field of Asian medical industries is vast, and so is the theoretical potential of scholarship concerning it. The present volume can only be a small step towards exploring this new territory, but if it manages to place Asian medical industries more firmly on the scholarly map and sketch, however provisionally, a possible conceptual approach to critically engage with them, its purpose is served.

Chapter outline

This book's ten main case studies are divided into three regional sections: East Asian medical industries, South Asian medical industries, and Sowa Rigpa industries. The first and largest section includes two chapters on Chinese medicines in different regions of China, as well as one chapter each on Kampo and *haichi* medicine in Japan. In Chapter 1, Liz Chee combines archival and ethnographic research on a pharmaceutical company in Guangzhou, South China, to explore the role of both modern science and the state in the invention and production of "authentic" Chinese medicines. She argues that while Chinese medicine is increasingly subject to scientific standards, the ambiguity of Mao's policies continues to shape pharmaceutical innovation, manufacturing, and regulation processes today, resulting in a plethora of non-pharmaceutical health product or food categories.

In Chapter 2, Manuel Campinas focuses on medicinal plants among Qiang ethnic minority communities in Sichuan to illustrate the connections between dwindling raw material supplies, the Chinese medicine industry, China's minority policies, and its agricultural development strategies. Assembling ethnographic data from a range of different contexts, he shows how efforts at creating a "Qiang" ethnic medicine industry are irrelevant or even detrimental to the rural communities and environments they are supposed to benefit. In Chapter 3, Ichiro Arai, Julia Yongue, and Kiichiro Tsutani trace the revival of Kampo medicine and its integration into Japan's national health care system since the 1960s. Analysing both domestic and international factors for the application of biomedical regulations ("Good Practices," or GxP) to Kampo medicines, they argue that this regulatory integration was central to the development of a successful Kampo industry. In Chapter 4, Tomoko Futaya and Calum Blaikie provide deeper historical insights into the evolution of the *haichi* pharmaceutical industry of patent household remedies including local herbs, Kampo formulas, and (later) biomedical ingredients in Japan's Toyama prefecture. They show how *haichi* medicines needed to be reinvented, transformed, and hybridised in order to maintain their legitimacy and marketability under changing political and economic conditions, laying the foundations for what would become the largest pharmaceutical production zone in Japan.

The second section, on South Asian medical industries, contains three chapters exploring different aspects of the Ayurveda industry in India. Chithprabha Kudlu's Chapter 5 offers a new perspective on Ayurveda's commodification, industrialisation, and globalisation, exploring how the Ayurvedic industry is affected by frictions between state-envisioned homogenising tendencies inherent in the global promotion of Brand India and the heterogeneous reality of Ayurveda's actual constitution and its domestic market. She argues that contemporary industrial Ayurveda no longer serves as an instrument for nation *building* (as it had as a medical system), but as a resource for nation *branding*, revealing the complex entanglements between politics, local and global markets, cultural identity and health care that shape Asian medical industries. Chapter 6 by Harilal Madhavan and Sajitha Soman explores some of these issues in the specific case of CARe Keralam, an Ayurvedic industrial cluster in the South Indian state of Kerala. Tracing the cluster from its inception through its top-down implementation to its ultimate failure, they argue that the under-achievement of its laudable aims can be explained by the structure of the Ayurvedic industry itself and a misunderstanding of the differential needs of small, medium, and large firms in terms of innovation, raw materials, and research and development. The case of CARe Keralam and its eventual failure thus provides an important look underneath Ayurveda's smooth official representations and grand development plans, reminding us of the complex local assemblages that constitute Asian medical industries. Remaining in Kerala, in Chapter 7,

Lucie Dejouhanet and Sreelakshmy M. provide a detailed analysis of the local and regional raw material supply networks the Ayurvedic industry existentially depends on. Describing the complicated itineraries of Ayurvedic plants from their wild collection to the factories, they show how new collection and procurement practices emerge as the industry's growth puts increasing pressure on limited natural resources. As a consequence, the generally close connection of the Kerala Ayurvedic industry to its social environment is counterbalanced by its progressive disconnect from its natural environment, providing an additional layer of complexity to an already entangled industry.

The volume's third section consists of three chapters on Sowa Rigpa industries in India, Nepal, and Mongolia. In Chapter 8, Jan van der Valk traces Tibetan medicinal plants back from the pharmaceutical factory to their suppliers in North India in order to highlight the complexities surrounding plant cultivation, trade, and conservation in Sowa Rigpa (and, by implication, other Asian medical) industries. Critically describing practices of corruption, bribery, and illegality that form the alter ego of the state-sanctioned herbal sector, he argues that raw material sourcing is often characterised by convoluted legislative and moral grey zones, giving a seemingly magical quality to what he calls "sourcery." In Chapter 9, Calum Blaikie and Sienna Craig explore the emergence and contemporary dynamics of a Sowa Rigpa cottage industry in Nepal. They argue that while Sowa Rigpa in Nepal offers a point of contrast to the much larger Sowa Rigpa industries in China, India, Bhutan, and Mongolia, it is also exemplary of the ambivalent attitudes vis-a-vis industrialisation among Sowa Rigpa practitioners throughout the region. Nepal's Tibetan medicine production thus offers a unique perspective on the Sowa Rigpa industry in Asia, in which skilful, personal involvement in all stages of medicine making remains highly valued despite an increasing transition to pharmaceutical mass production. Moving from the southern to the northern edge of the Sowa Rigpa world, Stephan Kloos's Chapter 10 provides historical and ethnographic insights into the development and status quo of the Sowa Rigpa industry in both Mongolia and Inner Mongolia. Following processes of Mongolian medicine's de- and reterritorialisation through different periods of communism, liberalisation, and industrialisation from the 1930s up to today, he argues that both the Mongolian and Chinese states have played a crucial but ambivalent role in the emergence of a Mongolian medicine industry.

In the conclusion, Calum Blaikie connects and compares the case studies presented in the ten chapters, and in doing so, revisits the main aims and arguments of this volume. In particular, he identifies the role of the state, regimes of regulation and reformulation, and raw material supplies as the three central domains cutting across all chapters as well as the various Asian medical industries they explore. In a final theoretical step, Blaikie asks what Asian medical industries – as a concept and a subject of inquiry – can contribute to broader fields of scholarship that exceed individual disciplines like anthropology, history, development studies, or economics, such as work on pharmaceutical and frontier assemblages or theories of industrialisation. In a productive way, the conclusion thus integrates the scholarship presented in this volume, which can be seen as an assemblage in and of itself, into broader conversations. At the most fundamental level, the contributions collectively show that the notion of Asian medical industries is more than just a new label for old wine. Rather, Asian medicines and their industries are an increasingly prominent reality that transforms healthcare, economic and sociocultural landscapes across contemporary Asia and the world, and it is high time to give them sustained and serious scholarly attention.

Bibliography

Adams V (1988) Modes of Production and Medicine: An Examination of the Theory in Light of Sherpa Medical Traditionalism. *Social Science and Medicine* 27(5): 505–513.

Adams V (1998) Suffering the Winds of Lhasa: Politicized Bodies, Human Rights, Cultural Difference, and Humanism in Tibet. *Medical Anthropology Quarterly* 12(1): 74–102.

Adams V (1999) Equity of the Ineffable: Cultural and Political Constraints on Ethnomedicine as a Health Problem in Contemporary Tibet. *Working Paper Series* 99: 283–305.

Adams V (2001a) Particularizing Modernity: Tibetan Medical Theorizing of Women's Health in Lhasa, Tibet. In: Connor L and Samuel G (eds) *Healing Powers and Modernity: Traditional Medicine, Shamanism, and Science in Asian Societies.* Westport, CT: Bergin & Garvey, pp. 197–246.

Adams V (2001b) The Sacred in the Scientific: Ambiguous Practices of Science in Tibetan Medicine. *Cultural Anthropology* 16(4): 542–575.

Adams V (2002a) Establishing Proof: Translating "Science" and the State in Tibetan Medicine. In: Nichter M and Lock M (eds) *New Horizons in Medical Anthropology.* London & New York, NY: Routledge, pp. 200–220.

Adams V (2002b) Randomized Controlled Crime: Postcolonial Sciences in Alternative Medicine Research. *Social Studies of Science* 32(5–6): 659–690.

Adams V (2005) Modernity and the Problem of Secular Morality in Tibet. In: Houben V and Schrempf M (eds) *Figurations of Modernity: Global and Local Representations in Comparative Perspective.* Frankfurt & New York, NY: Campus, pp. 105–120.

Adams V (2007) Integrating Abstraction: Modernising Medicine at Lhasa's Mentsikhang. In: Schrempf M (ed) *Soundings in Tibetan Medicine: Anthropological and Historical Perspectives.* Leiden: Brill, pp. 29–43.

Adams V (2013) Evidence-Based Global Public Health. In: Biehl J and Petryna A (eds) *When People Come First. Critical Studies in Global Health.* Princeton, NJ: Princeton University Press, pp. 54–90.

Adams V and Li FF (2008) Integration or Erasure? Modernizing Medicine at Lhasa's Mentsikhang. In: Pordié L (ed) *Tibetan Medicine in the Contemporary World: Global Politics of Medical Knowledge and Practice.* Oxon & New York: Routledge, pp. 105–131.

Adams V, Schrempf M and Craig S (eds) (2011) *Medicine between Science and Religion: Explorations on Tibetan Grounds.* Oxford and New York, NY: Berghahn Books.

Alter J (ed) (2005) *Asian Medicine and Globalization*. Philadelphia, PA: University of Pennsylvania Press.

Arai I (2009) The Current Situation of Japanese Medicinal Plants Industry and its Significance for the Pharmaceutical Industry. http://hdais.coa.gov.tw/htmlarea_file/web_articles/hdais/1354/980108_1.pdf

Attewell G (2005) *Refiguring Unani Tibb: Plural Healing in Late Colonial India*. Hyderabad: Orient Longman.

Banerjee M (2002) Power, Culture and Medicine: Ayurvedic Pharmaceuticals in the Modern Market. *Contributions to Indian Sociology* 36(3): 435–467.

Banerjee M (2008) Ayurveda in Modern India: Standardization and Pharmaceuticalization. In: Wujastyk D and Smith FM (eds) *Modern and Global Ayurveda: Pluralism and Paradigms*. Albany: SUNY Press, pp. 201–214.

Banerjee M (2009) *Power, Knowledge, Medicine: Ayurvedic Pharmaceuticals at Home and in the World*. Hyderabad: Orient Black Swan.

Bates DG (ed) (1995) *Knowledge and the Scholarly Medical Traditions*. Cambridge: Cambridge University Press.

Bhabha H (1994) *The Location of Culture*. Oxon and New York, NY: Routledge.

Biehl J (2007) Pharmaceuticalization: AIDS Treatment and Global Health Politics. *Anthropological Quarterly* 80(4): 1083–1126.

Biehl J and Petryna A (2013) Critical Global Health. In: Biehl J and Petryna A (eds) *When People Come First. Critical Studies in Global Health*. Princeton, NJ: Princeton University Press, pp. 1–20.

Blaikie C (2015) Wish-Fulfilling Jewel Pills: Tibetan Medicines from Exclusivity to Ubiquity. *Anthropology & Medicine* 22(1): 7–22.

Blaikie C (2019) Mainstreaming Marginality: Traditional Medicine and Primary Healthcare in Himalayan India. *Asian Medicine* 14(1): 145–172.

Blaikie C, et al. (2015) Coproducing Efficacious Medicines: Collaborative Ethnography with Tibetan Medicine Practitioners in Kathmandu. *Current Anthropology* 56(2): 1223–1238.

Bode M (2008) *Taking Traditional Knowledge to the Market: The Modern Image of the Ayurvedic and Unani Industry 1980–2000*. Hyderabad: Orient Blackswan.

Bold S (2013) History and Development of Traditional Mongolian Medicine (from Neolithic Age – Early 21st Century). *Third Revised and Enlarged Edition*. Ulaanbaatar: Sodpress Kompanid Khevlv.

Brass P (1972) The Politics of Ayurvedic Education. In: Rudolph S and Rudolph L (eds) *Education and Politics in India: Studies in Organization, Society, and Policy*. Cambridge, MA: Harvard University Press.

Chee LPY (2019) "Health Products" at the Boundary between Food and Pharmaceuticals: The Case of Fish Liver Oil. In: Coderey C and Pordié L (eds) *Circulation and Governance of Asian Medicine*. Oxon and New York, NY: Routledge, pp. 103–117.

Chee LPY (2021) *Mao's Bestiary: How Animal-Based Drugs Changed Chinese Medicine*. Durham: Duke University Press.

Cho BH (2000) The Politics of Herbal Drugs in Korea. *Social Science and Medicine* 51(4): 505–509.

Coderey C and Pordié L (eds) (2019) *Circulation and Governance of Asian Medicine*. Oxon and New York, NY: Routledge.

Cohen L (1998) *No Aging in India: Alzheimer's, the Bad Family, and Other Modern Things*. Berkeley, CA: University of California Press.

Collier S and Ong A (2005) Global Assemblages, Anthropological Problems. In: Ong A and Collier S (eds) *Global Assemblages: Technology, Politics, and Ethics as Anthropological Problems*. Malden, MA and Oxford: Blackwell Publishing, pp. 3–21.

Comaroff J and Comaroff J (2009) *Ethnicity, Inc*. Chicago, IL and London: University of Chicago Press.

Connor L and Samuel G (eds) (2001) Healing Powers and Modernity. *Traditional Medicine, Shamanism, and Science in Asian Societies*. Westport, CT: Bergin & Garvey.

Craig S (2007) A Crisis of Confidence: A Comparison Between Shifts in Tibetan Medical Education in Nepal and Tibet. In: *Soundings in Tibetan Medicine: Anthropological and Historical Perspectives*. Schrempf M (ed) Leiden and Boston, MA: Brill, pp. 127–154.

Craig S (2008) Place and Professionalization: Navigating Amchi Identity in Nepal. In: Pordié L (ed) *Tibetan Medicine in the Contemporary World: Global Politics of Medical Knowledge and Practice*. London and New York, NY: Routledge, pp. 62–90.

Craig S (2011) "Good" Manufacturing by Whose Standards? Remaking Quality, Safety, and Value in the Production of Tibetan Pharmaceuticals. *Anthropological Quarterly* 84(2): 331–378.

Craig S (2012) *Healing Elements: Efficacy and the Social Ecologies of Tibetan Medicine*. Berkeley, CA: University of California Press.

Craig S and Adams V (2008) Global Pharma in the Land of Snows: Tibetan Medicines, SARS, and Identity Politics across Nations. *Asian Medicine* 4: 1–28.

Dang H, et al. (2016) The Integration of Chinese Materia Medica into the Chinese Health Care Delivery System, an Update. *Phytotherapy Research* 30(2): 292–297.

Dejouhanet L (2014) Supply of Medicinal Raw Materials: The Achilles Heel of Today's Manufacturing Sector for Ayurvedic Drugs in Kerala. *Asian Medicine* 9(1–2): 206–235.

Deleuze G and Guattari F (1980) Mille Plateaux. *Capitalisme et Schizophrénie*. Tome 2. Paris: Les Editions de Minuit.

Ernst W (ed) (2002) *Plural Medicine, Tradition and Modernity, 1800–2000*. London and New York, NY: Routledge.

Farmer P, et al. (eds) (2013) *Reimagining Global Health: An Introduction*. Berkeley, CA and Los Angeles, CA: University of California Press.

Farquhar J (1994) *Knowing Practice: The Clinical Encounter of Chinese Medicine*. Boulder, CO: Westview Press.

Farquhar J (1996) Getting Rich and Getting Personal in Medicine after Mao. *American Ethnologist* 23(2): 239–257.

Fjeld H and Hofer T (eds) (2010–2011) Women and Gender in Tibetan Medicine. Special Issue: *Asian Medicine* 6(2).

Frost L and Sullivan D (2016) 民民族医药的春天 (The Spring of Ethnic Medicine). http://www.frostchina.com/?p=3061

Garrett F (2008) *Religion, Medicine and the Human Embryo in Tibet*. London and New York, NY: Routledge.

Gaudillière J-P (2014a) De la santé publique internationale à la santé globale. L'OMS, la Banque Mondiale et le gouvernement des thérapies chimiques. In: Pestre D (ed) *Le gouvernement des technosciences. Gouverner le progrès et ses dégâts depuis 1945*. Paris: Découverte, pp. 65–96.

Gaudillière J-P (2014b) Herbalised Ayurveda? Reformulation, Plant Management and the "Pharmaceuticalisation" of Indian "Traditional" Medicine. *Asian Medicine* 9(1–2): 171–205.

Gaudillière J-P and Sunder Rajan K (2021) Making Valuable Health: Pharmaceuticals, Global Capital and Alternative Political Economies. *BioSocieties* 16(3): 313–322.

Goldschmidt A (2008) *The Evolution of Chinese Medicine: Song Dynasty, 960–1200*. London: Routledge.

Gyatso J (2015) *Being Human in a Buddhist World: An Intellectual History of Medicine in Early Modern Tibet*. New York, NY: Columbia University Press.

Halliburton M (2011) Resistance or Inaction? Protecting Ayurvedic Medical Knowledge and Problems of Agency. *American Ethnologist* 38(1): 86–101.

Hanson M (2015) Is the 2015 Nobel Prize a Turning Point for Traditional Chinese medicine? *The Conversation* 5, October 2015, https://theconversation.com/is-the-2015-nobel-prize-a-turning-point-for-traditional-chinese-medicine-48643

Hanson M (2016) The Anthropology and History of Medicine in Korea. *Asian Medicine* 11(1–2): 1–19.

Hofer T (2018) *Medicine and Memory in Tibet: Amchi Physicians in an Age of Reform*. Seattle: University of Washington Press.

Hsu E (2008a) The History of Chinese Medicine in the People's Republic of China and Its Globalization. *East Asian Science, Technology and Society* 2: 465–484.

Hsu E (2008b) Medicine as Business: Chinese Medicine in Tanzania. In: Alden C, Large D and Soares De Oliveira R, (eds) *China Returns to Africa. A Superpower and a Continent Embrace*. Oxford: Oxford University Press, pp. 221–235.

Hsu E (2009) Chinese Propriety Medicines: An "Alternative Modernity?" The Case of the Anti-Malarial Substance Artemisinin in East Africa. *Medical Anthropology* 28(2): 111–140.

Hsu E (2015) Tu Youyou and the Nobel Prize. *Somatosphere*, 19. October 2015

Ibisworld.com (2021) Traditional Chinese Medicine Manufacturing in China Industries Statistics. https://www.ibisworld.com/china/market-research-reports/traditional-chinese-medicine-manufacturing-industry/

Islam N (2017) *Chinese and Indian Medicine Today: Branding Asia*. Singapore: Springer.

Janes C (1995) The Transformations of Tibetan Medicine. *Medical Anthropology Quarterly* 9(1): 6–39.

Janes C (1999) The Health Transition and the Crisis of Traditional Medicine: The Case of Tibet. *Social Science and Medicine* 48: 1803–1820.

Janes C (2001) Tibetan medicine at the Crossroads: Radical Modernity and the Social Organization of Traditional Medicine in the Tibet Autonomous Region, China. In: Connor L and Samuel G (eds) *Healing Powers and Modernity: Traditional Medicine, Shamanism, and Science in Asian Societies*. Westport, CT: Bergin & Garvey, pp. 197–221.

Janes C (2002) Buddhism, Science, and Market: The Globalisation of Tibetan Medicine. *Anthropology & Medicine* 9(3): 267–289.

Janes C and Hilliard C (2008) Inventing Tradition: Tibetan Medicine in the Postsocialist Contexts of China and Mongolia. In: Pordié L (ed) *Tibetan Medicine in the Contemporary World: Global Politics of Medical Knowledge and Practice*. London and New York, NY: Routledge, pp. 35–61.

Kang Y and Kim J (2016) Preface to the Compendium of People-Saving Prescriptions Made with Native Korean Herbs. *Asian Medicine* 11(1–2): 161–170.

Khalikova V (2017) The Ayurveda of Baba Ramdev: Biomoral Consumerism, National Duty and the Biopolitics of 'Homegrown' Medicine in India. *South Asia: Journal of South Asian Studies* 40(1): 105–122.

Khalikova V (2020) A Local Genie in an Imported Bottle: Ayurvedic Commodities and Healthy Eating in North India. *Food, Culture, and Society* DOI: 10.1080/15528014.2020.1713429.

Kilty G (2010) Translator's Introduction. In: Desi Sangye G (ed) *Mirror of Beryl. A Historical Introduction to Tibetan Medicine*. Somerville, MA: Wisdom Publications, pp. 1–25.

Kim J (2006) Korean Medicine's Globalization Project and Its Powerscapes. *Journal of Korean Studies* 11(1): 69–92.

Kim J (2009) Transcultural Medicine: A Multi-sited Ethnography on the Scientific-Industrial Networking of Korean Medicine. *Medical Anthropology* 28(1): 1–64.

Kloos S (2011) Navigating "Modern Science" and "Traditional Culture": The Dharamsala Men-Tsee-Khang in India. In: Adams V, Schrempf M, and Craig S (eds) *Medicine between Science and Religion: Explorations on Tibetan Grounds*. Oxford and New York, NY: Berghahn Books, pp. 83–105.

Kloos S (2013) How Tibetan Medicine Became a "Medical System." *East Asian Science, Technology and Society* 7(3): 381–395.

Kloos S (2015) Introduction: The Translation and Development of Tibetan Medicine in Exile. In: Ploberger F (ed) *Das Letzte Tantra, aus "Die vier Tantra der Tibetischen Medizin"*. Schiedlberg: Bacopa, pp. 28–35.

Kloos S (2016) The Recognition of Sowa Rigpa in India: How Tibetan Medicine Became an Indian Medical System. *Medicine, Anthropology, Theory* 3(2): 19–49.

Kloos S (2017a) The Pharmaceutical Assemblage: Rethinking Sowa Rigpa and the Herbal Pharmaceutical Industry in Asia. *Current Anthropology* 58(6): 693–717.

Kloos S (2017b) The Politics of Preservation and Loss: Tibetan Medical Knowledge in Exile. *East Asian Science, Technology and Society* 10(2): 135–159.

Kloos S (2020) Humanitarianism from Below: Sowa Rigpa, the Traditional Pharmaceutical Industry, and Global Health. *Medical Anthropology* 39(2): 167–181.

Kloos S (2021) From Buddhist Deities to the Spirit of Capitalism: Tibetan Medicine and the Remaking of Inner Asia. In: Gingrich A (ed) *Contemporary Anthropology in Austria: Continuities, Discontinuities, and New Agendas*. Canon Pyon: Sean Kingston, pp. 112–135.

Kloos S, Madhavan H, Tidwell T, et al. (2020) The Transnational Sowa Rigpa Industry in Asia: New Perspectives on an Emerging Economy. *Social Science and Medicine* 245: 112617.

Kloos S and Pordié L (2022) Introduction: The Indian Face of Sowa Rigpa. In: Pordié L and Kloos S (eds) *Healing at the Periphery: Ethnographies of Tibetan Medicine in India*. Durham and London: Duke University Press, pp. 1–21.

Kudlu C and Nichter M (2019) Indian Imaginaries of Chinese Success in the Global Herbal Medicine Market: A Critical Assessment. *Asian Medicine* 14(1): 104–144.

Kuo WH (2015) Promoting Chinese Herbal Drugs through Regulatory Globalisation: The Case of the Consortium for Globalization of Chinese Medicine. *Asian Medicine* 10(2): 316–339.

Lakoff A (2005) *Pharmaceutical Reason: Knowledge and Value in Global Psychiatry*. Cambridge: Cambridge University Press.

Lang C (2018) *Depression in Kerala: Ayurveda and Mental Health Care in 21st Century India*. Oxon and New York, NY: Routledge.

Langford JM (2002) *Fluent Bodies: Ayurvedic Remedies for Postcolonial Imbalance*. Durham and London: Duke University Press.

Lee, T (2016) The State-Centred Nosology: Changing Disease Names of Traditional Medicine in Post-Colonial South Korea. *Asian Medicine* 11(1–2): 100–132.

Lei XS (2014) *Neither Donkey nor Horse. Medicine in the Struggle over China's Modernity*. Chicago, IL and London: University of Chicago Press.

Leslie C (1968) The Professionalisation of Ayurvedic and Unani Medicine. *Transactions of the New York Academy of Sciences (Series 2)*, 30(4): 559–572.

Leslie C (1973) The Professionalizing Ideology of Medical Revivalism. In: Singer M (ed) *Entrepreneurship and Modernisation of Occupational Cultures in South Asia*. Durham: Duke University Press.

Leslie C (1974) The Modernization of Asian Medical Systems. In: Poggie J and Lynch R (eds) *Rethinking Modernization: Anthropological Perspectives*. Westport, CT: Greenwood Press, pp. 69–107.

Leslie C (1976a) The Ambiguities of Medical Revivalism in Modern India. In: Leslie C (ed) *Asian Medical Systems: A Comparative Study*. Berkeley, CA: University of California Press, pp. 356–367.

Leslie C (ed) (1976b) *Asian Medical Systems: A Comparative Study*. Berkeley, CA: University of California Press.

Leslie C (1989) Indigenous Pharmaceuticals, the Capitalist World System, and Civilization. *Kroeber Anthropological Society Papers* 69–79: 23–31.

Leslie C and Young A (eds) (1992) *Paths to Asian Medical Knowledge*. Berkeley, CA: University of California Press.

Li X, et al. (2013) Traditional Chinese Medicine in Cancer Care: A Review of Controlled Clinical Studies Published in Chinese. *PLOS One* 8(4): e60338

Lock M (1980) *East Asian Medicine in Urban Japan: Varieties of Medical Experience*. Berkeley, CA: University of California Press.

Lock M (1993) *Encounters with Aging: Mythologies of Menopause in Japan and North America*. Berkeley, CA: University of California Press.

Ma E (2015) Join or Be Excluded from Biomedicine? JOINS (R) and Post-Colonial Korea. *Anthropology & Medicine* 22(1): 64–74.

Ma E (2019) Science as a Global Governance and Circulation Tool? The Baekshuoh Disaster in South Korea. In: Coderey C and Pordié L (eds) *Circulation and Governance of Asian Medicine*. Oxon and New York, NY: Routledge, pp. 48–62.

Madhavan H (2009) 'Commercialising Traditional Medicine': Ayurvedic Manufacturing in Kerala. *Economic and Political Weekly* XLIV(16): 44–51.

Madhavan H (2017) Below the Radar Innovations and Emerging Property Right Approaches in Tibetan Medicine. *The Journal of World Intellectual Property* 20(5–6): 239–257.

Manderson L, Cartwright E and Hardon A (eds) *The Routledge Handbook of Medical Anthropology*. New York & Oxon: Routledge.

Meier Zu Biesen C (2018) From Coastal to Global: The Transnational Flow of Ayurveda and Its Relevance for Indo-African Linkages. *Global Public Health* 13(3): 339–354.

Meulenbeld GJ (1999–2002) *A History of Indian Medical Literature (in 5 volumes)*. London: Royal Asiatic Society and Wellcome Institute for the History of Medicine.

Meyer F (1995) Introduction. In: van Alphen J and Aris A (eds) *Oriental Medicine: An Illustrated Guide to the Asian Arts of Healing*. London: Serindia Publications, pp. 11–15.

Nandy A (ed) (1988) *Science, Hegemony and Violence. A Requiem for Modernity*. Delhi: Oxford University Press.

Nichter M (1996) Pharmaceuticals, the Commodification of Health, and the Health Care-Medicine Use Transition. In: Nichter M and Nichter M (eds) *Anthropology and International Health: South Asian Case Studies*. Amsterdam: Gordon and Breach, pp. 265–326.

Ong A and Chen N (eds) (2010) *Asian Biotech: Ethics and Communities of Fate*. Durham & London: Duke University Press.

Otsuka Y (1976) Chinese Traditional Medicine in Japan. In: Leslie C (ed) *Asian Medical Systems: A Comparative Study*. Berkeley, CA: University of California Press, pp. 322–340.

Park HL, et al. (2012) Traditional Medicine in China, Korea, and Japan: A Brief Introduction and Comparison. *Evidence-Based Complementary and Alternative Medicine* 2012: 429103.

Patterson TJS (1987) The Relationship of Indian and European Practitioners of Medicine from the Sixteenth Century. In: Meulenbeld GJ and Wujastyk D (eds) *Studies on Indian Medical History*. Groningen: Egbett Forsten, pp. 111–120.

Petryna A and Kleinman A (2006) The Pharmaceutical Nexus. In: Petryna A, Lakoff A and Kleinman A (eds) *Global Pharmaceuticals: Ethics, Markets, Practices*. Durham and London: Duke University Press, pp. 1–32.

Pordié L (ed) (2008) *Tibetan Medicine in the Contemporary World: Global Politics of Medical Knowledge and Practice*. Oxon and New York, NY: Routledge.

Pordié L and Hardon A (2015) Drugs' Stories and Itineraries. On the Making of Asian Industrial Medicines. *Anthropology & Medicine* 22(1): 1–6.

Pordié L and Gaudillière J-P (eds) (2014a) The Herbal Pharmaceutical Industry in India. *Asian Medicine* 9(1–2).

Pordié L and Gaudillière J-P (2014b) Introduction: Industrial Ayurveda – Drug Discovery, Reformulation and the Market. *Asian Medicine* 9(1–2): 1–11.

Pordié L and Gaudillière J-P (2014c) The Reformulation Regime in Drug Discovery: Revisiting Polyherbals and Property Rights in the Ayurvedic Industry. *East Asian Science, Technology and Society* 8: 57–79.

Pordié L and Kloos S (eds) (2022) *Healing at the Periphery. Ethnographies of Tibetan Medicine in India*. Durham and London: Duke University Press.

Prakash G (1999) *Another Reason: Science and the Imagination of Modern India*. Princeton, NJ: Princeton University Press.

Reuter KP, Weisshuhn TE and Witt CM (2013) Tibetan Medicine: A Systematic Review of the Clinical Research Available in the West. *Evidence-Based Complementary Alternative Medicine* 2013: 213407.

Sahoo N, Manchikanti P and Dey SH (2011) Herbal Drug Patenting in India: IP Potential. *Journal of Ethnopharmacology* 137(1): 289–297.

Sassen S (2008) *Territory, Authority, Rights: From Medieval to Global Assemblages* (Updated Edition). Princeton, NJ and Oxford: Princeton University Press.

Saxer M (2012) A Goat's Head on a Sheep's Body? Manufacturing Good Practices for Tibetan Medicine. *Medical Anthropology* 31(6): 497–513.

Saxer M (2013) *Manufacturing Tibetan Medicine: The Creation of an Industry and the Moral Economy of Tibetanness*. Oxford and New York, NY: Berghahn Books.

Scheid V (2002) *Chinese Medicine in Contemporary China*. Durham and London: Duke University Press.

Scheid V (2007) *Currents of Tradition in Chinese Medicine, 1626–2006*. Seattle: Eastland Press.

Schmidt Stiedenroth K (2020) *Unani Medicine in the Making: Practices and Representations in 21st-Century India*. Amsterdam: Amsterdam University Press.

Schrempf M (ed) (2007) *Soundings in Tibetan Medicine: Anthropological and Historical Perspectives*. Leiden: Brill.

Shankar D, Unnikrishnan PM and Venkatasubramaniam P (2007) Need to Develop Inter-Cultural Standards for Quality, Safety and Efficacy of Traditional Indian Systems of Medicine. *Current Science* 92(11): 1499–1505.

Smith A (2019) Negotiating Chinese Medical Value and Authority in the (Bio)polis. In Coderey C and Pordié L (eds) *Circulation and Governance of Asian Medicine*. Oxon and New York, NY: Routledge, pp. 83–102.

Smith, FM and Wujastyk D (2008) Introduction. In: Wujastyk D and Smith FM eds. *Modern and Global Ayurveda: Pluralism and Paradigms*. Albany: SUNY Press, pp. 1–28.

Sunder Rajan K (2006) *Biocapital: The Constitution of Postgenomic Life*. Durham: Duke University Press.

Sunder Rajan K (2017) *Pharmocracy: Value, Politics, and Knowledge in Global Biomedicine*. Durham and London: Duke University Press.

Taylor K (2005) *Chinese Medicine in Early Communist China, 1945–63*. Oxon and New York, NY: Routledge.

Tsing A (2015) *The Mushroom at the End of the World. On the Possibility of Life in Capitalist Ruins*. Princeton, NJ: Princeton University Press.

Umemura M (2011) Reviving Tradition: Patients and the Shaping of Japan's Traditional Medicines Industry. In Francks P and Hunter J (eds) *The Historical Consumer: Consumption and Everyday Life in Japan, 1850–2000*. Basingstoke: Palgrave Macmillan, pp. 176–203.

Unschuld P (1985) *Medicine in China: A History of Ideas*. Berkeley, CA: University of California Press.

van der Geest S, Whyte SR and Hardon A (1996) The Anthropology of Pharmaceuticals: A Biographical Approach. *Annual Review of Anthropology* 25: 153–178.

van Put I (1995) A Brief History of Medicine in Traditional Japan. In: van Alphen J and Aris A (eds) *Oriental Medicine: An Illustrated Guide to the Asian Arts of Healing*. London: Serindia, pp. 231–245.

Wang S (2019) Circumventing Regulation and Professional Legitimization: The Circulation of Chinese Medicine between China and France. In: C Coderey and L Pordié (eds) *Circulation and Governance of Asian Medicine*. Oxon and New York, NY: Routledge, pp. 139–156.

Wangchuk D (2008) Traditional Medicine in Bhutan. *Men-jong So-rig Journal* 1: 89–108.

Wangdue G (Go 'jo dbang 'dus) (2016) *Bod kyi gso rig lo rgyus thok gi slob grwa khag byung tshul rags tsam brjod pa dpyod ldan bung ba rtsen pa'i pad tshal zhes bya ba bzhugs so [Brief Outline of a History of Sowa Rigpa Schools]*. Lhasa: Bod ljongs lha ldan sman rtsis khang nas par du bskrun.

WHO (2008) *Beijing Declaration by WHO Congress on Traditional Medicine*. Beijing: World Health Organization.

WHO (2013) *Traditional Medicine Strategy 2014–2023*. Geneva: World Health Organization.

Whyte SR, van der Geest S and Hardon A (2002) *Social Lives of Medicines*. Cambridge: Cambridge University Press.

Wujastyk D and Smith FM (eds) (2008) *Modern and Global Ayurveda: Pluralism and Paradigms*. Albany: SUNY Press.

Wujastyk D (1998) *The Roots of Ayurveda: Selections from the Ayurvedic Classics*. New Delhi: Penguin Books.

Yang G (2014) The Origins of the Four Tantras and an Account of its Author, Yuthog Yonten Gonpo. In: T Hofer (ed) *Bodies in Balance: The Art of Tibetan Medicine*. New York, NY: Rubin Museum of Art, in association with University of Washington Press, pp. 154–177.

Yang J and Peng Y (2015) Traditional Miao Cures To Boost Health of Guizhou's Economy. *China Daily*, 18 March 2015. http://covid-19.chinadaily.com.cn/china/2015-03/18/content_19839959.htm

Zhan M (2009) *Other-Worldly: Making Chinese Medicine through Transnational Frames*. Durham and London: Duke University Press.

Zhang L, et al. (2009) Contemporary Clinical Research of Traditional Chinese Medicines for Chronic Hepatitis B in China: An Analytical Review. *Hepatology* 51(2): 690–698.

Zysk K (1991) *Asceticism and Healing in Ancient India. Medicine in the Buddhist Monastery*. Oxford: Oxford University Press.

Part I
East Asian medical industries

1 Discovering new drugs in "Traditional" Chinese Medicine

Inside Guangzhou Huahai pharmaceuticals

Liz P.Y. Chee

In 2015, Chinese pharmaceutical scientist Tu Yao Yao (or Tu You You) won the prestigious Nobel Prize in Physiology or Medicine for the discovery of the anti-malarial drug artemisinin. While Tu's win brought Chinese drug making and discovery to the world's attention, it generated at least two points of controversy within the Chinese medicine community. In the first instance, some challenged the jury's decision to confer the award to Tu and not to the many other Chinese researchers who, they argued, had jointly contributed to the study of *qinghao* (青蒿), the plant from which artemisinin was extracted. Tu had worked on *qinghao* during the Cultural Revolution (1966–1976), when she held the title "science worker," within a team whose mission was to find a cure for malaria using Chinese herbs. Scientific reports from this period did not carry names of individual scientists, since collective effort was supposed to define achievements in the early communist state. For the critics, the jury for the Nobel Prize (and for the 2011 Lasker-DeBakey Award, which she also won) had disregarded this historical and political context by singling out Tu for the act of discovery. There was even controversy in China as to whether Tu had isolated the active ingredient at all or had merely inspired others to do so (Su 2011; Li et al. 2013; Zhu 2016: 1485).

While disputes over priority in scientific discovery are common, a more subtle controversy regarding Tu's award, and one with little resonance outside the community of Chinese physicians and pharmacologists, was whether artemisinin was really an artifact of "Chinese medicine."[1] This was a central claim made in Tu's Nobel Prize lecture, entitled "Artemisinin: A Gift from Traditional Chinese Medicine to the World" (Tu 2015). Tu claimed to have drawn inspiration from the medical text *Zhou Hou Fang* (肘後方) by the famous Jin physician Ge Hong, who recommended that ingredients

---

1 I use "Chinese medicine/medicinals" to refer to what is more commonly called in English "Traditional Chinese Medicine" or TCM, as the former is a more direct translation from Chinese. This is also to recognize that Chinese medicine as currently organised and practiced is a modern hybrid, edited and systematised as a state medicine in the second half of the twentieth century, and replete with elements and influences imported from biomedicine.

DOI: 10.4324/9781003218074-3

from the plant *qinghao* be extracted using a particular process, which Tu replicated. Despite Tu's attempt to lay claim to Chinese medical heritage, however, the Nobel jury made no reference to *qinghao*'s long history of use in Chinese medicine, or Tu's use of pre-modern sources. The award was given for the discovery and synthesis of an active ingredient and not for research on the herb from which this ingredient was extracted. As Elizabeth Hsu (2006) points out, however, crucial details relating to the preparation which Tu had learned from pre-modern texts, such as using water "wringed out" of the soaked herb (rather than an extract produced by boiling), were by no means incidental to Tu's act of discovery, even if they were neglected in subsequent narratives of that event.

This concern over what might be called the *ethnicity* of artemisinin revived longstanding debates within Chinese medicine and pharmacology over its boundary with Western or biomedicine. In March 2016, three Beijing University professors co-authored a book of interviews with Tu, which included a section debating artemisinin's identity. Two contrasting positions were presented, the first proposing that "artemisinin is a non-Chinese drug (*yao* 药) but a plant-based extract with a well-defined singular structure, and so qualifies as a Western medicinal," and the second that artemisinin "is the result of [the longstanding movement to] combine Chinese and Western medicines." The authors themselves took a third view:

> Tu Yao Yao's recent win of the Nobel Prize triggered yet another debate on the problem between Chinese and Western medicines. It is important to note that we need to distinguish between Chinese Medical Theories (CMT) and Chinese Medicines (CM). We also need to refrain from using the generic term of Traditional Chinese Medicine (TCM) because it does not capture CMT and CM as two separate entities, and tends to be misleading. Even though the focus now is on CM, CMT has been weaved into the discussion which should not be the case.
> (Rao et al. 2016)

Despite their different emphases, all three positions acknowledged that artemisinin was something other than an unproblematic "gift from traditional Chinese medicine to the world" and that "the world" – in the form of biomedicine – was woven into the artifact from the time it was gifted.

In his study of an earlier anti-malarial drug, *changshan* (常山), Sean Lei described how the project of isolating active ingredients in Chinese herbs according to biomedical protocols has been of central concern to both the detractors and proponents of Chinese medicine since the Republican period, though for different reasons (Lei 2014). Lei sees the bioprospecting and laboratory analysis of Chinese herbs in the early to mid-twentieth century as an attempt to "re-network" them into Western medicine, minus the corpus of theory and practice surrounding their use. This was met with other strategies, however, which sought to "scientise" (inscribe science onto) Chinese medicine, and thus prove its efficacy to detractors, even as it was practiced and institutionalised as an alternative to biomedicine. How and to what purpose the research protocols of bioscience should be applied to Chinese medicine remained contested terrain throughout the early Communist period (Chee 2021) and, as the controversy over *artemisinin* demonstrates, into the current century as well.

The ambiguities surrounding modern Chinese medicine have not, however, prevented it from becoming a powerful – if not the most powerful – example of an *Asian medical industry*. Branded as "Traditional Chinese Medicine" (TCM) for an international public in the Mao period, it remains just "Chinese medicine" (CM) in China itself, though both terms belie its modern transformation into a platform for socialist revolution. Beginning in the 1950s, the early Communist regime reformulated many divergent health practices into an official state medicine, editing some out entirely, codifying and systematizing others while creating new textbooks, therapies, institutions, and professional roles. Moreover, Chinese medicine was tasked from the beginning with "combining" with Western medicine, which meant that the promotion of innovation and the creation of hybrid forms – rather than a conservative attachment to traditional practices, therapies, and materials for their own sake – was the order of the day (Taylor 2005; Andrews 2015; Chee 2021). Materiality was also stressed over theory. While some Asian medical industries discussed in this volume began the process of pharmaceuticalisation in response to globalisation (Kloos 2017; Kudlu, this volume), this trend began much earlier in China, for reasons both ideological and economic. In the latter category was China's continuing need for the foreign capital gained by marketing medicinals like deer antler, musk, and ginseng to its Asia-based diaspora, which continued despite the Cold War (Chee 2021). "TCM" also began to expand beyond China and Asia as an "alternative medicine" in the same period, initially in the form of foreign aid to other socialist states, mainly in Africa. Thus Chinese medicine had already been re-organised along industrial lines by the communist state prior to globalisation, with pharmaceuticals taking a prominent role alongside such practices as acupuncture. Strong state support for the drug-making sector continued as part of Deng Xiaoping's reforms in the 1980s and later, including efforts to open and expand overseas markets for TCM pharmaceuticals and to use Chinese medicine more generally as a lever of soft power and "nation-branding" (Kudlu, this volume).

This chapter explores how this twentieth-century legacy plays out in the contemporary process of making and marketing new "traditional" medicines both in China and abroad. I will use the Chinese pharmaceutical company Guangzhou Huahai Pharmaceuticals Co., Ltd. (hereafter Guangzhou Huahai) as an illustrative case. This company is part of what Pordie and Gaudillière (2014) call a "reformulation regime," developing and mass marketing "traditional" botanically based drugs in simplified and standardised forms to take advantage of expanded national and global opportunities. The firm is small but ambitious, one of an estimated 1500 in the Chinese medicinal industry as a whole. The combined products of these firms collectively constitute more than a quarter of the country's total pharmaceutical market and bring billions of dollars of export revenue into China on an annual basis. If one also factors in pharmaceutical firms operating outside the mainland (especially in Hong Kong, Taiwan, and Singapore) the Chinese medicine industry controls between 20 and 50 percent of the global market for herb-based medicinals, making it the largest of the Asian medical industries and the one with the greatest global reach (Lin et al. 2018; Ibisworld 2019; Zhou et al. 2019). China also supplies raw materials to other Asian medical industries, most notably those based in Japan (see Arai et al.; Futaya and Blaikie, this volume).

The TCM industry has rarely been studied comparatively, as its size and complicated political history make it an unwieldy "pharmaceutical assemblage" (Kloos 2017) even to those social scientists who make it their focus (Zhan 2009; Lei 2014). Pordie and Gaudillière (2014) see the TCM industry as "crossing the biomedical line" and thus "fail[ing] to provide the same kind of critical alternative" to biomedicine as the Ayurvedic industry of India that they primarily study. This is partly true, given that the Chinese pharmaceutical sector since the 1950s has been tasked by the state to "combine" Chinese medicine and biomedicine, rather than creating a binary or plural medical system. As we shall see, however, the flexible nature of Chinese regulatory categories allows for both the isolating and synthesizing of single active ingredients (the molecular model of drug development that produced *artemisinin*) and for the concoction of more complicated, multi-ingredient recipes, whose reformulation follows many of the same patterns observed in the Ayurvedic industry. While the new Chinese regulatory regime (particularly the reforms of 2007 and after) discourages many companies from registering and marketing their products as "drugs," the alternative categories "health product" and even "cosmetic" have not only proven profitable but are not necessarily viewed by firms and their customers as discordant with "tradition," given the history of unregulated Chinese "patent drugs." Some China-based companies have also moved to Hong Kong, where the even more lightly regulated category "food product" is also available. How a Chinese pharmaceutical company positions elements of its product line is strongly determined by these regulatory regimes, yet even non-drug categories are understood by companies and consumers to sustain the heritage of Chinese medicine, thus avoiding a crisis of relevance, or of marketing. By not strictly demarcating "drug" and "non-drug," and by creating many levels and shadings within each category, Chinese state regulations thus meet Chinese pharmaceutical companies halfway while still strengthening bioscience-based laboratory protocols.

The globalisation of markets has been considered the major driver in bioscience-based regulation of "traditional" medicines around the world, a process Wen-Hua Kuo (2015) calls "regulatory globalisation." While certainly important, this is only one factor shaping the industrialisation of Chinese medicine, which, as I have discussed, became a state project in a period when the market was not as global or controlling as it is today. The ambiguity of the Mao-era dictum to "combine" created internal tensions from an early date between the molecular regime of bioprospecting Chinese herbs for active ingredients (the process that produced artemisinin) and proponents of phytotherapies and multi-ingredient recipes who were not interested in that project, and sometimes hostile to it. These tensions played out within the community of Chinese pharmacologists but converged on the common goal of elevating Chinese medicine as a potent political and social force over and above strictly economic concerns (Taylor 2005; Lei 2014; Andrews 2015). The global market for Chinese drugs that has developed since the death of Mao and the beginning of Deng's reforms has changed the regulatory environment and the characteristics of the players but has not resolved differences in approach, nor necessarily de-politicised the larger and older project of "scientising" Chinese medicine, especially given its new global purchase.

In 2006, anthropologist Sjaak van der Geest commented that there were few studies of what he called "the first phase of the biography of medicines, namely the manufacture and marketing of pharmaceuticals" (Van der Geest 2006: 308). Access to pharmaceutical companies and their laboratories remains a challenge for medical anthropologists, despite recent pioneering work in this area (Pordie 2014; Kuo 2015; Kloos 2017; Kloos et al. 2020). Even when they are successful in gaining entry, scholars tend to write about pharmaceutical companies as "shrewd and greedy organisations interested only in selling and hardly concerned about people's health," to use van der Geest's formulation. He suggested instead to conduct a study from the viewpoint of the lab and the firm, which is one objective of this chapter, sections of which are based on interviews with the CEO and his research team, as well as figures connected to the regulatory regime in which his and other firms operate. This industry is quite divorced in time, intention, and organisation from the project which produced *artemisinin* in the 1960s, but it is influenced in fundamental ways by the Mao-period dictum to "combine Chinese and Western medicine."

This chapter animates these issues as they play out in Guangzhou Huahai and the regulatory milieu within which it and other modern-day pharmaceutical companies operate. I will start, however, with the "new drug" discovery process in Chinese medicine as it was established in the early Communist period.

"New Drugs" in Mao's China

Artemisinin was considered neither a Chinese nor Western drug when Tu conducted her lab research but was referred to as a "new drug" or *xinyao* (新药). Most "new drugs" were defined as imitations or substitutes for foreign products using native (Chinese) herbs, or animal tissue, as their base ingredients. This practice had its origins in the Republican era but expanded in the early Communist period at an unprecedented rate, as private medicinal companies became state owned and subject to state-directed policies and quotas. The Soviet Union had shown that it was possible to become nearly self-sufficient in local drug production by means of reverse engineering, and the new Chinese government drew on that example with the help of Soviet advisors. Bioprospecting occurred throughout the country in the 1950s and early 1960s, with numerous herbs brought to the laboratory with the hope of isolating their active ingredients, or at least producing single-herb-based formulas that could serve as substitutes for imported drugs. The many Soviet-inspired pharmaceutical factories built by the regime – designated by the names of their cities – often contained both laboratories and mass production facilities.[2] (Chee 2015, 2021)

These efforts in some sense continued the project Lei (2014) has described in Republican China of "re-networking" Chinese drugs into biomedicine. Under the slogan "Abandon Yi, Retain Yao" (*feiyi cunyao* 废医存药), the materiality of Chinese drugs had been isolated from the theory of Chinese medicine (*yi*), and herbs became the raw material for drug discovery based on western protocols. This was an early step in what Kloos (2017) has called "the process of pharmaceuticalisation" of traditional medicines, which held special relevance in a regime emphasizing industrial production and quotas, and which also inherited a "patent medicine" sector of long standing. But drug discovery under Mao would also have an ideological and political component, mandating that Chinese and Western medicine were to learn from one another if not be combined with each other. This allowed for the ambiguous identity of "new drugs," which neither fit the classic definition of a Chinese drug (*chengyao* 成药) nor counted as Western drugs (*xiyao* 西药). Soviet protocols were adopted in China, but the Chinese emphasis on the practical versus the theoretical and on "grass-roots" versus "elite" knowledge allowed room for many alternative interpretations of how Chinese and Western medicine were to achieve union under the banner of "science" (Lei 2014; Chee 2015, 2021).

The inability of Western laboratory protocols to account for drugs based on polyherbal formulas (*fufang* 复方) as opposed to formulas using single herbs (*danfang* 单方) became an issue early on for many Chinese physicians and pharmacologists. Traditionally, physicians had prescribed both, but remedies based on multi-herb recipes could not be reduced to single active ingredients. There was thus disagreement over the direction of drug discovery in Chinese pharmacology from an early date, despite the sense that medicinals were the platform on which Chinese and Western medicine could most easily "combine." This is evident in a statement by Fu Fengyong of the Institute of Materia Medica of the Chinese Academy of Medical Sciences during the Hundred Flowers Movement in 1963, which questioned the relevance of applying Western laboratory practices to analyzing fixed prescriptions involving multiple herbs, that is, *fufang*[3]:

---

2 E.g. Shanghai Number 1 Pharmaceutical Factory (Shanghai Di Yi Zhi Yao Chang).
3 The academy is called Zhongguo Yixue Kexue Yuan, and the institute is Yaowu Yanjiu Suo.

Chinese prescriptions are created based on such principles as negative qi (*xie* 邪), positive qi (*zheng* 正), syndrome (*zheng* 症), or aetiology (*yin* 因). Individual herbs are combined together so that they may effectively combat a disease. As such, there can be many active ingredients but each could be serving a different purpose. For instance, some take on a primary role while others are more secondary but nonetheless important. Compared to single-herb formula (*danwei yao* 单味药), categories for active ingredients in a multi-herb formula (*fufang*) are by comparison far more complicated. One ingredient may help to suppress another, while others may play complementary roles. There are also elements that are non-active by themselves but yet have a role to play alongside the main ingredient. And we call them the "related ingredient" (*youguan chengfen* 有关成分). It is therefore more complicated when analyzing *fufang* since we need to consider both the active and related ingredients ... Also, the final product from a *fufang* is not as concentrated as a single-herb formula. There are more residues (*zazhi* 杂质), and less of the [useful] ingredients. Not only that, it is also a complicated process to isolate and differentiate them.

(Zhonghua et al. 1963: 151–152)

Faith in the efficacy of multi-herb recipes by Chinese doctors and pharmacologists gathered momentum during the subsequent Cultural Revolution, despite the parallel project of synthesizing single active ingredients, which resulted in the *artemisinin* breakthrough. Ironically, the Cultural Revolution was the high-water mark for state interest in "folk remedies" and for drug discovery based on Soviet tissue therapy, which both separately and in combination dispensed with "Western" laboratory protocols altogether. Chicken Blood Therapy, which involved injecting blood from live chickens into humans as a rejuvenating agent, is only the most infamous of many attempts to fashion "miracle drugs" through "grass-roots innovation." The extreme eclecticism of drugs and drug discovery methods in this period doubtless had some influence on subsequent attempts to impose order on the Chinese pharmacy (Chee 2018, 2021).

Regulating Chinese medicinals and research protocols

Under Mao, and well into the subsequent Deng era, there was no central state control unit monitoring the efficacy nor even the safety of drugs. The strong political encouragement to achieve "breakthroughs" through experimentation was one factor. Even more important was the widely shared sense that Chinese medicine had been sufficiently tested by the centuries-long experience of the Chinese people. Both factors argued against such Western practices as animal testing and broad-based clinical trials. The State Drug Administration (SDA, later the State Food and Drug Administration [SFDA] and now the China Food and Drug Administration [CFDA]) was set up in 1985 as a comparatively small department within the Ministry of Health, before becoming a separate governing body in 1999. Until 2003, however, when the CFDA promulgated regulations mandating the central registration of new drugs, almost all decisions on Chinese medicinals were made at the provincial level and drug control "was haphazard," in the words of Professor Ye Zhuguang. Ye was the author of the 2007 "Supplementary Regulations on the Registration and Management of Chinese Medicine,"[4] which significantly tightened CFDA protocols for traditional drugs. In two earlier guidelines, instituted in 1987 and 2002 respectively, drugs that reproduced a known formula with only a change in dosage or mode of administration could be locally registered as "new drugs." For Chinese pharmaceutical companies, this was the easiest option and the market became saturated with "copy-cat" products. Ye cited the "worst" years as 2003–2005, when the concept of registration was still nascent and as many as 20,000 drugs of this kind were launched onto the market. This coincided with a boom in exports to (primarily) the Chinese diaspora, Korea, Japan, and the United States. It was with the intention of reducing the number of Chinese medicinal drugs on the market and tightening control over their development that the 2007 guideline was promulgated. With some exceptions, an applicant had now to document the Chinese ("traditional") medical basis for the research while at the same time providing evidence-based support for safety and efficacy using Western laboratory techniques, clinical trials, and other protocols, in order to register a product as a "drug."[5]

A clear intention of the early twenty-first century regulations has been to elevate the status of Chinese medicinals and thus better integrate them into the global drug market, a process occurring across many Asian medical industries (Pordie and Hardon 2015; Kuo 2015; Kloos 2017). In an influential 1998 report entitled "A Strategy to Modernize and Develop Chinese Drugs," Jia Qian (an official in the Ministry of Science and Technology) advocated that the standards of the US Food and Drug Administration (FDA) be used in China to assess drug-making and discovery for Chinese medicinals. Jia lamented that "Chinese drugs have never been sold as drugs in developed countries of the West, but only as 'health products' and 'food'" and offered the solution of applying US FDA standards to Chinese regulations (Jia 1998: 15). Jia would come to regret this stance years later, however, writing opinion pieces pointing out the differences between Chinese and Western medical theory and arguing that the search for active ingredients would undermine the status and even efficacy of Chinese medicine in the long run. He would also be among those who considered *artemisinin* nothing more than a Western drug (Jia 2016).

Although he used the term "health product," the Western marketing category that Jia was really warning against was "health supplement." As

---

4 "2007 *Ban Zhongyao Zhuce Guanli Buchong Guiding.*"
5 Author's interview with Professor Ye Zhuguang on 26th February 2018.

Professor Ye pointed out in an interview, "health supplement" literally means to supplement or make up for a nutritional deficiency such as a lack of Vitamin C, while "health product," as understood by himself and many other Chinese, refers to a substance with the ability to cure. Ye argued that Chinese health products play functional roles, such as boosting the immune system or combating aging, so they should also be considered *zhongyao* (Chinese drugs). Professor Ye suggests that Chinese pharmaceuticals that cannot pass the biomedical "drug" test should be registered as "health products," because the experience accumulated through generations of use of a prescription has likely already proven its efficacy.[6]

The current Chinese regulatory regime for traditional drugs is thus much more generous, broad, and flexible than the standards of the US FDA. Chinese drugs are arranged into nine different classes, from generic and traditional multi-herb "patent medicines" on the lower end to biomedicines synthesised from an herb-based active ingredient on the other (e.g. *artemisinin*). The regulations thus allow for a range of definitions of what a "Chinese medicinal" is, how and by whom it can be created, and how its efficacy should be judged. The multiplicity of categories also allows for hybrid formulations – such as those with "active fractions" (proven active components, making up more than 50 percent of extracts). In practice, however, the classificatory system is meant to accommodate two quite distinct drug development processes at either end: analyzing herbs (and animal tissue) for active molecules on the one hand and concocting multi-herb formulae from traditional recipes on the other. Significantly, they allow phase one and two clinical trials to be waived for so-called "classical prescriptions" (*jingdian fang* 经典方) and exempt their makers from naming the specific (biomedical) disease the drug is meant to treat. Traditionally, Chinese medicine targets the syndrome (*zheng hou* 证候) rather than a specific disease. To quote Ye, the new regulations "helped to bring out the unique characteristics of Chinese medicine" as much as to make Chinese medicine conform to biomedical protocols (Wu et al. 2014: 246–247).

In this sense the regulations bring forward into the twenty-first century the full range of early Communist period strategies for "scientising" or elevating the status of Chinese medicine while avoiding conflict between proponents of the "molecular model" of drug development and those who believe in the efficacy of multi-herbal formulae based on "the centuries-old experience of the Chinese people." For patent drug makers, however, the 2007 regulations significantly raise the bar in requiring "scientific proof" (based on laboratory practices and clinical trials, borrowed from biomedicine) for formulas that sufficiently deviate from classic prescriptions. There also remains the question of what counts as a "classical prescription." It was not the CFDA but a different

---

6 Ibid.

agency – the State Administration of TCM of the People's Republic of China[7] – that was tasked in 2007 with compiling the list of such classical recipes. Ten years on, however, the relevant authorities had still not approved a final list.[8]

Even within this generally favorable regulatory environment, some pharmaceutical companies producing new Chinese medicinals find it expensive and time-consuming to enter this regulatory process. Since the regulations have come into full force, only a handful of new Chinese medicinals have been approved under the category "new drug" (Wu et al. 2014: 242). Many firms have thus turned to utilizing the lesser-regulated categories "health product" and "cosmetic" to market products they still consider to be medicinals. In the following two sections, I provide insights into how one such company, Guangzhou Huahai Pharmaceuticals Co. Ltd, has created its drug research and development protocols, and arranged its product line, in accord with these new regulations.

Guangzhou Huahai Pharmaceuticals Co. Ltd

Guangzhou Huahai has been in business since 2002, though initially under a different name. Its president, Mr. Wu, pulled together resources from seven other collaborators to start the company, using an office originally located on the campus of what is now Guangdong Food and Drug Vocational College. "It was a small laboratory of about 100 square meters," Wu recalled, and he was the sole experienced scientist among the staff of four, the rest being fresh graduates or interns. By 2005, the company had moved to Guangzhou Science City (*kexue cheng* 科学城), and Wu had increased his staff to 20 full-timers. Today, he employs over 60. The firm's rise parallels the explosion of interest in Chinese drugs globally in the same period, and the Chinese government's increasing promotion of exports, though Guangzhou Huahai's primary market for the time being remains China (Mossialos et al. 2016: 23).

Like most pharmacologists of his generation, Wu was a product of the state drug manufacturing sector. After completing high school in 1984, he was "assigned [by the country]" to study at the *zhongyao* (中药) department of Nanjing Pharmaceutical Institute (*Nanjing Yaoxue Yuan* 南京药学院).[9] This was a four-year program, the first two years of which were spent studying Chinese medical principles and basic Western chemistry. From the third year onward, he studied *zhongyao* (Chinese drugs) in depth, including subfields such as drug analysis (mostly quality control), drug synthesis, biochemical pharmacology, and animal-based drugs. Prior to the 1980s, China

---

7 "*Zhongguo Renmin Gonghe Guo Guojia Zhongyiyao Guanli Ju.*"
8 It was only in 2016–2017, when a new guideline was promulgated, that authorities began efforts to create the list of classic prescriptions.
9 Author's interview with Mr Wu Zhinan on 21st February 2017

had no technology or expertise to "authenticate" (*jian ding* 坚定) a medicinal. It was the combined efforts of his teacher-researchers, Xu Luoshan and Xu Guojun, who established drug authentication as a legitimate subfield within *zhongyao* studies. Wu was thus from the beginning acculturated into a "Chinese medicine" which was both informed by and subject to protocols borrowed from biomedicine.

Upon graduation in 1988, Wu was assigned to work in the Number Two Drug-Making Factory (*Di Er Zhi Yao Chang* 第二制药厂) in Foshan, Guangdong, which focused on producing Chinese drugs in modern forms such as tablets and capsules. Number Two Drug-Making Factory was part of the larger Joint Pharmaceutical Factory (*Lianhe Zhiyao Chang* 联合制药厂), which was the result of merging all drug production workshops in Foshan in the 1950s. With the coming of economic liberalisation, the factory was renamed Foshan Dezhong Pharmaceuticals Co. Ltd while Wu was still in residence.[10] His responsibilities there included developing new drugs and reformulating existing ones using more modern forms of delivery.

Given this background, the language the firm uses to describe its approach to Chinese medicine is unabashedly forward-looking, paralleling in many respects that of biomedical drug firms. The company takes pride in its location in the "science and technology innovation base" of Guangzhou Science City and is described on one website as "a high-tech enterprise with innovative R&D at its core" (Guangzhou Huahai 2020). The firm has filed more than 30 patents related to lab-based technologies, and many of the technical or lab positions it recruits for would be found in any pharmaceutical firm in China, whether or not its products were TCM drugs or biomedicines (Guangzhou Huahai 2017).

Despite these convergences, Guangzhou Huahai considers itself not just a maker of Chinese medicine but a champion, promoting and shaping its ethos. The firm is currently striving to become the forerunner in developing painkillers made from Chinese medicinals. The reason, according to Wu, is "to challenge popular perception of what Chinese medicine can and cannot do." He wants to overturn the popular saying that Chinese medicine "cures the core [disease] but not superficial [symptoms]" (*zhiben bu zhibiao* 治本不治标). By demonstrating that Chinese drugs can also relieve pain, which is a superficial symptom, Wu hopes in this manner to "show the power and effectiveness of Chinese medicine." He was quick to recount in interviews how Chinese medicine has been denigrated from the Republican period onward. The company thus sees itself as not only serving a customer base who already believe in Chinese medicine but contributing to

---

10 For a history of Foshan Dezhong Pharmaceuticals Co. Ltd and Foshan Feng Liao Xing Pharmaceuticals Co. Ltd., refer to Yang Xionghui (2011), *Deng Zai Yao Zhong, Yao Wei Dazhong*, Guangzhou: Guangdong Keji Chuban She, 2011 and Wu Weixiao (2012), *Gu Jin Yin Zheng, Fo Yue Feng Liao Xing*, Guangzhou: Guangdong Keji Chuban She.

the longstanding project of "proving" the worth of that medicine to real and potential detractors using state-of-the-art laboratory processes. In that sense he and the company are not constitutionally opposed to the state regulatory regime, which shares some of the same basic goals.

Despite the intention of the 2007 regulations to raise the status of Chinese medicine, however, the increasing stringency of standards has caused Wu's company and many others to register and market many of their products as something other than "drugs." In fact, all the items I observed for sale in the shops of Guangzhou Huahai fell within the category of either "health product" or "cosmetic," though the company's "drugs" can only be sold through hospital pharmacies or clinics and not in its own shops. The registration process for Chinese drugs is long and expensive, typically taking 10–15 years, while a "health product" takes two to three years and "cosmetics" only one to two. CEO Wu claimed one could spend as much as 30 million yuan on developing a new drug, and given that the CFDA (China Food and Drug Administration) does not approve more than a few each year, this is a high-risk investment.[11] Companies like Guangzhou Huahai thus maintain product lines ranging across drug and non-drug categories, with the latter often being the most profitable. Yet they continue to invest significant capital and time in drug development, for reasons we shall subsequently discuss.

Inside the Laboratory of Guangzhou Huahai: The science of "New Drug" discovery

At Guangzhou Huahai, the steps taken to concoct new multi-herbal "traditional" drugs are roughly as follows, according to interviews with informants involved at various stages of this process. First, the company targets a particular condition it believes is undertreated by the Chinese drug market. Guangzhou Huahai has lately been conducting research into the condition known in Western medicine as Irritable Bowel Syndrome or IBS. The R&D team has first to match it to a known syndrome (*zhengxing* 证型) in Chinese medical literature, which in this case is "stasis of the liver qi" (*gan qi yu jie* 肝气郁结 or *gan yu* 肝郁 for short). The R&D team then locates a known prescription and modifies it by adding or reducing ingredients accordingly. In my interview with the Deputy General Manager, who also heads the R&D team, she used the phrase *jiajian* (加减, literally "plus-minus") to describe the process of modifying known recipes.[12] While she did not fully elaborate their method, it is the norm for Chinese pharmaceutical companies to consult with practicing physicians who have extensive "bedside experience" (*linchuang jingyan* 临床经验) in making and altering prescriptions.

---

11 The number of "new" traditional drugs approved across all classes by the CFDA decreased during the period 2009–2013 went from 81 to 12 (Wu et al. 2014)
12 Interview conducted on 26th February 2016.

Discovering new drugs in Traditional Chinese Medicine 43

There are also occasions when a physician offers his or her own original prescription to the company to be developed into a pharmaceutical. Such recipes were formerly obtained for free, with the understanding that the physician would profit through the resale of the pharmaceutical to customers. Under more recent regulations, however, companies are now obliged to pay physicians for rights over their prescriptions.[13]

The firm's research in IBS actually began through simplifying a doctor's existing polyherbal prescription and creating a standard form for its administration. The product was marketed as "Happy Intestine Granules" (*changle keli* 常乐颗粒). The manager commented that the conversion process did "change [the prescription into] a different medicine" but emphasised that this was an inevitable result of "the modernization of Chinese Drugs" (*zhongyao xiandaihua* 中药现代化). Conversion was not a simple matter of boiling the ingredients – which in this case consisted of six medicinals – and crushing and then hardening them back into the form of granules, but involved an intricate process of extraction.[14] Other possible modifications involve reducing a prescription to one or two essential medicinals, which is called *chai fang* (拆方) or literally "breaking down the prescription." While this would seem a product of cost-cutting and is in some instances, it is also considered by drug makers to have traditional sanction. Another informant, Professor Lyu Guiyuan, adopts the concept of clustering or *zu fen* (组分). To quote Lyu, *zu fen* involves removing and using a cluster of "effective parts" (*youxiao bu fen* 有效部分), which is different from Tu's method of singling out only one active ingredient. Lyu's experience, however, is that this method has been successful in his treatment of Western diseases but not Chinese syndromes. For instance, his laboratory has found wild chrysanthemum effective in treating high blood pressure by extracting the "effective part," called *huang tong* (黄铜). Traditionally, the plant has been known to "clear the liver" or *qing gan* (清肝), but Professor Lyu is not convinced that *huang tong* by itself can do the same. Another method is analyzing each ingredient separately and then removing and piecing together the separate active ingredients. This has been called by some researchers "the single extract" (*fen ti* 分体) and is popular among researchers with a strong background in bioscience.[15]

Once a recipe or prescription is finalised, the team then manufactures a prototype batch or *chengyao*. They also decide the mode of administration and the form the drug will take (e.g. granules, tablet, or capsule if via oral administration). There are two ways to extract ingredients from raw herbs.

---

13 This is called the "*chi you ren*" system which literally means "the person possessing [the rights]."
14 There are craft alternatives to extraction that are considered more "authentic" by some firms. For example, Hong Kong-based Ma Bai Liang, a medicinal shop with a 200-year history, has moved toward mechanisation to allow for mass production, but still uses whole ingredients rather than their extracts (author's visit to Ma Bai Liang, February, 2018)
15 Author's interview with Professor Lyu Guiyuan on 6th March 2018.

The first, more traditional, method is to boil them in water. This is called *shuiti* (水提) or "extracting using water." The other common and more modern method is to soak the herbs for a period in an ethanol-filled container. Substances that submerge to the bottom of the container are called "residues" and discarded, while those floating on the surface are retrieved. The final product is called *jin gao* (浸膏), because it has been soaked (*jin*) in ethanol and is sticky (*gao*). The R&D team then converts the substance into the desired mode or form for administration.

Before proceeding to clinical trials, the R&D team has to document for regulators the ingredients (*ding xing* 定性) and their quantities (*ding liang* 定量), and finally conduct a quality check (*zhiliang yanjiu* 质量研究) of their sample batch. The dosage for each individual sample (pill, capsule, or granule, etc.) also has to be made consistent throughout.

Until very recently, efficacy and safety trials for new Chinese medicinals normally began with patients. Under the bioscience-influenced regulatory regime, however, they are now preceded by animal testing, which takes an average of 18–24 months. The main purpose is to ensure safety of the drugs, however, rather than their efficacy. There has been much debate about the accuracy and relevance of using animals for testing efficacy in Chinese pharmaceuticals, and most of my informants considered it impossible to recreate in animal models the different syndromes or patterns (*zheng hou* 证候) seen in human patients.

Clinical trials themselves involve four stages, with the pool of human subjects increasing with each stage, from tens in the first to hundreds by the third. It is here that the company spends the most money, since it has to absorb the medical fees of all patients, including transport to and from the hospital or clinic. The company is also required to provide reports describing all the above processes – from R&D through to the clinical trials – to the CFDA for final approval. Once the new drug is approved for sale, the company still has to gather feedback from users, which counts as the fourth and final stage of clinical trials (Bian et al. 2012).

As mentioned earlier, very few "new drugs" in the Chinese medicine sector have been approved since the 2007 guidelines governing Chinese pharmaceuticals were promulgated, causing more and more companies to market medicinals as "health products" or "cosmetics." On the other hand, companies like Guangzhou Huahai continue to enter the drug approval arena with what they consider their most promising or important products. This is not only in order to profit from the sale of prescription drugs, as these are not necessarily as profitable as over-the-counter medications. Having an officially sanctioned drug gives the company legitimacy, in its own eyes and those of its customers, and elevates the status of the whole product line, including products in the lesser categories of health products and cosmetics. Despite the stringency of the new regulations, there is a sense in the industry that they are not being implemented in a draconian manner, that is, in order to marginalise or eliminate Chinese medicine as a sector. The Chinese regulatory arena is, to quote an informant, "more like a dialogue"[16] or, as one recent report put it, has a "strict entry and tolerant exit" approach, in contrast to the "tolerant entry and strict exit" process of the American FDA (Wu et al. 2014). Companies with the capital and facilities to embark on lengthy and expensive R&D and regulatory processes are generally encouraged, with the CDFA jury providing suggestions for improvement at various stages and allowing companies the chance to make amendments.

Chinese medicine as food: Healthy Medicine Holdings Ltd, Hong Kong SAR

For some companies, "food" is an even more accessible marketing category than "health product," given that food has traditionally been considered close to medicine in Chinese culture. There is even a saying *"yaoshi tongyuan"* (药食同源, literally "food and medicine have the same origin"). The contemporary boundary between food and medicine is rather strictly maintained by the CFDA, however, which has led a number of pharmaceutical companies to open branches and register their products in Hong Kong, which has a different regulatory regime that allows for such a translation.

In many respects, there are fewer barriers for a company seeking to bring a Chinese medicinal to market in Hong Kong SAR. During my visit to Hong Kong-based Healthy Medicine Holdings Ltd (hereafter Healthy Medicine), for example, the CEO discussed the ease with which she had set up her drug manufacturing business within a short period, in contrast to the longer development trajectory of Guangzhou Huahai. A Chinese national who has her own drug-making business in mainland China, the CEO gave various reasons for why Hong Kong was more attractive as a business location, including tax holidays, fewer regulations, and the ability to market medicinals across a broader range of categories, including food.[17] This is partly a result of a strategy launched in the late 1990s to make Hong Kong into a Chinese medicine hub, with Chinese pharmacological researchers from the mainland or overseas recruited to key positions under the Quality Migrant Admission Scheme. This initiative also paved the way for mainland Chinese drug firms to set up branches or register as new firms in Hong Kong. Moreover, it is not mandatory for pharmaceutical companies in Hong Kong to meet the GMP (Good Manufacturing Practices) standards of mainland China. Healthy Medicine has, however, chosen to build its

---

16 Author's interview with Mr Chen Weiwu on 9th March 2018. Mr Chen heads the research department of Gansu Qizheng Zangyao Youxian Gongsi, a company producing Tibetan pharmaceuticals. According to Mr Chen, drugs produced based on ethnic medical systems are judged by CDFA as though they are Chinese medicine. However, as there are theoretical differences between Tibetan and Chinese medicines, this has often been a point of contention with the CFDA jury.

17 The Chinese tax system has more colloquially been called "The Million Taxes."

Hong Kong factory according to GMP requirements for the sake of gaining consumer trust.

The most attractive pull factor, however, is the allowance to market Chinese medicine in Hong Kong as a food product. This is not a separate category from those in China, as all consumable "health products" are also considered food in Hong Kong and are governed directly by the Food and Environmental Hygiene Department. There are no procedures for testing the medical efficacy of health/food products, as long as they are digestible, but there is a two- to three-year waiting period for drugs. Healthy Medicine thus has only one drug item in its product line, which is its own version of the longstanding *Wuji Baifeng Wan* (乌鸡白凤丸, literally "Black Chicken White Phoenix Pill") – a post-menstrual nourishment pill.[18] Rather than considering the Hong Kong policy more lax, companies are more likely to respond, as did the CEO of Healthy Medicine, that: "There is an inextricable relationship between food and medicine in *zhongyi* (中医)," and this is simply better recognised in Hong Kong than in mainland China. The mainland prohibition on advertising medicinal functions (*gong neng* 功能) for products in the "food" category is thus considered outside of Chinese medicinal tradition by some informants and likely their customers.

It is an open question, however, as to how much longer companies like Healthy Medicine can benefit from Hong Kong's different regulatory regimes. According to Professor Ye, there are now plans to tighten pharmaceutical laws in Hong Kong to match those on the mainland. If that happens, it is the more established Hong Kong medicine companies that may be the most hard-hit, as everything from factory layout and lab protocols to the labeling of ingredients on packaging will have to be changed in compliance with the standards of the Chinese government.

Conclusion

Bioscientific protocols have been strengthened as benchmarks for assessing and proving how Chinese drugs work in China. Yet while the Chinese regulatory regime is part of a global process and trend, intent on building greater trust in Asian industrial medicines, it also embodies compromises and flexibilities that Chinese pharmacologists and pharmaceutical companies have been working out domestically since the mid-twentieth century. The search for active ingredients in Chinese herbs, for example, is now only one route which pharmacological practice in this field can allowably travel. Also, the flexibility with which Chinese regulations allow Chinese drugs to be differentially classed, in some instances as something other than "drugs," has given firms significant leeway. Some actors in this process even consider

---

18 Hong Kong companies are required to produce at least one drug before they can become GMP-certified.

the ongoing tension between bioscience and Chinese medicine to be a positive thing. To quote researcher You Yun from the Academy of Chinese Medical Sciences, "there will only be progress with conflict."[19]

Chinese companies like Guangzhou Huahai demonstrate some practices and patterns common across the Asian medical industries described in this volume yet differ in other respects. As in the Ayurvedic industry, Guangzhou Huahai reformulates polyherbal drugs by identifying symptoms in biomedical terms, prospecting among historic recipes (or those presented by physicians and other informants as historic), simplifying or otherwise altering such recipes to suit batch or mass production, and developing protocols to produce and test finished products (Pordie and Gaudillière 2014). The concern in the Ayurvedic and other Asian industries with property rights is much less pronounced in the Chinese case, however, for reasons requiring further study. Despite being known as "patent medicines," Chinese multi-herbal concoctions were historically not protected by patents, and there has been little sense that foreign companies were bioprospecting Chinese herbs, alleviating any need to protect natural resources under national ownership (Xu and Yang 2009: 134; Mossialos et al. 2016: 146). Like the Toyama-based *haichi* firms described by Futaya and Blaikie (this volume), Chinese medicine firms like Guangzhou Huahai directly market to consumers, continuing a tradition that pre-dates the communist revolution. However, they simultaneously supply prescription-only drugs to physicians and hospitals, given strong clinical support for Chinese medicine by the communist state. Chinese companies have not been as concerned with GMP as their counterparts in the Japanese Kampo industry, but both exist within a regulatory regime whose "complexity and multi-layered quality" (Arai et al., this volume) moderates the homage they also pay to "international standards."

Certain historic features of the Chinese medical industry influence its modern regulatory regime in ways that set China apart. The Mao-era dictum to "combine" Chinese and Western medicine, while creating a highly institutionalised and politically powerful Chinese medicine and drug discovery culture, limited its ability to reject – or consider itself a full alternative to – biomedicine. "Scientisation" was accepted even prior to globalisation as a positive goal, one that would make Chinese medicine better understood throughout the world. Recent regulations based on biomedical protocols have indeed greatly reduced the number of new "drugs," but not necessarily the number of marketable products understood by makers and users to constitute "Chinese medicinals."

The current regulations governing the registration of "new" traditional Chinese drugs thus preserve the earlier twentieth-century compromise between molecular and reformulation regimes. On the one hand, they

---

19 Author's interview with You Yun on 27th February 2018.

capture for Chinese medicine the type of biomedical protocols that allowed *artemisinin* to become a universally accepted drug. On the other hand, they allow arguments based on "the centuries-long experience of the Chinese people" to waive the need for animal testing and clinical trials in the case of certain new patent drug recipes. This flexibility of categorisation is taken even farther by allowing drug companies to market certain products in non-drug categories like "health products," "cosmetics" and "food." "Traditional Chinese Medicine" in this respect bends not only "tradition" but also the very concept of "medicine" to conform to the layered structure of a dynamic market. The burgeoning success of the Chinese medicine industry in the domestic and global marketplace thus does not depend on establishing itself as an "alternative" to biomedicine, nor to its selective adaptation of biomedical protocols, but to its ability to create varied product lines which satisfy a range of consumer and regulatory expectations as to what "Chinese medicine" is and can do. Ambiguity in this sense has long been, and continues to be, a strength for the industry rather than a weakness.

Bibliography

Andrews B (2015) *The Making of Modern Chinese Medicine, 1850–1960*. Honolulu, HI: University of Hawaii Press.

Bian Z, Chen S, Cheng CW, et al. (2012) Developing New Drugs from Annals of Chinese Medicine. *Acta Pharmaceutica Sinica B* 2(1): 1–7.

Chee LPY (2015) *Reformulations: How Pharmaceuticals and Animal-Based Drugs Changed Chinese Medicine, 1950–1990*. PhD Dissertation.

Chee LPY (2018) To Cure a Hundred Diseases: The Curious Case of Chicken Blood Therapy. *Science, Technology & Society* 23(2): 195–213.

Chee LPY (2021) *Mao's Bestiary: Medicinal Animals and Modern China*. Durham, NC: Duke University Press.

Guangdong Shipin Yaopin Zhiye Xueyuan Jianjie (2017) http://www.gdyzy.edu.cn/web/loadWebPage.do?4401401_440113222_0_4 (accessed 5 April 2017).

Guangzhou Huahai Pharmaceutical Co, Ltd., Company Profile (2020). https://www.qgyyzs.net/shangpu/4057/ (accessed 1 June 2020).

Guangzhou Huahai Pharmaceutical Co. Ltd. (2017). Pharmaceutical Production Operator Job Description. http://www.jobuy.com/jobs/81801.html (accessed 2 June 2020).

Hu Q (2015) TCM Safety Regulation in China (paper presented at the 12th World Congress of Chinese Medicine, Barcelona, 2015). http://www.chetch.eu/cms/index.php/dissemination/cat_view/34-dissemination/2-events/37-12th-world-congress-of-chinese-medicine.html (accessed 15 May 2018).

Hsu E (2006) Reflections on the "Discovery" of the Antimalarial *Qinghao*. *British Journal of Clinical Pharmacology* 61(6): 666–670.

Ibisworld (2019) Traditional Chinese Medicine Manufacturing in China Industry Trends (2015–2020). https://www.ibisworld.com/china/market-research-reports/traditional-chinese-medicine-manufacturing-industry/ (accessed 1 June 2020).

Jia Q (1998) *Zhongyao Xiandai Hua Fazhang Zhanlue*. Beijing: Kexue Jishu Wenxian Chuban She.

Jia Q (2016) Zhongyao Xiandaihua Jue Bushi Jiang Zhongyao Hua Wei Xiyao http://www.360doc.com/content/16/0303/01/30472303_538964528.shtml (accessed 23 March 2018).

Kloos S (2017) The Pharmaceutical Assemblage: Rethinking Sowa Rigpa and the Herbal Pharmaceutical Industry in Asia. *Current Anthropology* 58(6): 693–705.

Kloos S, Madhavan H, Tidwell T, et al. (2020) The Transnational Sowa Rigpa Industry in Asia: New Perspectives on an Emerging Economy. *Social Science and Medicine* 245: 112617.

Kuo W (2015) Promoting Chinese Herbal Drugs Through Regulatory Globalisation: The Case of the Consortium for Globalization of Chinese Medicine. *Asian Medicine* 10: 316–339.

Lei HS (2014) *Neither Donkey nor Horse: Medicine in the Struggle over China's Modernity*. Chicago, IL: University of Chicago Press.

Li R, Rao Y and Zhang D (2013) 523 Renwu Yu Qinghaosu Faxian De Lishi Tanjiu. *Ziran Bianzheng Fa Tongxun* 1: 107–121.

Lin AX, Chan G, Hu Y, et al. (2018) Internationalization of Traditional Chinese Medicine: Current International Market, Internationalization Challenges and Prospective Suggestions. *Chinese Medicine* 13(9). https://doi.org/10.1186/s13020-018-0167-z (accessed 1 June 2020).

Massialos E, Ge Y, Hu J, et al. (2016) *Pharmaceutical Policy in China: Challenges and Opportunities for Reform*. Geneva: World Health Organization.

Pordie L (2014) Pervious Drugs: Making the Pharmaceutical Object in Techno-Ayurveda. *Asian Medicine* 9(1): 49–76.

Pordie L and Hardon A (2015) Drugs' Stories and Itineraries: On the Making of Asian Industrial Medicine. *Anthropology and Medicine* 22(1): 1–6.

Pordie L and Gaudillière J-P (2014) The Reformulation Regime in Drug Discovery: Revisiting Polyherbals and Property Rights in the Ayurvedic Industry. *East Asian Science, Technology, and Society* 8(1): 57–80.

Rao Y, Li R and Zhang D (2016) *Xinsuan Yu Rongyao: Zhongguo Kexue De Nuojiang Zhilu*. Beijing: Beijing Daxue Chuban She.

Su J (2011) Tu Youyou, Controversial "Mother of Artemisinin"(2). http://www.ecns.cn/figure/2011/10-10/2876_2.shtml (accessed 28 November 2017).

Sunder Rajan K (ed) (2012) *Lively Capital: Biotechnologies, Ethics, and Governance in Global Markets*. Durham, NC: Duke University Press.

Taylor K (2005) *Chinese Medicine in Early Communist China, 1945–63: A Medicine of Revolution*. London: Routledge.

Tu Y (2015) Artemisinin – A Gift from Traditional Chinese Medicine to the World. https://www.nobelprize.org/nobel_prizes/medicine/laureates/2015/tu-lecture.pdf (accessed 28 November 2017).

Van der Geest S (2006) Anthropology and the Pharmaceutical Nexus. *Anthropological Quarterly* 79(2): 303–314.

Wu W (2012) *Gu Jin Yin Zheng, Fo Yue Feng Liao Xing*. Guangzhou: Guangdong Keji Chuban She.

Wu WY, Hou JJ, Long HL, et al. (2014) TCM-Based New Drug Discovery and Development in China. *Chinese Journal of Natural Medicines* 12(4): 0241–0250.

Xionghui Y (2011) *Deng Zai Yao Zhong, Yao Wei Dazhong*. Guangzhou: Guangdong Keji Chuban She.

Xu J and Yang Y (2009) Traditional Chinese Medicine in the China Health Care System. *Health Policy* 90(2–3): 133–139.

Zhan M (2009) *Other-Worldly: Making Chinese Medicine Through Transnational Frames*. Durham, NC: Duke University Press.

Zhonghua S, Hui K, Zhuanye Y, et al. (1963) *Xunzhao Xinyao De Lilun Jichu He Linchuang Shiji*, Shanghai: Shanghai Jishu Chuban She.

Zhou X, Li CG, Chang D, et al. (2019) Current Status and Major Challenges to the Safety and Efficacy Presented by Chinese Herbal Medicine. *Medicines (Basel)* 6(1): 14.

Zhu J (ed) (2016) *Bainian Zhongyi Shi A Century of Traditional Chinese Medicine 1912–2015 (Xia Ce)*. Shanghai: Shanghai Keji Chuban She.

2 Cultivation and paternalism in the service of the market

Medical industry and ethnicity in Southwest China

Manuel Campinas

At a national forum of the China Medical Association of Minorities (CMAM) in Chengdu, I witnessed first-hand both the collaboration and competition surrounding the development of proprietary medicines among China's ethnic minorities. The main theme of this "Sixth National Ethnic Medicine Inheritance and Innovation Development Forum" was the pervasive "One Belt One Road" (*yidai yilu*一带一路) initiative.[1] Han as well as Mongol, Yi, Dai, and Qiang (Ch'iang) doctors and academics took the stage to showcase their achievements on the research and production of different medicinal products. A few spoke of the theory behind their "system of ethnic medicine," the Mongols boasted of their "dialectical and logical thinking methods," while others summed up the challenges and opportunities they faced. The majority of speakers, however, focused on topics such as biomedical aetiology and pathology, compound prescriptions, active ingredient extraction, Crohn's disease and interferons, high performance liquid chromatography, mass spectrometry, and polymerase chain reaction, as well as the large investments they had secured. In the spirit of "One Belt One Road," their gaze was also fixed abroad on the partnerships being developed with countries such as Thailand, Vietnam, Laos, and Cambodia.

With the passing of the Chinese Medicine Law of 2016, the Chinese medicines industry now officially includes ethnic minority medicines (PRC Twelfth National People's Congress 2016). The push to expand this industry has increasing importance in China's policies, even as outputs continue to grow (Di Tommaso et al. 2017). Together with internationalisation linked to the "One Belt One Road" initiative, policy priority is given to standardisation and innovation (SATCM 2016; State Council of the PRC 2016). In

---

1 The "One Belt One Road" or "Belt Road" initiative refers to China's grand foreign policy and trade strategy announced in 2012 and launched as policy in 2015. This strategy has been described as a means of "promoting China's new vision of global governance" (Callahan 2016), while others see it as merely a new name for the solidification of international cooperation efforts running since the 1990s (Aoyama 2016). The initiative focuses particularly on relations with the rest of Asia, Europe, the Middle East, and Pacific Islands, while pushing also for wider global influence.

DOI: 10.4324/9781003218074-4

political-industrial-academic circles such as the CMAM, these aims are frequently brought together under the maxim of ensuring the "inheritance and development" of Chinese medicine and medicines. The main focus of ethnic medicine conferences tends to be proprietary medicines (*zhongchengyao* 中成药), as the market value for such products was four times the size of that for "herbal pieces" (*yinpian* 饮片), or crude medicinal plant materials, in 2014 (Di Tommaso et al. 2017). Such priority is framed as part of a "natural" developmental progression, with industrial pharmaceutical production and market entry at the pinnacle. In anthropological research, these pharmaceutical transformations have variously been referred to as "reformulation," with Chinese *materia medica* feeding into drug-discovery and industrial scale production (Chee 2015, this volume), as "re-networking," with Chinese medicine doctors giving way to scientists in the production of medicines (Lei 1999), and as the emergence of an "alternative modernity" (Hsu 2009).

I argue that in political-industrial-academic circles, this widely shared and rarely questioned vision of linear industrial development is closely tied to the notion of "lateness," reflecting frequent references to East Asian countries as "latecomers" to modernity and industrialisation (Wang 2016). This phenomenon has been explored by Science, Technology, and Society (STS) scholars working in East Asia, who rephrased Latour's famous "we have never been modern" quote (Latour 1993) as "we have never been latecomers" (Chen 2015; Lin and Law 2015) in an attempt to locate alternative knowledge spaces for local technosocial practices. Indeed, some see the conjoining of such modernist discourses, both from without and within, as key to the production of "modern China" (Yang 1994). However, it is notable that this sense of deficiency has not resulted in a completely one-sided push to copy "the West," nor hostility towards what is considered to be Chinese, but has instead allowed "for shifting and contested positions toward traditions, ranging from projects that would entirely destroy the 'old' to those that would preserve or even invent traditions as sources of modernization" (Meinhof 2017: 53). I argue that the ethnic minority pharmaceutical industry in China largely reflects the latter project. Reaction and compliance to external rules and standards emerge both when China faces the rest of the world and when ethnic minorities face Chinese institutions. In relation to Chinese medicine, the minorities developing their own ethnic medicines are considered the "latecomers." Among these, the Qiang are even further "latecomers" down the road, blaming missed opportunities for not (yet) having registered proprietary medicines for nationwide sale. I contend that a deeper understanding of such projects among Chinese ethnic minorities is crucial because it is among these stakeholders that the technosocial evolutionism that resides at the core of China's pharmaceutical development initiatives is laid bare.

The size of the Chinese medicines industry is hard to assess, not only due to over- and under-reporting for economic or political purposes but also due to the coexistence of various inclusion and exclusion criteria that reflect "partially overlapping pharmaceutical assemblages" (Kloos, introduction, this volume). This "overlapping" is particularly accentuated in ethnic minority pharmaceutical industries. Since 1992, Tibetan, Mongolian, and Uyghur medicines have acquired their own pharmaceutical centres within China, contributing to a "race between minorities" for the potential financial gains. However, it remains unclear which outputs fall within the ethnic minority domain and which are counted as part of "Chinese medicine." This blurriness has only increased with the recent law changes designating all ethnic medicines as part of Chinese medicine (PRC Twelfth National People's Congress 2016). Individual reports have accounted for 2.4 billion USD in 2013 from sales of Miao medicines (Yang and Peng 2015), 500.2 million USD from Tibetan medicines, and 162 million USD from Mongolian medicines in 2017 (Kloos et al. 2020), but overall sales values are very difficult to establish with any degree of certainty. This chapter focuses on the current foundational phase in the creation of a Qiang medical industry. Although not yet an established industry let alone a "pharmaceutical assemblage" (Kloos 2017), examining this aspirational stage renders visible the negotiations, conflicts, and pressures central to the endeavour of pharmaceutical industry development within the prevailing policy and market environment. There are less than two dozen self-entitled "Qiang medicine doctors" operating today, a small number of whom produce compound medicines in their clinics and at least one that outsources production. They are only allowed to sell their products within local medical institutions, not in pharmacies nationwide, but one research institution is attempting to develop "Qiang medicines" with a wider target market, in partnership with an established pharmaceutical company. There is also an overlap in the ethnic attribution of medicines circulating in the Chinese medicine market, which I examine in detail below.

While one cannot speak of a "Qiang medical industry" per se, there is an overwhelming push for industrialisation underway, as well as efforts to foment demand through the development and promotion of "Qiang" medicinal products, and to actively seek external investment to enable industrial expansion. Such imperatives were evident among the participants of this research and also reflect central government policies. However, given mounting recognition of the unsustainability of the present supply chains for Chinese medicines, both policy and practice must address the growing "contradiction between supply and demand" (State Council of the PRC, 2015a). At the policy level, the blame for unsustainable resource extraction is laid upon those collecting and trading in primary products rather than on the industry itself, which in turn is used to justify the rapid scaling up of cultivation initiatives and the advancement of a "protection through development" strategy (ibid.). This strategy is framed as essential for both environmental protection and economic growth, and is widely portrayed as a "win-win scenario." However, as medicinal products are increasingly marketed as "ethnic" and medicinal plant cultivation initiatives multiply, so do disconnects between the stakeholders in pharmaceutical enterprises, rural communities, and members of the minority groups in question. It is these interactions, collaborations and disjunctures that I explore in this chapter by focusing on the emergence of a vestigial Qiang medicines industry.

Researching human-medicinal relations in Sichuan

Based on long-term, multi-sited ethnographic fieldwork in Sichuan as well as the study of a wide range of Chinese policy documents, this chapter is composed of two parts. The first follows a plant species and a variety in their contested ethnic Qiang attributions. The species is *qianghuo* (羌活 *Notopterygium incisum* K.C. Ting ex H.T. Chang),[2] the name of which literally means "Qiang life" and has been in use for at least 2000 years. The variety is *wabu beimu* (瓦布贝母 *Fritillaria unibracteata* var. *wabuensis* (S.Y. Tang & S.C. Yueh) Z.D. Liu, Shu Wang, & S.C. Chen), which although "discovered" over 30 years ago, was given the name *qiang beimu* (羌贝母) by a pharmaceutical company in the two years prior to my interview with their representative. These two cases of ethnic label attribution raise several critical issues of relevance both within China and across other Asian medical industries.

In general, ethnicity has rarely been attributed to raw materials used in Chinese medicines. Such attributions have largely been reserved for registered proprietary medicines developed through research and industrial processes, thereby associating both the product and the ethnic group in question with "progress" and "development." However, because the Qiang do not yet have any nationally registered medicines, the two cases discussed here go against the prevailing trend, producing an articulation of Qiang medicines that in the first case is anchored in a shared imagined past, and in the second is malleable and exploited for marketing purposes. Throughout this chapter, I refer to "articulation" (Latour 1999) as the act of drawing from a variety of material aspects in order to arrive at artefacts, in this case "Qiang medicines."

I followed both *qianghuo* and *wabu beimu* in two villages, between Qiang medicinal herb collectors and dealers, among villagers who used them in their self-care, and in town and city Qiang medicine clinics. I also followed them into various research institutions, pharmaceutical companies, and ethnic medicine conferences. In institutional circles, I uncovered attempts to develop and grow cultivars that mimic their wild counterparts, struggles with pharmacopoeia restrictions, and the harnessing of morphological features as a way to assert the authenticity and ethnicity of cultivated *qiang beimu*. I also found Qiang medicine doctors drawing from ancient textual

---

2 The Latin nomenclature for botanical identification used in this chapter is that of the Chinese Pharmacopoeia (Chinese Pharmacopoeia Committee 2015). While aware of the inaccuracies surrounding state-sanctioned uniformisation and issues of species substitution, my intention is to use a categorisation that reflects local institutional definitions.

records of *qianghuo* in order to legitimise the Qiang medical discipline they promoted. These efforts contrasted with the preference of villagers for wild *qianghuo* and *wabu beimu*, as well as their disregard for the ethnic associations of either.

The second part of this chapter explores the motivations that lie behind current policies concerning medicinal plant sustainability and cultivation. It also shows the paternalism directed at medicinal herb collectors in institutional circles, where they are derided as the main cause of environmental degradation (see also Dejouhanet and Sreelakshmy, this volume).

Sichuan is one of the Chinese provinces with the biggest annual output of Chinese proprietary medicines and "herbal pieces" (*yinpian*), valued at around 8 billion USD (Di Tommaso et al. 2017). It is known colloquially as "the home of Chinese medicine, the treasury of Chinese medicines" (*zhongyi zhi xiang, zhongyao zhi ku* 中医之乡, 中药之库) for its abundance and variety of medicinal resources. The province's deep mountain valleys are also home to several ethnic minorities, the Qiang among them.

Apart from the Han majority, the Chinese government recognises 55 ethnic minorities, with many others considered sub-groups or remaining unrecognised. This categorisation appeared with the ethnic classification project of the 1950s, which was a consciously political exercise aiming not to accurately describe existing communities but to outline plausible ones, preparing the ground for future governance (Mullaney 2011). Guided by ideas of social evolutionism but under the guise of "development," this identification project strove for a particular vision of national political unity (Dreyer 1993; Mullaney 2011). The development and promotion of ethnic medicine and medicines reinforce this notion of *duoyuan yiti* (多元一体), which can be translated as "ethnic diversity within national unity" (Wang 2015: 35), while also serving political objectives. The definition and mobilisation of ethnicity are complex processes in China and particularly for the Qiang, as the term Qiang itself carries deep historical baggage as a synonym for "otherness" (Wang 1999).

Those who are nowadays officially classified as Qiang live in the Northwest of Sichuan, both in the "Aba Tibetan and Qiang Autonomous Prefecture" (where most of my fieldwork was conducted) and in the "Beichuan Qiang Autonomous County." According to the 2010 census, the Qiang number is 309,576 (National Bureau of Statistics of China, n.d.). Many speak a Tibeto-Burman language in local dialects that vary greatly, making Chinese (Sichuan dialect) the preferred medium of communication between many Qiang communities (Wang 2002). The Qiang have gathered particular visibility in the country at large following the devastating earthquake of 2008, which tragically killed around 10 percent of the Qiang population (Companion and Chaiken 2017).

The earliest record of the ethnic label Qiang (羌) is a pictograph from the mid-Shang period (ca. 1300 BCE). Throughout history, Qiang was used as a blanket term for a wide range of peoples inhabiting the vast area on the eastern fringe of the Tibetan plateau (Wang 1999). This label is thus considered the oldest, blurriest, and least stable boundary delineating the Han (ibid.). Over time, many western non-Han populations were classified into new ethnic groups and so removed from the category of Qiang.

China's ethnic classification project attributed many minority groups ethnonyms that differed from their autonyms. In the case of the Qiang, the autonym *Rma* equates to the concept of "us." This meant that before the 1950s, most of the people in question had never heard the term "Qiang" (Wang 1999). To complicate things further, even *Rma* was not a mutually agreed upon denomination because communities identified themselves and those inhabiting the same valley as *Rma* but excluded those upstream as *tshep* (barbarians) and those downstream as *erh*, or "crafty Chinese" (ibid.). Their state categorisation under the common denomination Qiang in the 1950s was foremost a matter of practical governance, which refashioned the ethnic boundary between Han and Qiang in a more accommodating manner, under the spirit of "ethnic diversity within national unity."

Over recent decades, those Qiang who proceed into further studies in some sense come to "learn about themselves" through historicised narratives of descent. Many of the medical practitioners I met mentioned several historico-mythical figures that they were convinced were "Qiang." They gained legitimacy by claiming Qiang medicine as the ancestor of Chinese medicine, positioning themselves as both the inheritors of "ancient" knowledge and as "the oldest ethnic minority in China." This medical ethno-nationalism is performed while borrowing standards, materia medica, and practices from the state-approved medical system, in this way demonstrating integrity within the state framework, rather than opposition to it (Lai and Farquhar 2015). Such a stance provides a way to navigate China's sociopolitical landscape and carve out a potentially valuable space within Chinese society and its burgeoning healthcare market. It also offers the means to consolidate an ethnic identity. Hence, although expressions of Qiang identity have only emerged recently, they are performed as if they had been so since time immemorial.

Following "Qiang" medicinal materials

Qianghuo – the weight of "history" and legends (chuanshuo 传说*)*

During a conference of the Qiang medicine branch of CMAM, a group of participants encircled a large hotel dinner table and discussed the following question: "Is *qianghuo* a Chinese medicine or a Qiang medicine?" The most influential practitioner of Qiang medicine at the government level, whom I refer to as Dr Zhang, argued forcefully that it was Qiang, but a few colleagues working in the pharmaceutical industry disagreed. The discussion was finally wrapped up by Guang De, a Qiang medicine development strategist, who equivocated by stating: "it is both Chinese and Qiang."

Endemic to Sichuan and surrounding provinces, the medicinal use of *qianghuo* in China dates back at least to the time of the "Divine Farmer's Materia Medica Classic" (*shennong bencao jing* 神农本草经). Compiled from various sources between 200 and 250 CE, this is considered the oldest Chinese pharmaceutical body of written work available (Unschuld 1986). *Qianghuo* appears later in the sixteenth century "Compendium of Materia Medica" (*bencao gangmu* 本草纲目) (Zhang and Unschuld 2014) and is still widely prescribed right across the country today, mainly for treating colds and "wind damp" (*fengshi* 风湿) or rheumatism (Li 2010). Its high therapeutic status is verified by its appearance in 262 Chinese proprietary medicines produced at 694 pharmaceutical factories (Jiang et al. 2017), as well as its recent inclusion in a formulation recommended nationwide for the treatment of COVID-19 (Xin and Hsu 2020).

Guang De's way of settling the argument over *qianghuo*'s origins reflected both its high medicinal value and the recent policy changes that have incorporated minority medicine into Chinese medicine. However, for Dr Zhang, this was no ordinary medicine but "a very famous medicine among Qiang medicines." Its mention in the "Divine Farmer's Materia Medica Classic" as the "protector of the Qiang envoy" and "protector of the Qiang king" (Sun and Sun 2010) made him consider it as "the core medicine" in this medical canon that lists over 300 medicinal herbs. According to him, no other medicinal plant has such a long and minutely detailed Chinese literary record. Another doctor explained the connection between the Qiang and *qianghuo* differently:

> A tribal leader was seriously ill and we had a doctor here who told him that if he took this medicine he would be cured. At that time, there was no name for this medicine (...) but he asked the doctor what the medicine was called. He said he didn't know, but then the leader told him to call it *qianghuo*, because he was the king of the Qiang. The king of the Qiang, who took this medicine to survive, named it *qianghuo*. It's a legend, a beautiful legend.

Yet another Qiang medicine doctor argued that back in the time when the Qiang lived a nomadic hunting life, they often caught colds (*ganmao* 感冒) and learned that *qianghuo* could help with this:

> Because of the wind and cold attack (*fenghan de qinxi* 风寒的侵袭), it was very easy to get headaches, body aches, to develop dampness (*chansheng shiqi* 产生湿气), so *qianghuo* would be the first medicine to use. Because Qiang people were the first to use it, this endowed it with the name *qianghuo*. Because this medicine has solved most of the pain and hardship of the Qiang people, made them active and allowed them to survive, so it is named *qianghuo*. Its name originated this way.

Only one town doctor disputed the ethnic attribution of *qianghuo*, pointing out that its name in the Qiang language was *sigea*. Among the (entirely Han) academic members of the Qiang branch of CMAM, some saw the ethnicity of *qianghuo* as relative and dependent on whatever ethnic medical theory was used while employing it therapeutically. While accepting that the Qiang were the first to use *qianghuo*, another referred to it as a "multi-ethnic cross-use medicinal material" and an "authentic medicinal material of Sichuan" that "hasn't had the *chuan* character added to it."[3] In this highly ethnically diverse region, the preference for regional rather than ethnic attributions has been previously documented (Springer 2015) and I return to examine it further below. Outside institutional circles, however, such debates are largely irrelevant, as we shall now see in the case of medicinal herb collectors.

Collecting qianghuo

Climbing up to about 3100 m, we passed grazing yaks while eagles hovered above us. I followed the four women, all in their forties, as they moved up the mountains at impressive speed, clearing the way through the mud and thorny bushes with their adzes. They collected *qianghuo* from dawn to dusk, making what was extremely hard work seem easy with songs, chatter, and laughter. One collector asked if I was tired and I asked the same question back, to which she replied "can't do anything about it, need to make money."

Although other collectors had told me that *qianghuo* was best harvested while flowering, on all occasions I witnessed both flowering and non-flowering plants collected. The collectors were skilful at spotting both, even when the plants were hidden among other foliage or under trees. They dug the soil with one to three strokes of their adzes, grabbed the plant by the root, snapped it off, and smacked it on the adze handle to loosen the earth, before stuffing it into a bag or apron pouch. All this was done in a repetitive, almost automatic fashion. The women frequently checked how much each had collected as a means of comparison. Just before lunch, one of them realised she had collected a lot less than the others, so did not stop to eat until she had collected what she thought was a fair amount. The other ladies moved the roots to plastic bags and then into bigger bags so that they were kept dry. "Today we got less than usual" one said. They could sell each *jin*[4] of *qianghuo* for a few dozen yuan.

---

3 The construction of a Sichuan authentic medicine certification service is one of the objectives of the *Sichuan Province Chinese Medicine Industry Development Plan 2018–2025* (SATCM 2019). Outside of China, regional denomination for the creation of brands is a central feature of the European Union's Common Agricultural Policy (CAP) and Protected Designations of Origin (PDO) – see Higgins (2018).

4 One *jin* is approximately equivalent to 1.1lb.

In Qiang villages, the "representativeness" of *qianghuo* seems very much an external representational device. A local doctor told me bluntly that people here do not see any relation between *qianghuo* and the Qiang, again remarking that *sigea* was its Qiang name. However, the herb collectors that I accompanied referred to it by its Chinese name, as they do with all the herbs they collect, even while speaking to one another in the Qiang language. Other villagers told me that they did not know the Qiang name for *qianghuo*, or that such a name did not exist. Together with the fact that very few medicinal herbs were used in peoples' homes, the use of the Chinese name suggests collection predominantly destined for sale to Han people, at least since the late Qing dynasty (Bian 2017). In one instance, I asked collectors whether there was a relationship between *qianghuo* and Qiang people and was met with an indifferent silence. I continued, asking "do you think it's your medicine?," prompting one to laugh and in a joking manner reply "sure, it's our thing." Despite the absence of any sense of ethnic ownership, *qianghuo* is commonly kept in Qiang homes and used to treat common colds. For example, I have seen *qianghuo* brewed together with ginger in a pot on the stove, to treat the cough of my host's youngest son.

One thing that all interlocutors agreed on was that every year, during the summer collection period, less and less *qianghuo* is available and it is necessary to travel further and climb higher to find it. My host in the second village where I conducted fieldwork told me how that year had been the first when he did not collect *qianghuo*, because there were now "too few and too far away."

Cultivating "fake" and "real" *qianghuo*

"Broad-leaved *qianghuo*" (*kuanye qianghuo* 宽叶羌活 Notopterygium franchetii H.Boissieu) grows at lower altitudes, often by the side of the road. Known to germinate very easily and therefore simple to cultivate, villagers in my first fieldwork location grew it themselves, which was not possible with "real" *qianghuo*. Referred to as *luyazi*, "fake *qianghuo*," or "stinky Qiang" (*chouqiang* 臭羌) due to its strong aroma, the villagers argued that it was a totally different plant to standard *qianghuo* "with a very different flavour." Villagers did not consider it as medicine, insisting that it was far inferior to the one growing high in the mountains, which was confirmed by the fact that they were only able to sell it for a third of the price. Indeed, in general, the association between cultivated and "fake" was, for most villagers, overarching.

When it comes to what villagers considered to be "real" *qianghuo* (*Notopterygium incisum* K.C. Ting ex H.T. Chang), the inability to transplant it to low altitudes as well as its increasing scarcity in the wild inspired the "*Qianghuo* research group" at the Sichuan College of Chinese Medicine to spend the past 20 years working on a way to grow a particular cultivar of the plant. Bringing biologists, pharmacists, and soil specialists together, they conducted dozens of cultivation projects all over Aba prefecture with the final aim of training villagers to cultivate it themselves. While they insisted that the plants were identical in terms of chemical composition, their biggest obstacle was correcting morphological problems with the cultivar they worked with, which meant that its market value remained much lower than its wild counterpart. In place of long, individualised roots, their cultivar presented a large mass of fibrous roots.

While attempting to solve this particular problem, the university researcher who headed the research group drew a distinction between "medicine" and "medicinal material." As he saw it, although the quality of their cultivar as "medicine" was identical to the wild variety, its quality as "medicinal material" was not, for two main reasons. Firstly, the morphological differences could be too large for the cultivar to match the current description of *qianghuo* in the Chinese Pharmacopoeia. Secondly, pharmaceutical enterprises could encounter problems when processing this raw material. The morphological differences, lower market prices, and lack of previous use in local self-care contributed to such cultivars retaining labels of "fakeness," "inferiority," or "ineffectiveness," at least in the eyes of the villagers who could not, or would not, cultivate it. I return to explore the variety of motivations and implications surrounding these cultivation initiatives in the second part of this chapter.

Qiang Beimu – new ethnic possibilities

Commonly used across China in the treatment of coughs, *beimu* (贝母 *Fritillaria*) earned its name, which also means "mother-of-pearl," for the morphological resemblance of its bulbs to white shells (Cunningham et al. 2018). An important ingredient in more than 200 Chinese medicines (Li et al. 2013), about 100 tons of these small medicinal bulbs were used each year in China alone in the mid-2000s. However, the real market demand is much higher than the available supply (ibid). In Qiang language it is called *gvubgea*. As part of a marketing strategy by a particular pharmaceutical company, the character *qiang* (羌) was added in recent years to make the name *qiang beimu*, even though this variety was not recognised by anyone else as having any particular connection to the Qiang.

During CMAM's Qiang branch meetings, there are always a couple of stalls outside the conference auditoriums run by enterprises associated with the organisation, promoting medicinal materials or herbal extracts. It was at one of these stalls that I found *beimu* in its raw material state, labelled as "Qiang medicinal material label, *wabu guobuge, qiang beimu*." *Wabu* stood for the variety *wabu beimu* (*Fritillaria unibracteata* var. *wabuensis* (S.Y. Tang & S.C. Yueh) Z.D. Liu, Shu Wang, & S.C. Chen), and *guobuge* for the Chinese transliteration of the Qiang name of *gvubgea*. *Wabu beimu*'s bulbs are considerably larger than those of the *beimu* most commonly collected and consumed in China. It was first registered as a new species in the early 1980s (Tang and Yueh 1983) and in the 1990s was recognised as a variety of *Fritillaria unibracteata* (Liu et al. 2009). The name *wabu* comes from the fact that it was "first found" in the mountains of Waboliangzi (瓦钵梁子). Next to the bulbs, long sachets sat on display, containing a powder preparation of *qiang beimu* that was easy to drink and could be swallowed directly as well.

I began chatting with the pharmaceutical representative at the stall, an acquaintance of Dr Zhang, whom I will call Mr Luo. I showed him a photograph of the *wabu beimu* that grew in the cultivation base outside my first fieldwork village. After looking carefully, he replied that it looked "fake": the bulb did not open as it should and the cloves stayed close together. According to him, even at one year of age, the bulbs that he grew would already be opened. Another difference was that his *beimu* did not grow in a greenhouse, but outdoors. Each bulb took a minimum of three years before it could be sold, being at its best at five years of age. The reason for naming it *qiang beimu* was attributed to the suggestion of a professor whom I will refer to as Professor Zhou. This was someone I knew and who Mr Luo claimed had been working with his company.

Like Mr Luo's *beimu*, the bulbs in the village cultivation base that I visited were shipped to the city for processing. This particular company advertises on their website that they were the first in China to achieve Good Manufacturing Practice (GMP) standards for medicinal herbs and that their products were "sold to excellent factories of Chinese proprietary medicines, hospitals and chain drugstores nationwide and exported to countries and regions such as Korea, Japan, the US, Singapore, Hong Kong and Taiwan, etc." According to Mr Luo, the domestication of *chuan beimu* (a broad range of *beimu* types including *wabu* and several other species that grow mostly in Sichuan province) had not been successful for many years. However, at a later stage, a combination of factors provided the perfect opportunity for his company to start operations, as others had already done. The first was the inclusion of *wabu beimu* in the Chinese Pharmacopoeia in 2010 (Chinese Pharmacopoeia Committee 2010). The second was the increasing difficulty pharmaceutical firms were facing in meeting their demand for *beimu*, due to the depletion of wild stocks. The third was Mr Luo's encounter with a Qiang farmer with plenty of experience in *wabu beimu* cultivation, who became his technical consultant. The main reasons his company chose *wabu beimu* over other varieties and species were its larger output volumes and "more mature planting technology."

The morphology of authenticity

With a major stake in the promotion and development of *wabu beimu*, Mr Luo took the fact that his product matched previously documented morphological descriptions as a token of authenticity, quality and superiority over other varieties that did not. With several different domesticated cultivars appearing in the past 20 years, individual variations abound and morphological details are increasingly being used by certain producers as a way to claim authenticity. However, because most *wabu beimu* bulbs are both much larger than the more commonly used *anzi beimu* (暗紫贝母 *Fritillaria unibracteata* P.K. Hsiao & K.C. Hsia) and have only recently entered the market, they are not yet widely accepted.

The recognition of *wabu beimu* in the Chinese Pharmacopoeia opened the doors of the market to it. However, there were particular reasons for its use. According to an academic researcher, although tests had shown there was no difference in "curative effect" (*liaoxiao* 疗效) between the two, patients preferred the small *anzi beimu* and Chinese medicine doctors also considered *anzi beimu* more effective. This generated controversy between doctors and certain academics, the latter who thought they were both of the same clinical value. Meanwhile, pharmaceutical producers were increasingly choosing to use the bigger and cheaper *wabu beimu*, as this significantly increased the profit margins on their proprietary medicines.

Furthermore, through selective breeding, some cultivators started producing *wabu beimu* bulbs that were far larger than the parameters defined in the Pharmacopoeia. This left several Sichuan enterprises with a high output of artificially cultivated, enlarged *wabu beimu* and struggling to find a market. This did not seem to affect Mr Luo, since he claimed that his *wabu beimu* was in line with the legal requirements of the Pharmacopoeia. The Qiang doctors I knew did not express a strong preference for either *anzi* or *wabu beimu*, but none of them referred to the larger variety as *qiang beimu*.

Villagers were largely sceptical of the bigger *wabu beimu*, with many stating that its efficacy (*gongxiao* 功效) was not as good as that of *anzi beimu*, either in the relief of coughs or as an alcoholic solution to stop bleeding and heal wounds. The doctor at the first village explained that among the many kinds of *beimu*, the one growing on their mountains was both "normal" and best. In his view, important distinctions were not only morphological but also between that which was wild and that which was cultivated.

The marketing of qiang beimu

Mr Luo's enthusiasm over the relabelling of *wabu beimu* as *qiang beimu* was not shared by Professor Zhou, to whom he attributed the initial idea. When I asked her about their collaboration, she dismissed it as a few meetings at conferences, suggesting that "deep level cooperation" had not yet begun. She did not seem aware of the *qiang beimu* label, despite having been present at the conference where this product was promoted:

> If they've given it this name, the country will not recognise it. It is originally a "multi-ethnic species". Han, Tibetan, Yi (…) in Sichuan, many nationalities use *beimu* (…) but it must be included in the Pharmacopoeia,

so it can't be called like that. (...). The government will not recognise it. Because it just states that it has the characteristics of the Qiang minority. Once so unified by the state, then you can't have Tibetans calling it Tibetan *beimu*, Han calling it whatever, the Yi minority calling it whatever kind of *beimu*: this is impossible.

While I was unable to verify what had actually taken place in meetings between Professor Zhou and Mr Luo, it was clear that the former wanted to distance herself from the attribution of ethnicity to a medicinal material. By invoking the unfeasibility of such labelling in the eyes of the government, she positioned herself on the safe side of any ethnic or legal disputes. When I spoke with two other researchers with no stakes in this marketing move, the picture they painted was more nuanced than one of stark governmental rejection. While not recognising *wabu beimu* as *qiang beimu* themselves, they saw certain benefits in such labelling with regard to the market. One was especially relaxed about the ethnic labelling of medicines. After repeating the name *qiang beimu* twice, as if to get a feel of how the words sounded, she continued:

> How to look at it ... If someone wants to promote our brand of Qiang medicine, to find some special entry points, to add some colour to the medicine behind our nationality culture, I think this is not a bad thing; it's very good.

Although this was simply a raw material in powder form, sold alongside whole bulbs, the entire process of creating, developing, and promoting this "ethnic product" was driven by the aim of entering the proprietary medicines market and thus becoming available in pharmacy chains all over China. This particular "reformulation regime" (Pordié and Gaudillière 2014) was using place of origin, assumed "historical use" and Qiang-led cultivation in order to materialise Qiang ethnicity in a medicinal product, specifically for marketing purposes. Furthermore, this approach worked with the format of direct-to-consumer advertising, thus bypassing the potential role of doctors in devising or prescribing the product in question.

Although most Qiang doctors were enthusiastic about the development of Qiang proprietary medicines, for which single herb preparations appeared as a first step, this feeling was not shared by all. One Qiang doctor in particular strongly rejected materialising ethnicity in such a way. He articulated Qiang medicines differently, arguing that "real Qiang medicines can be produced anywhere" and what mattered most was how such medicines were used. He assigned little value to proprietary medicines in general, or to single-component preparations such as powders and granules, as these did not require people to prepare and boil their own medicines. Instead, he centred ethnicity in the role of Qiang medicine among practitioners and lay Qiang people alike, claiming that one could only refer to "Qiang medicines" if they were used within "Qiang medicine." Using a label to crystallise a particular medicine as "Qiang," regardless of how it was going to be used, ran counter to this logic. The idea of ethnic medicines as artefacts that are packaged and labelled solely to boost their circulation in the market was therefore contested, as in this alternative articulation "Qiang medicines" only come into being when they are prescribed and used.

Competing in Sichuan and beyond

With demand for *beimu* far outweighing supply and with each bulb taking years to become medically useful, Professor Zhou viewed the disappearance of wild *chuan beimu* species as inevitable, despite her claims that the government had given it high priority by designating it a "heritage authentic Sichuan medicinal material" (*chuancheng daodi yaocai* 传承道地药材).[5] She saw wild *anzi beimu* as growing under fragile ecological conditions and producing very low yields, both factors that were "very difficult for human beings to influence in a short time." For her, the major advantages of *wabu beimu* cultivars were that they could be cultivated on a commercial scale at lower altitudes, and that their large size resulted in much bigger output volumes. From this perspective, the fact that the Pharmacopeia had still not changed its legal description to accommodate larger *beimu* bulbs was a contradiction that had not yet been resolved.

The growing scarcity of *beimu* bulbs in the wild imbued corporate cultivation and production initiatives with a particular tone of care for the environment and benevolence towards local populations. Cultivation initiatives were portrayed as the saviours of nature, pharmaceutical companies and local communities alike, while wild herb collectors were accused of wrecking the environment, an issue that I explore in more detail below. Mr Luo spoke of him and other companies producing *wabu beimu* in the region as developing high-quality medicines, in areas free of pollution and with good soil quality. Although Mr Luo's company was at a very early stage in production, he spoke of opening more cultivation bases in the future, of combining their operations with China's poverty alleviation policy (*fupin zhengce* 扶贫政策), and of solving local unemployment problems.

This rosy vision of a network of high-output, ethical, socially and environmentally responsible cultivation bases was later called into question when a patient at a Qiang medicine clinic joined a conversation that I was

---

5 For the list of medicinal material resources monitored under the *Sichuan Province Chinese Medicine Industry Development Plan (2018–2025)*, see SATCM (2019).

having with one of the doctors. According to him, a *beimu* cultivation base nearby was using hormone fertilisers indiscriminately in order to increase production by two or three-fold, thus "eating up resources meant for local people" while "eating up millions in targeted poverty alleviation efforts (*jingzhun fupin* 精准扶贫)."

Beneath these competing interests and opinions, one thing that all my interlocutors agreed upon was the regional superiority of the *chuan beimu* group. Despite including many different species and varieties, everyone agreed that *chuan beimu* were far superior to their historical "competitor," *zhe beimu* (浙贝母 *Fritillaria thunbergii*), originally from the eastern coastal province of Zhejiang. Doctors and academics all mentioned the latter's "poor antitussive effect" and its consequently low market price. With wild *beimu* resources at risk of disappearing altogether and industrial demand at an all-time high, the domestication of different varieties of *beimu* offered excellent profit prospects for enterprises, as long as they could keep their products within the morphological parameters described in the Pharmacopoeia. Various locally specific but nationally significant ecological, economic, and social considerations were portrayed as going hand-in-hand with such endeavours. However, with each base employing only a handful of people and with the spectre of dubious cultivation practices being involved, the real benefits to each of these fields remain unclear. Ethnic labelling occupies a similarly ambiguous place in this process. Although Mr Luo claimed that his company based the attribution of *qiang beimu* on a "realisation" rather than a concrete marketing effort, it was not universally accepted and was clearly at odds with most Qiang people's preference for the smaller, wildcrafted *anzi beimu*. Even so, the majority of those involved were able to justify this unofficial ethnic attribution as a beneficial marketing move for the promotion of Qiang medicine.

Articulating Qiang medicines for a growing market

> If minority medicine wants to develop, it is medicines, not medicine, that will really contribute the most to its development. (...) One doctor sees a few patients, but medicines are different, (...) the one that circulates in the market, the one that has a registration number, is targeting a group of more than a billion people in China.
> (Guang De, interlocutor working on "Qiang medicine development strategy")

As the Chinese medicines industry grows and proprietary medicines become increasingly central to it (Hsu 2009), contests over the ethnic attribution of raw materials look likely to diminish. I argue that as such compound preparations are formulated, developed, and labelled as ethnic on their commercial packaging, they follow a different mode of articulation that distances them from questions around the ethnicity of raw materials. Furthermore, materialising ethnicity through combining claims to authentic "traditional" knowledge with the results of industrial design processes embraces tropes of "advancement" and "development," while feeding inter-ethnic competition over the registration and sale of novel pharmaceutical products.

The articulation of *qianghuo* and *qiang beimu* as Qiang medicines among academics, some practitioners and pharmaceutical industry actors appear as highly artificial and manipulative. The first case claimed the legitimacy of "history," based on the widespread use of *qianghuo* by villagers in the region, but despite the fact that no one accepted any ethnic connotations when referring to *qianghuo*. This confirmed such an ethnicised designation as a recent phenomenon, harnessed by people living elsewhere and holding particular interests. Regular use over time in these villages did not translate into any overarching affinity between *qianghuo* and one ethnic group, especially since "the Qiang" were only unified as a single ethnic minority seven decades ago and this move was entirely engineered by the Chinese state.

The case of *qiang beimu* revolves around contemporary marketing practices, as well as combined medicinal plant cultivation and development strategies. It is notable that the new possibilities that emerged for the ethnic denomination of this *beimu* cultivar did not reflect initiative or interest from Qiang people themselves, as they were not directly involved in this enterprise. Neither did it draw upon the practices, uses or preferences of the majority of the contemporary Qiang. This case shines light on the way the articulation of materials, properties, and history operates by singling out certain geographic areas and then designating certain individuals to represent the whole ethnic group. In this way, whatever is said on behalf of the Qiang and that suits those directing the process is mobilised for marketing purposes, while the rest is overlooked. The inner workings of this process are practically oriented, with actors moving quickly between abstract and historical arguments, rejecting or approving certain labels. It is this pragmatic wish to promote and develop Qiang medicine and medicines, within China's contemporary policy, market, and industrial frameworks, which enabled those involved to justify such attributions without necessarily accepting their veracity. Finally, under the guise of poverty alleviation, job creation and biodiversity conservation, the engine driving the entire process was the prospect of entering the vast Chinese and international markets for raw materials, medicines, and supplements, which gave impetus to the tremendous efforts underway to develop a Qiang medical industry.

The fact that not a single Qiang formula has been granted a "national medicine registration number" (*guoyao zhun zihao*国药准字号) means that, for the time being, these medicines cannot be sold nationwide. The main reason invoked to explain this absence was missed opportunities in the

1980s and 1990s. This was a period when the registration of medicinal products was far more straightforward, as the state would approve and register formulas easily as long as a practitioner's prescription was declared "to have very good effect" (see Chee, this volume). This period preceded the 2002 implementation of a centralised system for drug registration by the State Food and Drug Administration (SFDA), later renamed the National Medical Products Administration (NMPA), which introduced extensive requirements including scientific studies of safety and efficacy (Saxer 2013). Drugs registered locally before 1997 were exempt and passed onto the new system, but the ones registered later required re-registration according to the new protocols (ibid.). This new registration called for pre-clinical (animal) testing and three phases of clinical trials (Craig 2012). Dr Zhang claimed that, in contrast to other minorities like the Miao (Yang and Peng 2015), Qiang doctors did not receive comprehensive or timely information concerning the process of drug registration during the 1980s and 1990s, due to poor coordination between government bodies and grassroots workers. He views the much more stringent current regulatory requirements as a major bottleneck hindering the development of Qiang medicine, complaining that even if the government was supportive, there are simply too many barriers in place to enable the smaller ethnic medical disciplines to develop and register new medicines and products.

It is clear that catering to the imaginations of the Han majority is paramount within contemporary attempts to develop and market ethnic minority medicines and health products. Interestingly, the category "Qiang," by virtue of being a historically Han-defined "other," reflects as much on the majority as it does on the Qiang themselves. As an externally constructed group definition, it loops back to appeal to the Han majority through the allure of "ethnic medicines," "ethnic clothing" and "ethnic places." Overall, emerging ethnic attributions are contingent to particular markets, whether relating to medicines or tourism, within an "ethno-preneurialism" (Comaroff and Comaroff 2009) that manages and markets minority "cultural" products and practices in symbiosis with the country's ethnic majority.

Raw materials, sustainability, and paternalism

Another hindrance holding back the development of a Qiang medical industry, and a major one restricting the expansion of the Chinese medicines industry as a whole, is the question of resource sustainability. Indeed, the fundamental contradictions between constant demand growth, industrial expansion and dwindling raw material supplies are increasingly problematic across Asia's herb-based medical industries, as many of the chapters in this volume attest. This dimension relates directly to the cultivation initiatives being developed in Sichuan to feed China's burgeoning pharmaceutical industry, which were introduced in the first part of this chapter and are examined in greater detail below.

Environmental sustainability initiatives in Sichuan are framed within China's "Western Development Plan" (*xibu da kaifa* 西部大开发), launched in 1999 and still the largest regional development plan in the country so far (Jeong 2015; Lai 2002). Its long-term planning is divided into three stages: "Laying the foundations" from 2001 to 2010, "Accelerating development" from 2010 to 2030, and "Comprehensively promoting modernisation" from 2031 to 2050 (China Development Gateway 2021). This plan was ostensibly designed to reduce the economic gap between coastal China and the interior that appeared with the post-Mao market reforms. However, by distributing significant state resources to selected minority areas for particular purposes, such policies can also be seen as a mechanism for controlling social and ethnic unrest (Jeong 2015). Although civil unrest has not affected Qiang areas, in Tibetan regions and Xinjiang, past isolated outbreaks are used as justification by the state for its proactive attempts to mitigate against further troubles.

As well as reducing regional income inequalities, the Western Development Plan was designed to provide the industrialised coast with resources, while simultaneously tackling the social and environmental problems that have accompanied economic transformation (Flower 2009). In the process, it has strengthened market penetration, state capacity, and regulatory infrastructure (McNally 2004). A major consequence of pushing Sichuan to supply ever-larger quantities of herbal material to growing domestic and foreign medicinal industries is that several species have become endangered and are being monitored, including *qianghuo* and those classified as *chuan beimu* (SATCM 2019).

Research conducted in Sichuan and Tibet has shown that the bulbs of one of the *chuan beimu* species, *Fritillaria Cirrhosae,* are reducing in size and growing deeper underground in response to over-collection (Li et al. 2017). Ironically, this change makes for even more desirable *chuan beimu*, given the widespread preference for smaller bulbs. As Landecker (2016) points out, political and industrial shifts can produce visible and lasting biological manifestations and material outcomes, for good or ill.

The political solution proposed for these mounting problems is the "Plan for the Protection and Development of Chinese Medicinal Materials 2015–2020" (State Council of the PRC 2015a). This was hailed as the "first national special plan to alleviate the supply and demand conflict of endangered Chinese herbal medicines within five years" (State Council of the PRC 2015b). Far from being a simple plan for biodiversity conservation, it is built around the premise of "protection through development" (State Council of the PRC, 2015a). It uses this premise to justify the massive expansion of cultivation initiatives, focusing on the "construction of standardised, large-scale, and industrialised production bases" to supply the expansion of an industry of "innovative Chinese medicine and medicines with ethnic characteristics" (ibid.). The "disorderly development of authentic medicinal materials" is blamed for offsetting the "sustainable and healthy development of Chinese medicine" (SATCM 2018). Thus, without ever questioning rising (arguably already excessive) industrial demands, this approach places firm conviction in "rational," technologically driven and market-led methods of restoring economic-ecological balance (see also van der Valk, this volume).

The "orderly development" proposed under the "Sichuan Province Chinese Medicine Industry Development Plan 2018–2025" (SATCM 2019) focuses on several initiatives including those concerning Tibetan and Yi medicines. However, it also promotes "research on the transformation of wild varieties and the industrialisation of artificial planting" for "four to six representative Qiang medicines," as well as the creation of a regional brand of Qiang medicines. Thus, the plan stresses sustainability and ecological protection while simultaneously underscoring the potential financial gains of expanded raw material production and industrial consolidation. Through "vigorously promoting standardised and large-scale production bases," the development targets for the province were for 7 million planted acres of medicinal materials, with an annual output value exceeding 20 billion RMB for 2020. These targets then rise to 8.5 million acres and 30 billion RMB for 2025.

Accompanying these impressive agricultural targets are industrial and marketing goals such as "deepening industrial integration" and "internationalising industrial brands" (SATCM 2019). These national and regional plans clearly show that conservation is equated to cultivation and is seen, foremost, as instrumental to continuous industrial expansion. By focusing both on large-scale cultivation and brand creation, the aim is to simultaneously increase supply and foster demand (Blaikie 2009). Proposing such solutions to a crisis of scarcity illustrates how environmental impediments can themselves constitute the source for novel forms of accumulation (Brockington and Duffy 2010; Brockington, Duffy and Igoe 2012; Cons and Eilenberg 2019; Tsing 2015; van der Valk, this volume).

In practice, there are three main formats for medicinal plant cultivation in Sichuan. The first involves individual farmers who cultivate their own land, the second local cooperatives closely linked to the companies buying their produce, and the third companies employing workers to cultivate land that they control (as in the cultivation base mentioned above). The "*Qianghuo* research group" trained people to work in all three formats, as well as employing individuals without farming knowledge who found ways to grow *qianghuo* in forest areas. The researchers saw their mission as reversing environmental degradation by convincing collectors to cultivate instead, so as "not to destroy the wild resources." Mr Luo, the pharmaceutical representative, spoke highly of the second format. He worked with a cooperative set up by local farmers who supplied land and labour, while his company was in charge of management, "expanding the market and solving the problem of marketing the local agricultural products." He saw this as a great model for "solving the problems of idle land and unemployment, while increasing farmers' income." In general, my questions as to who benefited most from such initiatives were answered confidently by most non-villager interlocutors with reference to a "win-win situation" (*shuangying*双赢).

Brockington and Duffy (2010) advise caution with regard to the resolutely positive, win-win rhetoric of market-based solutions to "saving nature." Such images of benevolence are accentuated in the case of medicinal herbs through the nobility attributed to the act of healing. Referring to the local "Min River lily" (*Lilium regale* E.H. Wilson, *minjiang baihe*岷江百合),[6] a Qiang doctor illustrated perfectly how industrial solutions can "solve" industrial problems:

> If we make good use of local varieties and develop industries, planting in the original ecology of the "common people", then it will benefit the people. The benefit for the country is in treating the lung diseases of many people. If our lungs are healthy, there will be more genes resisting smog, and our immunity will be improved. As a result, many medical costs will be reduced for the country, which will benefit the country. In this way, a company also develops and achieves win-win results.

Instead of questioning the causes of industrial pollution, this practitioner had already interiorised the problem of smog as an unavoidable reality, distant as it was in hilly Aba prefecture. Therefore, industrialising the Min River lily for the sake of "multiplying smog resistant genes" appeared a feasible solution to industrial pollution, while reducing medical costs nationwide.

One pharmaceutical technologist stood out as the only researcher I spoke to who was not enthusiastic about private cultivation initiatives. Echoing others' concerns over the abuse of fertiliser, he felt that companies and cultivators would pursue economic benefit above all other concerns. If they saw that the price per weight was not moving in the right direction, they would surely use technological and chemical inputs to increase production volumes and reduce planting times, which would inevitably lead to contamination and quality degradation. He was also of the opinion that the benefits of such initiatives were biased in favour of companies to the detriment of local people, whether employees or independent cultivators. At the other end of the spectrum, questions of imbalance frustrated one of the leaders of the "*Qianghuo* research group." For her, a farmer was simply dealing with a commodity and selling it at a price that was contingent to the market demand.

> On the one hand, he sells it as a commodity to respect the market demand. On the other hand, he is at a relatively backward agricultural

---

6   *Minjiang baihe* does not feature in the Chinese Pharmacopoeia and so I have used the Latin denomination of eFloras (2008).

level, so the government has many supporting policies to help him, one is to help him learn (planting) technology, the other is to help him with costs. For example, give him seeds of medicinal materials, then give him some inputs needed for agriculture, and then help him to develop this. It's meaningful for the industry, and it's also good for farmers so as to improve their living conditions. So, is China not helping the poor? In this aspect, it is the best in the world at doing it.

In her view, beneficiaries could not be polarised into winners and losers, since each individual would earn their due portion from the business process, adding that "a company is not a welfare institution." Overall, those working with cultivation initiatives held mixed attitudes towards herb collectors, involving blame but also a willingness to "help."

Many companies took pains to claim social responsibility for their work, often linked to their involvement in the government's poverty alleviation programme. This was named "Targeted Poverty Alleviation" in 2013 (Liu et al. 2018) but has run since the mid-1980s, with priorities shifting gradually from relief provision to income generation (Croll 1994). Participating companies can receive tax relief, land transfers and financial support from the government if they invest in an area, usually rural, deemed to be poor by the state (Yan 2015). They can also partake in specific "social responsibility" activities. In relation to Qiang communities, even claiming to be involved in these programmes constituted a marketing effort, the more so after the 2008 Sichuan earthquake, when donations poured in from all over the country to help the survivors. The state also gave funds and resources to post-earthquake reconstruction projects, resulting in the Qiang being regarded as a "fortunate" state-rescued ethnic minority, whose living conditions and "traditional culture" were immediately supported and promoted (Zhang 2016).

The "cause of Qiang medicine" also received plenty of attention after the earthquake, as Zhang et al. (2014) illustrate through the paternalistic Chinese idiom: "a child who can cry has milk to drink" (*hui ku de haizi you nai chi*, 会哭的孩子有奶吃). They argue that minority medicine had been "a child who wasn't able to cry," but this situation changed for the Qiang after the earthquake. As many pushed for a Qiang medical industry, one large and well-established pharmaceutical company was invited to join the CMAM Qiang branch by the Sichuan Administration of Chinese Medicine in order to support these efforts. This company found a way to capitalise on that "cry" in the marketing of the medicinal herb extracts that they produced, specifically through a promotional video portraying a rescue worker with a company badge rescuing Qiang villagers from the earthquake. Upon meeting two company representatives, they claimed to have cultivation bases in Qiang areas and to participate in the government's poverty alleviation programme, but did not disclose details of their "social responsibility" activities.[7] One thing I am positive of is that they did not have a rescue team at the earthquake site, and thus their advertisement is a purely allegorical and highly paternalistic portrayal of "saving the Qiang."

I have shown how responsibility for the depletion of medicinal herbs in Sichuan is placed squarely on collectors, rather than being linked to excessive and growing industrial demand. I have also illustrated how cultivation initiatives are increasingly being portrayed as the solution not only to the question of sustainability, but also to issues of rural unemployment, poverty, inequality, and industrial underdevelopment, despite the many inconsistencies and contradictions such convenient elisions raise. In the next section, I give an overview of how China's efforts to standardise cultivation initiatives are failing to achieve their desired effect, even as these initiatives continue to multiply.

Good Agricultural Practices and the workings of standardisation

The standardisation of Chinese medicine's raw material cultivation is ensured by China's Good Agricultural Practices (GAP). These were developed along the lines of the WHO's Good Agricultural and Collection Practices (GACP), but did not constitute a binding set of standards when Saxer elaborated on them in the context of Tibetan medicines (2013) and still do not today. It is notable also that so far, only 177 GAP approved cultivation sites have been established across the whole of China (WHO 2019).

The views of Mr Luo, the Sichuan-based pharmaceutical company representative, on this matter are both instructive and revealing. He agreed that the early stage of Chinese medicine cultivation should be standardised, to make sure that pesticides, fertilisers and "rotten medicines" were controlled, and that soil composition was suitable. However, the standardisation that he advocated was one that dispensed with official, centralised accreditation. In fact, his company was not GAP certified and he did not see a need for it to be so, as they followed their own internal quality control processes. Moreover, while supporting some sort of a company-enforced standardisation at the initial stages of production, he was against the strict GMP standard controls in place for final products. He was convinced of a hierarchy within the industry that set level standards of production and determined the price of medicines accordingly, rather than this being decided by whether it had a high content of a particular component. Therefore, he saw raising the bar on the latter to be pointless. In this way, he thought it was important for companies themselves to ensure that only high quality and uncontaminated raw materials entered the Chinese medicine supply chains,

---

7 For anthropological approaches to corporate social responsibility, see Rajak (2011) and Dolan and Rajak (2016).

but saw little value in the additional levels of standardisation for finished products required by GMP.

Because Chinese pharmacopoeial parameters were initially based on wild medicinal materials, subsequent standardisation efforts inadvertently serve to protect the interests of those collecting and trading in wild-crafted herbs, while also forcing cultivation initiatives to emulate those same parameters, both in morphology and chemical composition. On the one hand, this creates problems for those developing cultivars that do not match the pharmacopoeia description due to their enlarged size, such as with *wabu beimu*, or their fibrous roots, such as with *qianghuo*. On the other hand, these parameters offer some protection against the use of materials containing high levels of pollutants such as pesticides. The abuse of pesticides and fertilisers is a growing problem and has been recognised by the Chinese government in the "Plan for the Protection and Development of Chinese Medicinal Materials (2015–2020)" (State Council of the People's Republic of China, 2015a). However, so long as GAP remains an optional requirement, these problems are likely to persist, even with the flash inspections that Professor Zhou claims are now routinely performed by the government. Regarding the safeguarding aspects of standardisation towards the industry, Tsing has a point when she asks bitingly "why not live for the moment and throw away all our plans? Who needs standards when the prizes are so close to hand?" (2009: 364).

Therefore, as one looks closer, the standardisation of Chinese medicines loses its inherently positive or negative connotations. As pharmaceutical companies complain of regulatory hurdles, medicinal herb collectors manage to hold some advantages over cultivation initiatives, and some Qiang practitioners hope for investment so that their family recipes can be standardised and move on to nationwide distribution. However, the advantage of medicinal herb collectors is a fragile one, since they collect finite resources and therefore work on a thin margin of possibilities. They are also dependent on unstable market prices that spur rushes for whatever raw material is suddenly profitable to collect, at times facing increasing demands as the industry continues to grow, while at other times halting collection due to certain medicinal resources becoming too scarce in a particular region to justify their labourious gathering, or due to price drops induced by new cultivation initiatives. Such initiatives thus appear once more as eco-saviours, supplying pharmaceutical companies in a supposedly sustainable manner, while herb collectors are once again accused of wrecking the environment.

Conclusion: an industrial disconnect

Considerable effort has been invested in the creation of a Qiang medical industry over recent years by a wide range of actors, even though all those involved are fully aware of the unsustainability of current raw material supply chains. My interlocutors regularly mentioned how demand far outweighed supply and many important resources were increasingly depleted.

The Chinese state used this predicament to justify a "protection through development" strategy, focusing on swift and extensive scaling up of medicinal plant cultivation. Despite the WHO's guidelines on GACP, which state that "small-scale cultivation is often preferable to large-scale production" (WHO 2003: 9), industrial scale cultivation initiatives are being rolled out across Sichuan, ostensibly in coordination with national and international policies and strategies aiming for sustainable resource management (WHO 2002, 2013). These enterprises claim widespread benefits in terms of high marketable product volumes, rural employment, and income generation, as well as enhanced safety, quality, and accessibility of the health products that emerge from them. However, as I have shown, the actual impacts of such initiatives in each of these fields are questionable at best and their implications require careful unpacking.

China's role in steering WHO strategies that promote the production and consumption of mass produced herbal proprietary medicines has both domestic and international dimensions (Saxer 2013). The purpose of China's "One Belt One Road" initiative is not limited to expanding its export market, even though it clearly seeks further overseas sales of Chinese products, including materia medica and medicines. The initiative also explores local resources abroad to import for the production of new products, much of it under the guise of international aid and development, and in search of international political endorsement (Callahan 2016).[8] The country's relationship with Tanzania offers a good example. In addition to becoming an important market for Chinese medicines (Hsu 2015), Tanzania has been the recipient of considerable Chinese investment for the development, industrialisation, and export of its own medicinal raw materials (Langwick 2011). This dynamic fits well within the priorities of the WHO "Traditional Medicine Strategy 2014–2023" (WHO 2013), which is geared towards the development and harmonisation of "traditional" medical industries around the world.

In institutional circles in Sichuan, there is a pervasive assumption of mutual benefits for industrial firms, researchers, state actors, consumers, and local farmers related to such an approach. The enterprise of Chinese minority medical industry development is portrayed as benefitting everyone along its production chain, taking the form of a ubiquitous and largely unquestioned win-win scenario that is powered by a notion of "lateness" as it strives to reach national and international markets. Scratching beneath the surface, however, it appears that the WHO and Chinese state's push to develop "traditional" medical industries fundamentally misunderstands the real circumstances of people at the village level in China, including medicinal plant cultivators and collectors. For many in the villages where I conducted fieldwork, proprietary medicinal products were of minimal

---

8 Such foreign policy strategies are by no means exclusive to China – see Peluso (1995) and Black (2018).

relevance to their daily lives and thus there was little local interest in the development of "Qiang medicines." Such a predicament suggests the need for further research among other communities who are portrayed as benefitting from initiatives focused on the development of "traditional medicine" and its associated industries. These industries, products and services rely on the growing trend of pharmaceuticalisation, which gives centre stage to industrially mass produced medicines, both at the industry level and at the level of consumers, especially through direct-to-consumer advertisements. This reconfiguration is supported by influential actors who are aware of the potential that the development and sale of ethnic minority medicines can hold to financially enable further initiatives, such as the building of minority medicine institutions, clinics, and hospitals. The result is a fine balancing act in which minority medicine practitioners are aware of being bypassed by pharmaceutical producers and markets, as these medicines reach consumers directly, but still concurrently attempt to harness medicinal products as vehicles for the legitimation and promotion of their practices.

Central to the emergence of these ethnic minority medical industries is the concept of "authenticity" of medicinal materials that appeared in institutional circles. I argue that such notions were not only the product of specific environmental and sociocultural conditions, which local stakeholders could associate with and draw from, but also of a particular constellation of economic and political circumstances. These conditions facilitate the marketing of ethnic and locality-associated products and emerge from a particular "market-state nexus" (Hardon and Sanabria 2017), which acquires peculiar contours in the context of China. Its uniqueness resides in Marxist-inspired technosocial evolutionism combined with a postcolonial sense of emancipation, which Chinese government actors and academics insist is a "socialist market economy" at work, rather than a capitalist one (He 2007; Ong 2006). Such a political and academic stance underpins an automatic assumption of the beneficence of the market and of industry. Thus, this market-state nexus is pervaded with "altruistic" nationalist and communist undertones, and so portrayed as a necessary configuration for the prosperity of the nation and the masses (Campinas 2020). However, the predominant way Qiang medicines are articulated in institutional circles shows how far the development of these "ethnic" products is removed from the realities of health, illness, and healing in Qiang villages. Medical knowledge, medicinal resources (and arguably aspects of ethnicity itself) were created, captured, reshaped, capitalised, and marketed in order to nourish the unquestioned technosocial evolutionism that lies at the heart of China's medical industry. This state-industry-market configuration leads to the rolling out of large-scale cultivation initiatives that transfigure medicinal materials through the development of cultivars, while tacitly acknowledging that it is only a matter of time before endangered wild varieties disappear altogether. Through local academic and industry intermediaries, the same configuration encourages a Qiang medical industry to "take off" and join the well-established industry of Chinese medicines. This predicament takes place despite a regulatory system that significantly hinders such development paths and market conditions that offer limited benefits to the Qiang at large, who remain largely uninterested in such an enterprise even if these hurdles could be overcome.

Bibliography

Aoyama R (2016) "One Belt, One Road": China's New Global Strategy. *Journal of Contemporary East Asia Studies* 5(2): 3–22.

Bian S (2017) *Mountains, Gods and modernity – Resilience and adaptations in the Sino-Tibetan borderland of Northwest Sichuan*. Unpublished PhD thesis. University of Oslo, Norway.

Black M (2018) *The Global Interior: Mineral Frontiers and American Power*. Cambridge, MA: Harvard University Press.

Blaikie C (2009) Critically Endangered? Medicinal Plant Cultivation and the Reconfiguration of Sowa Rigpa in Ladakh. *Asian Medicine* 5(2): 243–272.

Brockington D and Duffy R (2010) Capitalism and Conservation: The Production And Reproduction of Biodiversity Conservation. *Antipode* 42(3): 469–484.

Brockington D, Duffy R and Igoe J (2012) *Nature Unbound: Conservation, Capitalism and the Future of Protected Areas*. London: Routledge.

Callahan W (2016) China's "Asia Dream" the Belt Road Initiative and the New Regional Order. *Asian Journal of Comparative Politics* 1(3): 226–243.

Campinas M (2020) *Stones, demons, medicinal herbs, and the market: ethnic medicine and industrial aspirations among the Qiang of Western Sichuan*. Unpublished PhD thesis. University of London.

Chee L (2015) *Re-formulations: how pharmaceuticals and animal-based drugs changed Chinese medicine, 1950–1990*. Unpublished PhD thesis. National University of Singapore – University of Edinburgh.

Chen D (2015). We Have Never Been Latecomers: A Critical Review of High-Tech Industry and Social Studies of Technology in Taiwan. *East Asian Science, Technology and Society: An International Journal* 9(4): 381–396.

China Development Gateway (2021) *Great Western Development*. In Chinese. Available at: http://cn.chinagate.cn/economics/xbkf/node_7082836.htm

Chinese Pharmacopoeia Committee (2010) *Chinese Pharmacopoeia*. 2010 ed. Beijing: Traditional Chinese Medicine Science and Technology Press of China.

Chinese Pharmacopoeia Committee (2015) *Chinese Pharmacopoeia*. 2015 ed. Beijing: Traditional Chinese Medicine Science and Technology Press of China.

Comaroff J and Comaroff J (2009) *Ethnicity, Inc*. Chicago, IL: University of Chicago Press.

Companion M and Chaiken M (2017) *Responses to Disasters and Climate Change: Understanding Vulnerability and Fostering Resilience*. New York, NY: CRC Press.

Cons J and Eilenberg M (eds) (2019) *Frontier Assemblages: The Emergent Politics of Resource Frontiers in Asia*. Oxford: Wiley.

Craig S (2012) *Healing Elements: Efficacy and the Social Ecologies of Tibetan Medicine*. Berkeley and Los Angeles: University of California Press.

Croll E (1994) *From Heaven to Earth: Images and Experiences of Development in China*. New York, NY: Routledge.

Cunningham AB, Brinckmann JA, Pei SJ, et al. (2018) High Altitude Species, High Profits: Can the Trade in Wild Harvested Fritillaria cirrhosa (Liliaceae) be Sustained? *Journal of Ethnopharmacology* 223: 142–151.

Di Tommaso M, Huang M, Yue Q, et al. (2017) The Chinese TCM Industry: Growth, Changes, and Policies. In: Mucelli A and Spigarelli F (eds) *Healthcare Policies and Systems in Europe and China*. Singapore: World Scientific Publishing.

Dolan C and Rajak D (eds) (2016) *The Anthropology of Corporate Social Responsibility* (Vol. 18). New York, NY: Berghahn Books.

Dreyer JT (1993) China's Minority Peoples. *Humboldt Journal of Social Relations*, 19(2): 331–358.

eFloras (2008) Published on the Internet http://www.efloras.org. Missouri Botanical Garden, St. Louis, MO & Harvard University Herbaria, Cambridge, MA.

Flower J (2009) Ecological Engineering on the Sichuan Frontier: Socialism as Development Policy, Local Practice, and Contested Ideology 1. *Social Anthropology* 17(1): 40–55.

Hardon A and Sanabria E (2017) Fluid Drugs: Revisiting the Anthropology of Pharmaceuticals. *Annual Review of Anthropology* 46: 117–132.

He P (2007) On the Phenomenon of "Return to Marx" in China. *Frontiers of Philosophy in China* 2(2): 219–229.

Higgins D (2018) *Brands, Geographical Origin, and the Global Economy: A History from the Nineteenth Century to the Present*. Cambridge: Cambridge University Press.

Hsu E (2009) Chinese Propriety Medicines: An "Alternative Modernity"? The Case of the Anti-malarial Substance Artemisinin in East Africa. *Medical Anthropology* 28(2): 111–140.

Hsu E (2015) From Social Lives to Playing Fields: "The Chinese Antimalarial" as Artemisinin Monotherapy, Artemisinin Combination Therapy and Qinghao Juice. *Anthropology & Medicine* 22(1): 75–86.

Jeong J (2015) Ethnic Minorities in China's Western Development Plan. *Journal of International and Area Studies* 22(1): 1–18.

Jiang SY, Sun H, Wang, HL, et al. (2017) Industrialization Condition and Development Strategy of Notopterygii Rhizoma et Radix. *China Journal of Chinese Materia Medica* 42(14): 2627–2632.

Kloos S (2017) The Pharmaceutical Assemblage: Rethinking Sowa Rigpa and the Herbal Pharmaceutical Industry in Asia. *Current Anthropology* 6: 693–717.

Kloos S, Madhavan H, Tidwell T, et al. (2020) The Transnational Sowa Rigpa Industry in Asia: New Perspectives on an Emerging Economy. *Social Science & Medicine* 245: 112617.

Lai H (2002) China's Western Development Program: Its Rationale, Implementation, and Prospects. *Modern China* 28(4): 432–466.

Lai L and Farquhar J (2015) Nationality Medicines in China: Institutional Rationality and Healing Charisma. *Comparative Studies in Society and History* 57(2): 381–406.

Landecker H (2016) Antibiotic Resistance and the Biology of History. *Body & Society* 22(4): 19–52.

Langwick S (2011) *Bodies, Politics, and African Healing: The Matter of Maladies in Tanzania*. Bloomington, IN: Indiana University Press.

Latour B (1993) *We Have Never Been Modern*. Cambridge, MA: Harvard University Press.

Latour B (1999) *Pandora's Hope: Essays on the Reality of Science Studies*. Cambridge, MA: Harvard University Press.

Lei SH (1999) From Changshan to a New Anti-malarial Drug: Re-networking Chinese Drugs and Excluding Chinese Doctors. *Social Studies of Science* 29(3): 323–358.

Li S (2010) *Bencao gangmu: Chinese Classic Collection Edition (*本草纲目：中国古典名著珍藏版*)*. Jilin: Time Art Publishing House.

Li S, Liu J, Gong X, et al. (2013) Characterizing the Major Morphological Traits and Chemical Compositions in the Bulbs of Widely Cultivated Fritillaria Species in China. *Biochemical Systematics and Ecology*, 46: 130–136.

Li X, Liu L, Gu X, et al. (2017) Heavy Collecting Induces Smaller and Deeper Fritillariae Cirrhosae Bulbus in the Wild. *Plant Diversity* 39(4): 208–213.

Lin W and Law J (2015) We Have Never Been Latecomers!? Making Knowledge Spaces for East Asian Technosocial Practices. *East Asian Science, Technology and Society* 9(2): 117–126.

Liu Y, Guo Y and Zhou Y (2018) Poverty Alleviation in Rural China: Policy Changes, Future Challenges and Policy Implications. *China Agricultural Economic Review* 10(2): 241–259.

Liu ZD, Wang S and Chen SC (2009) A Taxonomic Note of Fritillaria wabuensis (Liliaceae). *Acta Botanica Yunnanica* 31(2): 182.

McNally C (2004) Sichuan: Driving Capitalist Development Westward. *The China Quarterly*, 178: 426–447.

Meinhof M (2017) Colonial Temporality and Chinese National Modernization Discourses. *InterDisciplines. Journal of History and Sociology* 8(1): 51–80.

Mullaney T (2011) *Coming to Terms with the Nation: Ethnic Classification in Modern China*. Berkeley, CA: University of California Press.

National Bureau of Statistics of China (NBS) (n.d.) *Tabulation on the 2010 Population Census of the People's Republic of China. Distribution by age, sex, and ethnic groups*. In Chinese. Available at: http://www.stats.gov.cn/tjsj/pcsj/rkpc/6rp/excel/A0201.xls

Ong A (2006) *Neoliberalism as Exception: Mutations in Citizenship and Sovereignty*. London: Duke University Press.

Peluso NL (1995) Whose Woods are These? Counter-mapping Forest Territories in Kalimantan, Indonesia. *Antipode* 27(4): 383–406.

People's Republic of China Twelfth National People's Congress (2016) *People's Republic of China, traditional Chinese medicine law*. Promulgated December 25. In Chinese. Available at: http://www.satcm.gov.cn/e/action/ShowInfo.php?classid=140&id=23573

Pordié L and Gaudillière J-P (2014) The Reformulation Regime in Drug Discovery: Revisiting Polyherbals and Property Rights in the Ayurvedic Industry. *East Asian Science, Technology and Society: An International Journal* 8(1): 57–79.

Rajak D (2011) *In Good Company: An Anatomy of Corporate Social Responsibility*. Stanford, CA: Stanford University Press.

Saxer M (2013) *Manufacturing Tibetan medicine: The Creation of an Industry and the Moral Economy of Tibetanness*. New York, NY, Oxford: Berghahn.

Springer L (2015) Collectors, Producers, and Circulators of Tibetan and Chinese Medicines in Sichuan Province. *Asian Medicine*, 10(1–2): 177–220.

SATCM - State Administration of Traditional Chinese Medicine of the People's Republic of China (2016) *Outline of the strategic plan for Chinese medicine development (2016–2030)*. In Chinese. Available at: http://www.gov.cn/zhengce/content/2016-02/26/content_5046678.htm

SATCM - State Administration of Traditional Chinese Medicine of the People's Republic of China (2018) *National authentic medicine production base construction plan (2018–2025)*. In Chinese. Available at: http://bgs.satcm.gov.cn/zhengcewenjian/2018-12-24/8631.html

SATCM - State Administration of Traditional Chinese Medicine of the People's Republic of China (2019) *Sichuan province Chinese medicine industry development plan (2018–2025)*. In Chinese. Available at: http://www.satcm.gov.cn/d/file/p/2019/07-22/5c3acdc7b2eea7e7e58e88fda4c39e0e.pdf##15635076197432c-740cfc38600c9e11589d9d23633ec51563507595.pdf##1.32%20MB

State Council of the People's Republic of China (2015a) *Plan for the protection and development of Chinese medicinal materials (2015–2020)*. In Chinese. Available at: http://www.gov.cn/zhengce/content/2015-04/27/content_9662.htm

State Council of the People's Republic of China (2015b) *Endangered Chinese medicinal materials supply and demand conflicts ease within 5 years*. In Chinese. Available at: http://www.gov.cn/zhengce/2015-04/28/content_2853867.htm

State Council of the People's Republic of China (2016) *Outline of the "healthy China 2030" plan*. In Chinese. Available at: http://www.gov.cn/zhengce/2016-10/25/content_5124174.htm

Sun XY and Sun FY (2010) *Shennong bencaojing (神农本草经)*. Taiyuan: Shanxi science and Technology Press.

Tang S and Yueh S (1983) Three New Species of Fritillaria Linn. *Acta Academiae Medicinae Sichuan* 14: 327–334.

Tsing AL (2009) Beyond Economic and Ecological Standardisation. *The Australian Journal of Anthropology* 20(3): 347–368.

Tsing A (2015) *The Mushroom at the End of the World: On the Possibility of Life in Capitalist Ruins*. Princeton, NJ: Princeton University Press.

Unschuld, P (1986) *A History of Pharmaceutics*. Berkeley, CA: University of California Press.

Wang M (1999) From the Qiang Barbarians to the Qiang Nationality: The Making of a New Chinese Boundary. In: Huang S and Hsu C (eds), *Imagining China: Regional Division and National Unity*. Taipei: Institute of Ethnology.

Wang M (2002) Searching for Qiang Culture in the First Half of the Twentieth Century. *Inner Asia*, 4(1): 131–148.

Wang G (2015) Ethnic Multilingual Education in China: A Critical Observation. *Working Papers in Educational Linguistics (WPEL)* 30(2): 3.

Wang FL (2016) *Institutions and Institutional Change in China: Premodernity and Modernization*. Berlin: Springer.

WHO (2002) *WHO traditional medicine strategy 2002–2005*. World Health Organisation, Geneva, pp. 1–74. Available at: http://www.wpro.who.int/health_technology/book_who_traditional_medicine_strategy_2002_2005.pdf

WHO (2003) WHO guidelines on good agricultural and collection practices [GACP] for medicinal plants. World Health Organization.

WHO (2013) *WHO traditional medicine strategy 2014–2023*. Alternative and integrative medicine. pp. 1–76. Available at: http://apps.who.int/iris/bitstream/

WHO (2019) WHO global report on traditional and complementary medicine 2019. World Health Organization.

Xin S and Hsu E (2020) Translation of Beijing's Recommendations for Traditional Chinese Medicine (TCM) Treatment of Covid-19. *Cultural Anthropology*. https://culanth.org/fieldsights/translation-of-beijings-recomendations

Yan K (2015) *Poverty Alleviation in China: A Theoretical and Empirical Study*. Berlin: Springer.

Yang MM-H (1994) *Gifts, Favors, and Banquets: The Art of Social Relationships in China*. Ithaca, NY: Cornell University Press.

Yang J and Peng Y (2015) Traditional Miao cures to boost health of Guizhou's economy. *China Daily*, Beijing. 18 March, 2015. https://www.chinadaily.com.cn/china/2015-03/18/content_19839959.htm

Zhang Q (2016) *Making disaster zones into "scenic sites", homelands into "gardens", and peasants into "grateful survivors": The Chinese state in Qiang village earthquake recovery*. Unpublished PhD thesis. Tulane University.

Zhang Z and Unschuld P (2014) *Dictionary of the Ben cao gang mu, Volume 1: Chinese Historical Illness Terminology* (Vol. 1). Berkeley, CA: University of California Press.

Zhang D, Zhang J and Zhang Y (2014) Analysis on the Institutionalization of Ethnic Civilian Medicine: A Case Study on the Institutionalized Veteran Qiang Doctors. *Journal of Guangxi University for Nationalities* 36(6): 17–20.

3 The development of the Kampo medicines industry

"Good Practices" and health policy making in Japan

Ichiro Arai, Julia S. Yongue, and Kiichiro Tsutani

The roots of Kampo medicine date back to the sixth century CE when Chinese medicine was first imported into Japan. It was then "localised," in some cases by substituting foreign with indigenous plants, during the late Edo period (1603–1868) to suit local preferences and needs (Tsutani 2006). Influenced by various schools (such as Kohō 古方, Gōse 後世, Sechū 折衷), this localised Chinese medicine gradually became known as *Kanpō* (漢方) or "Han method" medicine (Kitajima 2017). Today the term *Wakanyaku*, which combines the Chinese characters of 和 (wa) signifying Japan, 漢 (han, often pronounced kan in modern Japanese) or Han China, and medicine 薬 (yaku), can be translated as "Japanese and Chinese crude drug." Since 1976, however, *Kanpo seizai* (漢方製剤) or "Kampo" has become the official term employed in Japan's modern healthcare system, a distinctive feature of which is the integration of biomedicine and Kampo medicine into one single medical system.[1] Accordingly, any physician licensed to practice in Japan can prescribe either type of medication to a patient, who can then expect equal coverage – regardless of the type – under the country's National Health Insurance (NHI). Moreover, in addition to NHI coverage, both types of medicine are subject to the same systems of pharmacovigilance, relief for the sufferers of adverse drug reactions (ADRs), and new drug approval procedures.[2] Within Japan's regulatory

---

1 In Japan, only physicians are legally permitted to provide prescription Kampo medicines. South Korea has a dual system, while the Chinese medical system recognises four types of physician licenses (see Tu and Tsutani 2007). Shim (2015) summarises the three institutional approaches of East Asian medicine as "unification in China, equalization in Korea, and subjugation in Japan."
2 In the 1990s, WHO also began introducing various guidelines to ensure herbal medicine quality, safety, and efficacy such as Guidelines for the Assessment of Herbal Medicines (1991), Research Guidelines for Evaluating the Safety and Efficacy of Herbal Medicines (1993), Guidelines for the Manufacture of Herbal Medicinal Products (1996), Quality Control Methods for Medicinal Plant Materials (1998), General Guidelines for Methodologies on Research and Evaluation of Traditional Medicine (2000), etc.

DOI: 10.4324/9781003218074-5

82 *Ichiro Arai et al.*

framework, therefore, Kampo medicines are technically no different from biomedicines.[3]

This single system has not always existed in Japan but is rather the outcome of long and complex processes of regulation and industrialisation of both biomedicine and Kampo medicine, which had two major, parallel dimensions. Thus, one crucial aspect of this development is the political dimension of Japan's regulatory history and its changing health policies over time (Sakuma 1988). Simultaneously, significant technological advances in factories and research hospitals led to the introduction of higher standards for pharmaceutical production, new drug approval, and the evaluation of safety and efficacy of both kinds of medicine. Both dimensions – the political-regulatory and the technological-industrial – come together in the field of "good practices" or GxP, which consist of the procedures and protocols for ensuring pharmaceutical quality (Good Manufacturing Practices or GMP), safety (Good Post-Marketing Surveillance Practices or GPMSP), and efficacy (Good Clinical Practices or GCP). Indeed, these "good practices" and standards, mandatory for all pharmaceutical products in use in Japan including Kampo medicines,[4] were key to the integration of Kampo medicines into the country's modern healthcare system, as well as their widespread prescription by Japanese physicians to their patients (JKMA 2011).[5]

If one cannot understand contemporary Kampo medicine outside the context of its integration into Japan's national healthcare system, then this integration similarly cannot be understood without considering the fundamental role played by GxP in bringing both Kampo and biomedicine within a single regulatory framework. This chapter therefore examines the introduction of GxP and its effects on Kampo medicine in order to trace the

---

3 The transliteration of Kampo follows the conventions of WHO International Standard Terminologies on Traditional Medicine in the Western Pacific Region, World Health Organization (2012), and Japan Pharmacopeia (JP). Regarding the transliteration of Japanese names, they appear in the Japanese order with the family name first. Japanese names of works in English follow the order in which they appear in the publication. Macrons are used except for well-known place names, company names, the term Kampo (as opposed to Kanpō), and Kampo medicines (shosaikoto rather than shōsaikotō).

4 Japan was the first Asian nation to adopt GxP, and Japanese government and industry representatives were directly involved in international negotiations with European and American lawmakers to devise and harmonise regulations on clinical trials, which would also apply to Kampo medicines. The early application of GxP to the Kampo medicines industry is symbolic of the importance that Japanese regulatory authorities have placed on introducing scientific, internationally recognised standards, and they have served as a fundamental tool for integrating the two different medicinal traditions into a single, modern regulatory system.

5 A JKMA survey of 627 physicians showed that 89 percent prescribed both types of medicines. Among them only two percent had never prescribed Kampo medicines, while 17 percent prescribe them exclusively (see https://www.nikkankyo.org/serv/pdf/jittaichousa2011.pdf).

emergence and development of today's Kampo industry in Japan. In doing so, the chapter addresses a dearth of academic work on Japan's herbal medicines industry as a sub-category of its pharmaceutical industry, which has attracted little interest among historians and medical anthropologists so far.

There exist, of course, useful overviews and accounts – mostly in Japanese – of the history of Japan's (biomedical) pharmaceutical industry, which grew out of the herbal medicines business in pre-Meiji Japan (Tanabe 1983; Takeda 1984; JSHP 1995). Thus, in a seminal work on the roots of the Japanese pharmaceutical industry, Yamada Hisao (1995) describes the import, types of medicines (including patent medicines) in circulation, and the regulations in place prior to the Meiji Restoration of 1868. Futaya and Blaikie (this volume) provide a new dimension to the history of the development of Japan's medical industry in their exploration of *haichi* medicines, for which Toyama prefecture is the most well-known. Another important study examines the formation of traditional medicine trading routes through the port of Nagasaki (Tong 2014). Entering the country during the "period of national isolation," these medicines were traded by medical merchant houses in Doshōmachi (central Osaka), the country's largest centre for the herbal medicines trade, and in Honchō (located in Nihonbashi in Tokyo, then known as Edo). Following the Meiji government's decision to dissolve the medical merchant guilds and introduce modern biomedicine, the networks on which this trade depended weakened, though the two medical marketplaces in Doshōmachi and Honchō adapted and were able to become the two principal locations of today's pharmaceutical industry (Tong 2014).[6] What all these studies show is the diversity, complexity, and continuity of Japan's medical traditions, as well as how they have contributed to the formation of its modern pharmaceutical industry.

Margaret Lock's *East Asian Medicine in Urban Japan* (1980), a classic on the modern uses of Kampo medicine, helps situate Kampo medicine within Japan's modern biomedicine-based medical system from the perspectives of practicing physicians, patients, and pharmacists. Exploring the effects of the so-called "Kampo boom," she notes that this boom attracted the interest of the modern biomedicines industry and served as an incentive for existing producers to enter this "new" and potentially lucrative sector. Furthermore, it also prompted a shift among academics and regulators to adopt a more scientific approach towards Kampo medicine. Maki Umemura (2012) shows how the exploding demand for Kampo medicines was driven by consumers and physicians, sustaining Kampo medicine's revival and the development of its industry after a long period of decline from the Meiji period onwards. Taking a different approach, this chapter focuses not on

---

6 Some of Japan's largest biomedical manufacturers such as Takeda and Tanabe started as herbal medicine businesses but transitioned to biomedicine during the Meiji (1868–1912) and Taisho (1912–1926) periods.

the role of consumers but on the so-far unexplored role of modern drug evaluation methodologies in the Kampo industry's development. Tracing how a scientific approach – specifically in the form of GxP – took root, as Lock suggested, this chapter explores its influence on the Kampo industry's development, as well as its long-term implications in providing greater legitimacy to Kampo medicine as part of mainstream Japanese healthcare.

To better understand the distinctive features of the regulatory policy environment for Kampo medicines in Japan, it is useful to situate this industry in a wider Asian context. As explored in other chapters in this volume, the introduction of GxP elsewhere reveals appreciable cross-country variations, which is particularly evident in the realm of globalisation. As Kudlu (this volume) asserts, globalisation was the key impetus for the introduction of standards for Ayurveda in India, where market and industry forces played a more important role than the state in their implementation. Similarly, globalisation was an important driver for the introduction of scientific standards in China, a move that revived a long-standing policy debate over the boundaries between Chinese and Western biomedicine (Chee, this volume). In Japan, however, there is no evidence of a concerted strategy among regulators or industry officials to globalise the Kampo industry overseas. Japan's Kampo medicines industry is, and will likely remain, relatively small in scale, being comprised mainly of small- and medium-sized manufacturers whose primary concern is to maintain domestic market share. The motivation to introduce scientific, internationally recognised standards grew out of the decision to extend NHI coverage of Kampo medicines, for which it was required that they be subjected to the same rigorous global GxP standards of safety, efficacy, and quality as biomedicines. Thus the main driver of "globalisation" in the Japanese context was not the market, as was the case in other countries examined in this volume, but the underlying goals of the regulatory regime.

Overview of the Kampo medicines industry and its development

Before examining GxP and its role in the development of the Kampo medicines industry, a brief overview of the industry is necessary to compare its relative size and value with the others covered in this volume. According to the most recent Japan Kampo Medicines Manufacturers Association (JKMA) statistics, the market for biomedicines in Japan in 2015 was 66 billion USD, or 97.6 percent of all sales of pharmaceuticals, while herbal medicines sales stood at just 2 billion USD (1 USD = 100 JPY), a mere 2.4 percent of the total market. According to the same data, a breakdown of the herbal medicines sector shows that prescription Kampo medicines is the largest category at 81 percent or 1.45 billion USD. Given their connection to GxP, namely GCP and GPMSP, this category is the focal point of this chapter. Sales of other herbal medicines include (1) over-the-counter (OTC) Kampo medicines with 19 percent or 346 million USD, (2) crude drug pieces for decoction with two percent or 98 million USD, and (3) other herbal products with five percent or 88 million USD (JKMA 2019). The low ratio for crude drug pieces for decoction can be explained by the fact that, in Japan, approximately 98 percent of all Kampo medicines are consumed as dried extracts, which are mass produced and packaged in factories, as opposed to China and Korea where decoctions are preferred.[7]

As the figures above demonstrate, though Kampo medicines are subject to NHI coverage, the weight, size, and earnings of the Kampo industry are much smaller than those of the biomedicines industry. At the same time, the number of Kampo medicines producers remains relatively large: as of 2018, JKMA was comprised of 66 member companies; among them, some manufacture both biomedicines and OTC Kampo medicines.[8] Tsumura & Co. (hereafter Tsumura) is by far the largest producer with over 80 percent of the market share, including sales of both prescription and OTC Kampo medicines.[9] It is followed by Kuracie, which occupies a 10 percent share.[10] The remaining 10 percent is comprised of numerous small-scale, often family-owned enterprises. One such company is Kotaro, founded in 1929, which though small compared to Tsumura, was key in developing extract technologies. Although most of these enterprises are members of JKMA, conducting a comprehensive survey of the industry is challenging as many are unlisted, meaning that they have no obligation to make their financial data or other pertinent information public. Some large biomedicine manufacturers also market Kampo medicines; however, it is not possible to discern their sales information from their financial statements.[11]

---

7 Official statistics on the use of decoctions and extracts are unavailable for the Chinese market. Nonetheless, the ratio is thought to be approximately 50 percent for each type. In Korea, however, the use of decoctions is much higher than for extracts.
8 Takeda and Daiichi Sankyo used to be JKMA members; however, in 2020 only their OTC-producing subsidiaries were. Another large biomedicines manufacturer, Taisho is a JKMA member, whose *overall* sales including biomedicines, exceeds Tsumura. If one considers earnings derived exclusively from the sale of Kampo medicines, Tsumura is Japan's largest Kampo medicines manufacturer.
9 Tsumura was founded in 1893 in Tokyo as Tsumura Juntendo (Tsumura 1964).
10 Kuracie's roots can be found in Kanegafuchi Spinning Company, established in 1887. Kanebo (now part of Kao), originally a spin-off of Kanegafuchi Spinning, entered the soap manufacturing in 1936 followed by entry into cosmetics sector for which it was once one of Japan's top brands. Research on medicine development began at Kanebo in 1934 when an R&D centre was established. However its entry in earnest began in the 1960s and 1970s with the acquisition of two pharmaceutical companies, Yamashiro in 1966 and Nakataki in 1971.
11 Though no statistics are available on unlisted firms, it is estimated that there are as many as several thousand Kampo medicines companies. According to Japanese government statistics for 2012, the biomedicines industry alone is comprised of some 801 firms. Due to policies regarding pricing, the number of small medicine companies in Japan is larger than most Western nations where medicines are supplied mainly by large multinationals. Other associations with Kampo medicine producing members are the Home Medicine Association of Japan (https://www.hmaj.com/english/), the Tokyo and Osaka Crude Drugs Associations (http://www.tokyo-shoyaku.jp; http://osakasyouyaku.jp), and the Japan Self-Medication Industry Association (http://www.jsmi.jp/english/index.html).

According to Kosoto Hiroshi (2014), it was not until the middle of the Meiji period (1868–1912) that the term *Oriental medicine* (*tōyō igaku* 東洋医学), used to signify traditional medicine or Wakanyaku, came into general use as distinct from Western medicine (*seiyō igaku* 西洋医学), also called *rampō* (Dutch medicine).[12] During this period, Kampo was identified and recognised as a specific form of medicine, but it also faced a major crisis. Under the Meiji government's mandate to modernise the nation according to a Western model, the Medical Affairs Bureau headed by Nagayo Sensai (1838–1902) introduced biomedicine as Japan's only officially recognised form of healthcare. The underlying impetus for fully embracing a Western model of medicine from an early date was the concern on the part of policy-makers that by not doing so, Japan – just as some of its Asian neighbours – could risk losing its sovereignty as a nation. This early example, as in other chapters in this volume, provides a vivid illustration of the crucial role played by the national government in shaping not only Japan's medical history but also the perception and status of Kampo medicine within the country's evolving medical system.

Among the many new measures that the new bureau enacted, the national medical examination system, introduced in 1883, dealt Kampo medicine its greatest blow. According to this measure, all those wishing to enter the medical profession were required to receive a Western medical education and pass an examination in order to receive official authorisation to practice. However, to prevent shortages and avoid strong resistance from the existing medical establishment, a concession was made, which allowed doctors to continue to practice Kampo medicine and/or *rampō* simply by registering themselves under the new system. In other words, they were permitted to continue their practice without having to pass the new (Western) medical examination. Family succession through apprenticeship, however, was no longer permitted (Bowers 1970; MHW 1988).

Lacking official recognition by the state as certified professionals and unable to devise a standardised set of procedures to use as the foundation for legitimising their activities, Kampo medicine practitioners gradually fell out of favour. Moreover, with the rise in imports of new and more effective biomedicines, combined with the growing acceptance of Western ideas among the general populace, Kampo medicine gradually earned a reputation as inferior, unscientific, and backward. In 1895, a group of Diet members put forth a bill opposing the exclusion of Kampo medicine from the medical system. However, despite strong political support for the bill by some key members of the existing medical establishment, including the Meiji emperor's personal physician, it failed to receive approval. Bereft of an official status within the new medical system, Kampo medicine entered

---

12 Dutch doctors residing in Japan, as well as Japanese translators of Dutch medical texts, first introduced Western medicine to Japan.

a long period of decline (Yamada 1996). While the number of Kampo medicine practitioners dwindled to near nil, *baiyaku* or patent medicines comprised of the same or similar crude materials as Kampo medicines were readily available at pharmacies. *Baiyaku* remained in general use at that time in much the same way as OTC medicines are today (Nishikawa 2010). Similar observations are made by Futaya and Blaikie (this volume), who show that legislative changes had a significant impact on the development of the *baiyaku* (*haichi* medicines) industry in the early 1900s and beyond.

From the 1950s and 1960s, Kampo medicine began to experience a gradual revival, which can be tied to four factors. The first was the institutionalisation of some elements of Kampo medicines into Japan's health coverage system, which began with the introduction of NHI in 1961 (Campbell and Ikegami 1998).[13] Though the system's foundations were clearly established on the principles of biomedicine, in 1960, just prior to its official implementation, regulators decided that a small number of crude drugs would be included. Four Kampo medicine extracts were subsequently added in 1967.[14]

The second factor was the resurgence of scholarship on traditional medicines. In 1950, the Japan Society for Oriental Medicine (JSOM) was established, with a total of 98 members. The founding of such a society was in itself significant, as decades later it would be at the forefront of promoting modern drug evaluation methodologies, referred to as the "scientisation" (or *kagaku-ka*) of Kampo medicine (Special Committee for Evidence-based Medicine 2002; Akiba 2010).[15] In the 1960s and 1970s, the creation of new institutes within existing pharmaceutical and medical schools also spread across Japan. The first was founded in 1963 at Toyama University (initially Research Institute of Wankanyaku, now Institute of Natural Medicine), followed by the Kitasato Institute (Oriental Medicine Research Institute) in 1972 (Hattori 2006). It is notable that Toyama University is a public (national) university.[16] From this development, one can infer that the central government had decided to provide indirect, limited support for the study of herbal and Kampo medicine via subsidies and grants from the Ministry of Education. As seen in Futaya and Blaikie's study (this volume) on the reshaping of the Toyama Medicines industry,

---

13 Precursors of NHI had been put in place in the pre-war period, but were not universal.
14 The first official drug pricing system, mentioned in the subsequent sections, was introduced in World War II to prevent sharp rises in drug prices and to help ration medicines. It was abandoned at the end of the war, then subsequently reinstated.
15 The "scientisation" or *kagaku-ka* of medicine eventually led to the establishment of the evidence-based medicine (EBM) committee within the JSOM in 2001. According to the society's website, its membership has grown significantly (8,518 persons), as has the importance of KM within Japan's medical system.
16 Although Toyama University is now a national university, it began as a vocational school founded by the local *baiyaku* industry.

the Toyama prefectural government, working alongside local actors, was far more cooperative. A treatment facility opened in 1979, while Toyama Medical and Pharmaceutical University Hospital (now Toyama University Hospital) became the first national university to establish a Wakanyaku Clinic. Like the JSOM, these institutions would come to play an important role in introducing modern drug evaluation methodologies through their clinical research and publications on Kampo medicine. The Ministry of Education, however, would not issue any formal medical school guidelines regarding standards for physician training in Kampo medicine until much later, in 2001.

Third was the introduction of new manufacturing technologies, enabling Kampo medicine to develop as an advanced, modern industry. Research on new production technologies was initiated as early as 1944, when researchers at Japan's largest biomedicine company, Takeda, undertook experiments to produce dried extracts of herbal medicines. It was not until 1957, however, that Kampo medicines manufacturer Kotaro would become the first company to develop dried extracts (Arai 2015). Contributing to these innovations was research on spray-drying technologies that could be applied across a variety of industries. Applications included not only the instant coffee and processed foods industries, whose demand increased exponentially during Japan's economic "takeoff" or High Growth Period (1954–1973) but also the Kampo medicines industry. Tsumura, which received approval in 1976 for products using this technology, serves as an early example. The technologies used to mass-produce Kampo medicine extracts have had important long-term implications for the development of Kampo medicine as a modern industry. Moreover, the introduction of industrial standards contributed to improved quality assurance.

The fourth and most significant factor was a 1976 regulatory reform. According to this measure, 38 prescription medicines were officially approved as Kampo medicine formulations, making them eligible for NHI reimbursement (Kikutani 2001). Of particular note is that this was carried out without any clinical validation studies (Tsutani 1993). The reform gave birth to a new category of medicine, which would officially be known as *kanpō seizai* (Kampo formulation).[17] It also made Kampo medicines more affordable and thus more accessible to patients, particularly the elderly. As examined below, the elderly received NHI coverage of treatments and medications free of charge from 1973 to 1983, which

---

17 38 Kampo medicine formulae were included as a result of the reform. Prior to this, only four were approved for inclusion but were categorised as *anti-inflammatory, analgesic* and *gastrointestinal drugs,* since an official category for Kampo medicines had not yet been introduced via NHI.

led to a decade of especially high market growth for Kampo medicines (Shimazaki 2009).

There were two sociocultural factors that contributed to this reform. First, in the 1960s and 1970s, a number of synthetic drugs had been identified as the source of serious side effects. Although the thalidomide disaster is perhaps the most well-known worldwide, in Japan, subacute myelo-optic neuropathy (SMON) caused by clioquinol had particularly devastating effects, leaving some 30,000 victims paralyzed or blind (Katahira 1997). With the succession of these widely publicised reports in the media, patients and physicians alike came to believe that Kampo medicines offered a safe alternative to synthetic drugs and began to lobby for their inclusion in NHI. This belief was at the root of the so-called "myth of Kampo medicines safety" discussed below.

Accompanying the wave of iatrogenic afflictions was a second factor, what might be termed as the "de-personalisation" of Western medical care, which was in sharp contrast with the "soft and humanised image of Kampo medicines." According to Otsuka Yasuo (1976), the growing acceptance of Kampo medicine described above can be traced to "the analytic nature of modern medicine" and "disregard of patients' complaints in modern medicine." Kampo medicine's approach offered more personalised, patient-focused medical care based on diagnostic methods entailing a lengthy consultation to determine the root cause of the patient's illness (Lock 1980).[18] For patients, Kampo medicine's use of classical decoctions, even in a modernised, dried form, conveyed an image of their being more "humanised goods" than synthetic drugs.

Political and economic factors were also at work. The sponsor of the 1976 legislation was a powerful Liberal Democratic Party (LDP) supporter and physician, Takemi Tarō (1904–1983), who served as the president of the JMA (Japanese Medical Association) from 1957 to 1982 (Campbell and Ikegami 1998). One can identify two personal connections that influenced Takemi's choice to sponsor this major legislative change. The first was Otsuka Keisetsu (1900–1980), a leading Kampo medicine specialist, one of the founders of JSOM and an early leader in the promotion of the Kampo medicine revival. As Takemi's physician, Otsuka had prescribed Kampo medicines to him in his treatments. Takemi received his medical degree from Keio University, known for its strong academic cliques. The second personal connection was a graduate of Keio and son of the founder of Tsumura, Tsumura Jūsha II

---

18 Consultations in Japan are short compared to the length of time one must wait to see a physician as a 1999 MHW survey shows. Most patients who visited a medical institution as an outpatient were required to wait from 30 minutes to an hour and received a 3- to 10-minute consultation. According to Lock's study, patients may in some cases wait up to one hour to see a KM doctor, though consultations generally take approximately 30 minutes.

(1908–1977). Takemi knew Tsumura and, according to the corporate history, was sympathetic to the development of Kampo medicine as a modern Japanese manufacturing industry (Tsumura 1982). At the time of the 1976 reform, Takemi received strong endorsement from the Kampo medicines industry, which stood to profit considerably from its inclusion.

Another influence was the nature of the universal health coverage system and its emphasis on equal access (Campbell and Ikegami 1998). One can find examples where Japanese health authorities have intervened to reduce the financial burden of medical care to patients and promote equal access by providing subsidies or by extending NHI coverage (Akazawa et al. 2014).[19] The 1976 legislative change corresponds to the latter. Thanks to their inclusion in NHI, patients could procure Kampo medicines from their physicians at a lower cost burden, while elderly patients could receive them free of charge. Coupled with the reform was an increase in the industry's marketing of Kampo medicines to physicians, the dramatic effects of which are shown below in Figure 3.1. Over time, the use of Kampo medicines rose, providing a favourable environment for the industry's development as a manufacturer of prescription drugs.

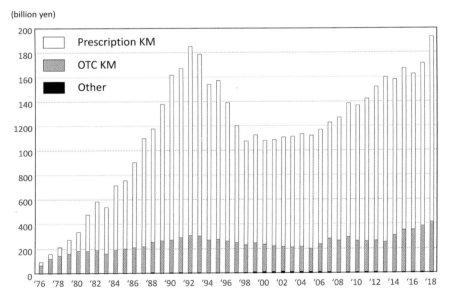

Figure 3.1 A comparison of prescription and OTC Kampo medicines sales in Japan (1976–2018). Source: Japan Kampo Medicines Manufacturers Association (2019).

19 Because some prefectures were offering vaccination free of charge while others were not, the government provided subsidies to ensure that all citizens would have equal access to vaccines, regardless of where they resided. A similar situation could be witnessed when free healthcare for the elderly was first introduced.

The reader should note the marked decrease in demand after 1992 followed by a levelling off from 2000 and a gradual rise from 2010, the reasons for which are dealt with below.

The effects of GxP on the manufacturing of Kampo medicines

Changes in international regulatory regimes tend to have a significant effect on Japan's domestic healthcare policies and regulations. Such was the case for Japan's manufacturing standards. The Food and Drug Administration (USFDA) first introduced GMP in 1963, followed by the World Health Organisation (WHO), which drafted its first GMP document in 1967 (WHO 2014). Japan's health ministry (Ministry of Health, Labour, and Welfare, MHLW), then known as Ministry of Health and Welfare (MHW), began applying GMP to the pharmaceutical sector in 1976 (MHW 1998).[20] Since then, Japanese regulators have continued to broaden the scope of GMP so as to encompass an ever-wider variety of quality-related standards, ranging from production facility specifications to employee training.

Japan's regulatory regime for Kampo medicines manufacturing

One important feature of Japan's regulatory regime for Kampo medicines manufacturing is the pervasiveness of voluntary or "quasi" standards, which are initially introduced by manufacturers, but often later become regulatory policies. One example is GMP. In the early 1970s, individual Japanese pharmaceutical manufacturers had already begun to put in place their own GMP on a trial basis, even before it became mandatory under the Pharmaceutical Affairs Law (PAL) in 1976 (Yamakawa 1995). By 1980, GMP was applicable to all types of pharmaceuticals manufactured and sold in Japan. While this included Kampo medicines, they were subject to exemptions due to the special features of herbal medicines as natural products, which unlike synthetic drugs, can vary in potency across lots. Just as pharmaceutical manufacturers had done prior to the official introduction of GMP, the Kampo medicines industry put in place voluntary, "quasi" quality standards. This section describes the circumstances under which these standards were implemented and the roles played by three main actors – regulators, industrial associations, and individual Kampo medicines manufacturers – in the process.

A major feature of the regulatory regime for Kampo medicines manufacturing is its complexity and multi-layered quality. The first of its four layers is the foundation for all medicinal manufacturing in Japan, the PAL, which incorporates not only GMP but also the standards listed in the Japan Pharmacopeia (JP). As national standards, these regulations are legally

---

20 The MHW became the MHLW in 2001.

binding and must be applied throughout the production process by all manufacturers. The second layer is comprised of voluntary, "quasi" standards devised by JKMA member companies. Though not legally binding, all the members of JKMA carefully respect their own self-imposed, mutually agreed-upon rules. This behaviour can be explained by the important roles of the JKMA and the industry's umbrella organisation, the Federation of Pharmaceutical Manufacturers Association of Japan (FPMAJ), which includes Kampo medicines and biomedicines manufacturers' associations, as lobbies in negotiations with regulatory authorities, as well as vectors of information collection and dissemination.[21] Member companies that do not comply with their recommendations risk harsh sanctions, the worst being ostracism from the associations. Non-compliance can also have highly negative repercussions on a firm's business operations and result in the withholding of vital industry and regulatory information. The third layer is the individual manufacturer's own in-house standards, which are firm-specific. The fourth and most recently added layer is international standards.

GMP and other Kampo medicine extract standards in the 1980s and beyond

As mentioned above, in Japan, most Kampo medicines are consumed as dried extracts. However, when the first extract products were launched in Japan in the late 1950s, there were no quality specifications designed to ensure potency equivalency for extracts vis-à-vis decoction formulations. Manufacturers only became aware of potential equivalency-related problems decades later, and by the early 1980s had begun to search for ways to remedy them. In 1982, the Advisory Committee for Kampo medicine Extract Products was founded, which cooperated with regulators in the Pharmaceutical Affairs Bureau of MHW to improve quality (i.e. equivalency of extracts to decoctions). This was followed by the establishment of a working group to set manufacturing standards for quality assurance. Also in the 1980s, regulators decided to conduct their own tests to verify whether extract formulations were component-equivalent to standard decoctions.[22] Their tests revealed two important quantity- and quality-related findings: they were not equivalent and the content of constituents found in dried extracts was generally inferior to standard decoctions.

21 For further information on the organisation and functions of FPMAJ, see: http://www.fpmaj.gr.jp/fpmaj_HPenglish.pdf#search=%27Federation+of+Pharmaceutical+Manufacturers+Association+of+Japan%27
22 To ensure the equivalency of standard decoctions and mass-produced extracts, each Kampo medicines company was first asked to prepare a decoction using standard crude herbs according to the classical decoction method. The decoction the company produced was then designated as the *standard decoction* for that particular company. Tests followed to verify whether the company's mass-produced extract was equivalent to its "standard decoction." The company's mass-produced dried extract is considered "equivalent" if the marker component amounts are the same (within a range of ±50 percent) as its standard decoction.

In response to these findings, a national directive was introduced in 1985 (MHW 1985). In accordance with this directive, at least two chemical markers of a given Kampo medicine were selected, followed by comparative trials of the Kampo medicine extract against the standard decoction. The purpose of these trials was to ensure the quality of the Kampo medicine extract by verifying that the quantity of the selected chemical markers found in the extract was equivalent to the standard decoction across batches. In these trials, the variation between the Kampo medicine and the standard decoction was to be at least within a 50 percent range, though 30 percent was considered preferable. Regulatory authorities also recommended performing "biological investigations of the pharmacological action," which when subject to verification, can be expected to be clinically in accordance with the contents, indications, and effects of the formulation. Though this directive was issued, no manufacturer actually performed any biological investigations, and quality standards varied across companies. To remedy such disparities, national quality standards have been gradually introduced starting from 2006 and are now in place for 37 types of Kampo medicine extracts.[23] All of them can be found in the Japanese Pharmacopeia 18th edition and its supplements, published in 2019.

Following the full integration of GMP into the PAL in 1988, JKMA members introduced additional self-imposed quality assurance standards. One example is the special monitoring system in place at firms' production sites, which are overseen by experienced crude drug control managers who inspect the external features (form, colour, odour, etc.) of the crude herbs used in prescription Kampo medicines. Though all firms have their own on-site drug control managers, the scope of their duties is not standardised and is thus to some extent firm-specific. In 1993, similar "quasi" standards were introduced for OTC Kampo medicines, signifying that *all* Japanese producers of Kampo medicines – prescription and OTC – currently adhere to their own self-imposed regimes.

Finally, international standards were added to the existing domestic regime in July 2014, when Japan became a member of the Pharmaceutical Inspection Co-operation Scheme (PIC/S). Founded in 1995, PIC/S aims to "harmonise GMP standards and quality systems of inspectorates in the field of medicinal products." Many herbal medicine producers, which include the Kampo medicines industry, have adopted these standards.[24] At the time of writing this chapter, Japan, South Korea, Taiwan, Hong Kong, Thailand, Indonesia, and Malaysia had joined the list of PIC/S participating authorities, while China and India – both large manufacturers of traditional

---

23 This was included the eighteenth edition of the Japanese Pharmacopoeia. Retrieved 7 June 2021, https://jpdb.nihs.go.jp/kyokuhou/index_e.html#jp18
24 PIC/S grew out of PIC, established in 1970 by EFTA (European Free Trade Association) as "The Convention for the Mutual Recognition of Inspections in Respect of the Manufacture of Pharmaceutical Products."

medicines with strong aspirations to market their products globally – had yet to adhere. Though the number of Asian PIC/S members is limited to those mentioned above, the Chinese and Indian herbal medicines industries apply their own respective domestic GMP standards, but non-members are not subject to PIC/S inspections (WHO 2012; He et al. 2015).

GMP regulations in the 1990s and 2000s

In the early days of Kampo medicine use in the sixth century, Japan relied heavily on imports of Chinese raw materials. Although efforts are now being made to substitute Chinese imports with the same or similar raw materials procured domestically, even today approximately 80 percent of all the raw materials used in Kampo medicine products are imported from China (JKMA 2015). This strong dependence on imports has had a significant impact on production costs and prices. Large companies such as Tsumura have put in place their own supply chains, mainly in East Asian countries, by establishing contracts with specific overseas growers as a means of ensuring a steady supply of raw materials and a high level of quality in their finished products. For their part, Japanese health, agriculture, and international trade ministries have strived in recent years to reduce the nation's dependence on Chinese imports by increasing the volume of medicinal herbs produced domestically, mainly through subsidised farming projects with local growers in various parts of the country.

The dependence on imports has indirectly affected regulatory policies regarding manufacturing safety standards. Crude drugs as well as finished Kampo medicine products are now tested for residual pesticides, heavy metals, and arsenic, as well as microorganisms. As was the case for GMP, in 2005 and 2006, JKMA established their own standard limits on contaminants for Kampo medicine extract formulations and non-Kampo medicine crude drug products. Taking private companies' initiatives into consideration, regulatory authorities followed suit by adding new GMP specifications for Kampo medicine extract products, as well as supplementary information to the 2006 JP regarding the level of purity (Arai 2009). Some large manufacturers have introduced traceability systems and regularly engage in data collection. The latter has helped to reduce the risk of incidents caused by high levels of contaminants and thus contributed to overall product safety.

As shown above, one can find numerous examples of cooperation between regulators, industry associations, and individual firms to improve Kampo medicine products. While GMP and JP standards are legally binding and must be implemented by all companies, many examples of voluntary "quasi" standards initiated by the industry associations also exist and have shown to strongly influence policy-makers' decisions when introducing new regulations. The fact that the quality and safety assurance standards mentioned apply to all types of medicines – be they biomedicines or Kampo medicines – is a factor that has served to strengthen Japan's single medical system. From an industrial and regulatory perspective, it has also contributed to a blurring of the boundaries that once existed between the two distinctly different medical traditions.

Post-marketing practices and their impact on the Kampo medicines industry

As shown in Figure 3.1, the 1976 reform, in combination with other factors, sparked a sharp rise in demand for prescription Kampo medicines. By the early 1980s, sales figures for prescription Kampo medicines had surpassed those of OTC Kampo medicines, which reached a plateau, then fell in the early 1990s. Yet despite the relative decline, the ratio of prescription drugs still far exceeds OTC Kampo medicines. This section traces the institutional and market-related factors leading to the rise in demand, as well as their effects on post-marketing standards for the Kampo medicines industry.

The rise in prescription Kampo medicine use: Institutional factors

The three institutional causes of the post-1976 "Kampo boom" were (1) drug dispensing practices, (2) NHI drug pricing policies in the 1970s and 1980s, and (3) health coverage policies for the elderly (defined as persons over 65 years of age). While the effects of these policies are relatively recent, the first cause, dispensing practices, has historical antecedents dating back to the pre-Meiji period when medical practitioners received payments for the medicines they provided rather than for their diagnoses.[25]

When Meiji period policy-makers first devised and implemented the medical system in the 1870s, their aim was to emulate those found in Western nations where for ethical reasons (i.e. a potential conflict of interests for doctors) a division of labour existed between those who prescribed (physicians) and those who dispensed (pharmacists) medicines (Yamakawa 2000).[26] As the notion of a separation of the two roles did not exist in Japan, Meiji policy-makers created a new term for it, *iyaku bungyō* (hereafter *bungyō*). In order to institutionalise this foreign practice, they also introduced a "new" supporting profession, that of pharmacy. However, as the existing medical practitioners knew that *bungyō* would result in a significant drop in their earnings, they strongly opposed it. Meiji government

---

[25] Edo period medical practitioners were known as *kusushi*, written with the characters, *drug* (薬) and *master* (師); today, *medical doctor* or *ishi* is written using the character for *medicine* (医) and *master* (師).

[26] Since the thirteenth century, doctors in Western nations were not permitted to dispense medicines. Due to the rising economic value of medicines in the preceding centuries, the separation of the role of the doctor and the pharmacist was made to ensure that doctors would prescribe medicines in the interest of treating the patient rather than a means of supplementing their incomes.

officials eventually conceded to their demands, a decision that was taken in part to deal with an initial shortage of trained pharmacists. Policy-makers thus "temporarily" amended the medical system so as to allow physicians to continue to dispense medicines until the shortage of pharmacists could be remedied. This "temporary" fix was lasting: all future attempts to introduce *bungyō* have failed (Akiba et al. 2012). Today, Japan remains one of the few countries in the world where physicians are allowed to prescribe as well as dispense (sell) medicines. As shown below, this feature would have an important influence on the rise in Kampo medicine use.

To understand the second factor contributing to the "Kampo boom," NHI drug pricing policies, a brief mention of the workings of Japan's official drug-pricing system is in order. In Japan, unlike in the United States, the government rather than the market determines drug prices, or *yakka*. In Japanese, the difference between the drug purchasing price and the officially set NHI drug price is known as *yakka-sa*. Viewed from the perspective of the medical institutions/physicians who purchase medicines, *yakka-sa* translates into profits derived from the sale of medicines. Due to the drug price calculation methods in place at the time of the 1976 reform, the difference was relatively high (Howells and Neary 1995). Moreover, not having a strong division of labour (*bungyō*) between prescriber (physician) and dispenser (pharmacist) provided an added incentive for physicians to prescribe – and in some cases over-prescribe – medicines covered by the NHI, including Kampo medicines (Wada 1997).

However, since the introduction of new policies, particularly in the 1990s, designed to curtail healthcare expenditures by lowering official drug prices and by extension reducing the difference between the purchasing price and the official price, or *yakka-sa*, regulators have largely succeeded in removing physicians' incentive to prescribe without officially depriving them of the right to dispense. As operating their own pharmacies has become an increasingly unprofitable undertaking, today, with the exception of large-scale hospitals, which have strong negotiating power vis-à-vis medicinal distributors, the majority of Japan's small and medium-sized medical institutions have voluntarily adopted *bungyō*.[27]

The third cause is health coverage policies for the elderly. In 1973, it was decided that all healthcare for the elderly, including medications, would be provided free of charge, while the co-payment for salaried workers would be 10 percent. Today, however, due to the rising financial burden stemming from the growing number of persons over 65 years of age, the elderly must, in principle, cover 10 percent of their healthcare expenses, while the co-payment for salaried workers has risen to 30 percent. There are two

---

27 The ratio was 9.7 percent in 1986, while in March 2016, it stood at just over 70 percent (https://www.nichiyaku.or.jp/activities/division/faqShinchoku.html).

explanations why providing free healthcare to the elderly contributed to a rise in the use of Kampo medicines.

The first reason, mentioned above, relates to the change in perceptions of Kampo medicines since the series of drug-induced disasters. Following these tragedies, many physicians came to believe that Kampo medicines offered a benign alternative to synthetic drugs. The so-called "myth of Kampo medicine safety" strongly influenced physicians' prescribing practices, and fuelled, as the case of *shosaikoto* below demonstrates, the over-prescribing of Kampo medicines to elderly patients with chronic illnesses or terminal diseases for which there were few if any effective treatments. The second reason relates to cultural factors, namely a more distant physician-patient relationship than in Western nations. As a result, patients, particularly elderly ones, rarely question their physicians' treatment choices or seek a second opinion. Because all healthcare for the elderly was provided free of charge, they rarely objected to receiving large quantities of medicines, including Kampo medicines.

"The myth of Kampo medicine safety" and their decline in use

As mentioned above, from 1976 to the early 1990s, Japan's market for Kampo medicines grew considerably, and until the early 1990s, the "market leader" was one Kampo medicine, *shosaikoto*, which according to MHLW statistics, accounted for approximately 36 percent of all Kampo medicine sales at its peak in 1992. The figure would plummet to 10 percent in 1999, then fall to just three percent in 2004 (JKMA 2019).[28] This medicine's gradual rise in popularity began in the mid-1980s, sparked by the publication of clinical trials in combination with more aggressive Kampo medicines industry marketing activities (Mizuta et al. 1983; Ishii and Shibuya 1985; Kawaguchi and Wada 1985; Oka et al. 1984; Wakahara et al. 1985). The clinical findings provided an indirect endorsement for *shosaikoto* as a treatment for hepatitis, which, by the end of World War II, was referred to as a "national disease" due to its high prevalence (Yatsuhashi 2016). The popular press took notice, and in 1987, articles appeared in major Japanese newspapers, one being the Asahi, whose headline read: "Kampo medicine *shosaikoto* effective in the prevention of liver cancer" (Asahi Newspaper 1987). As the popularity of *shosaikoto* grew, however, so did the number of ADRs reported via Japan's pharmacovigilance system. ADRs, including

---

28 *Shosaikoto* (小柴胡湯) showed the highest ratio followed by *saibokuto* (柴朴湯, 4.9 percent); *hochuekito* (補中益気湯, 4.9 percent); *hachimijiogan* (八味地黄丸, 3.3 percent); *kamishoyosan* (加味逍遙散, 3.2 percent); *rikkunshito* (六君子湯, 2.7 percent); *shoseiryuto* (小青龍湯, 2.4 percent); *saikokeishito* (柴胡桂枝湯, 2.4 percent) *daisaikoto* (大柴胡湯, 2.3 percent); *tōkishakuyakusan* (当帰芍薬散, 2.1 percent); other (35.7 percent).

deaths caused by interstitial pneumonia, began to raise regulators' concerns regarding the drug's safety.[29]

Over the years, regulatory authorities have implemented a raft of measures to prevent ADRs. Largely in response to the SMON scandal, new requirements for collecting information on ADRs and infections were introduced in 1979, followed by a revision of the PAL in 1980, which placed the responsibility on the pharmaceutical industry for reporting any ADRs caused by their products. Though voluntary, monitoring systems were also put in place at hospitals and pharmacies (Tsutani 1993). In 1993, post-marketing surveillance (PMS) was incorporated into GPMSP, which became legally binding in 1997. GPMSP requires all manufacturers to continue to monitor the safety of their products even after approval and in cases where ADRs have occurred, they must provide various types of safety warnings to physicians according to the level of risk. Good Vigilance Practices (GVP) require that manufacturers issue a *Yellow Letter Warning* and revise package inserts for physicians when necessary. These measures have been applied to all medicines, including Kampo medicines. Thus in 1991, in response to ADRs relating to *shosaikoto*, manufacturers began placing precautions regarding interstitial pneumonia in their package inserts, followed by the issuing of contraindications in 1993 against using *shosaikoto* in combination with interferon.

In 1996, another article appeared in the Asahi, based on information obtained from the MHW. The writer reported that since 1994, 10 deaths had resulted from *shosaikoto*, which had been administered in combination with interferon (Asahi Newspaper 1996). These deaths were caused by an immunological reaction to *shosaikoto* and would have two significant repercussions on demand. First, they cast strong doubt on the long-held assumption that Kampo medicines were a safe and benign alternative to synthetic drugs. Second, they greatly influenced prescribing patterns, the effects of which would be devastating for the operations of Kampo medicines manufacturers. Following media reports, sales of *shosaikoto* dropped significantly, as did the total market value for both prescription and OTC Kampo medicines. As shown in Figure 3.1, this downward trend would not show any sign of a recovery until the early 2000s.

Incorporating the special features of Kampo medicines into drug re-evaluations

In 1973, the MHW issued the first drug re-evaluation requirements, which applied to all medicines marketed before 1967, the year in which the Pharmaceutical Affairs Bureau of MHW issued the *Basic Policy for New*

---

29 As seen in Eunjeong Ma's study (2019) of the *baekshuoh* disaster in South Korea, Japanese health authorities were not alone in having to find ways to deal with safety-related issues. In both cases, the problems surfaced in a context where demand had risen sharply for a particular product.

Drug Approval, requiring that manufacturers submit clinical data to support the efficacy and safety of their drug candidates and perform controlled (double-blind) trials[30] (Sakuma 1988). This measure came in the wake of the implementation of the 1962 Kefauver Harris Amendments in the United States (Temin 1980). The purpose of the re-evaluations was to review, according to the most current standards of medicine and pharmaceutical science, the efficacy and safety of drugs already approved for use.

Regulatory officials began the re-evaluation process by collecting existing data on the safety and efficacy of all registered prescription drugs approved for use in Japan before 1967; however, over time, the scope of their review expanded to incorporate all prescription drugs (Tsutani 1993).[31] The government's decision also applied to Kampo medicines; however, their inclusion was postponed due to a number of practical considerations. Devising specific clinical evaluation methodologies was particularly problematic, not only because of their fundamental differences with biomedicines but also because of trial-related issues such as patient selection based on Western versus traditional diagnoses, placebo formulation, etc. (Tsutani 1985, 1993; Terasawa 2004). To consider how to address these specific issues, working groups were established in 1989 and 1990.

In accordance with a 1988 Pharmaceutical Affairs Director-General Notification, all prescription medicines were subject to a screening process every five years, in order to determine the type of re-evaluation they would undergo: "regular re-evaluation" or "special re-evaluation." It was decided that Kampo medicines would be subject to the latter. According to the "special evaluation" requirements, regulators, in consultation with the Central Pharmaceutical Affairs Council, determined the most appropriate re-evaluation procedures for cases where overseas and/or domestic studies on a particular Kampo medicine had suggested that a review of the efficacy and safety was necessary.

In 1991, according to a second Pharmaceutical Affairs Director-General Notification, eight Kampo medicine formulae with a total of 14 formula-indication sets became the subjects of the first of two series of re-evaluations. JKMA established two teams to sponsor the trials, which were headed by two Kampo medicine companies. Double-blinded randomised controlled trials (DB-RCTs) were then carried out for each formula-indication set. However, in some cases where sufficient data was available from previous trials, regulators could conduct their re-evaluations based on that data, while in others where there was an insufficient number of volunteers, the trials were interrupted. The full results of the re-evaluations would not be announced

---

30 In 1991, new terminology for EBM was introduced, and by the mid-1990s the term, "double-blind trial" had been replaced by "double-blind randomised control trial."
31 Evaluations for drugs approved before 1967 were made public after 1973, while those approved between 1967 and 1980, were made public after 1988.

until 2012. In 1996, however, the preliminary findings for *shosaikoto* and *shoseiryuto* were made public, as were the full results for *daiokanzoto*.

According to the "special re-evaluation" requirements, DB-RCT data from studies conducted on *shosaikoto* (indicated for liver dysfunction), *shoseiryuto* (allergic nasal inflammation), and *daiokanzoto* (constipation) were gathered (Agenosono 2001). Trials were conducted according to the more lenient Japanese GCP in place until 1998. Of note is that government transparency regarding the re-evaluations was extremely limited. Regulatory authorities did not make public even basic information such as the protocol, number, and length of the trials, despite moves during the same period by the WHO, in coordination with other large international entities, to devise guidelines for assessing the safety and efficacy of traditional medicines (Tsutani 1998). While authorities' motives for not making pertinent information public are unclear, as Vincanne Adams points out, a lack of transparency is not limited to Japan (Adams 2002). Moreover, no details regarding regulators' decisions were disclosed, despite the recommendations of a committee established in 1998 by the MHLW specifically to consider ways to prevent future "drug-induced suffering," or *yakugai* (MHLW 2008).[32]

Official notifications followed the announcement of the re-evaluations, confirming that regulators did not have any doubts regarding the efficacy of the three Kampo medicines under investigation, namely *shosaikoto*, *shoseiryuto*, and *daiokanzoto*, for their assigned indications, given in parentheses above. As for *shosaikoto*, this decision was based on an existing pool of data (Agenosono 2001). Thus no *new* DB-RCTs were commissioned for *shosaikoto* as indicated for liver dysfunction, as there was already ample published data to support its efficacy including that of Kanebo (now Kuracie) (Hirayama et al. 1990). Following these re-evaluations, in some cases, product labels were modified slightly to reflect the findings. However, only one Kampo medicine, *shoseiryuto*, was withdrawn as a treatment for renal disease, renal inflammation, and nephritis.

The results of drug re-evaluations

On 7 April 2014, some 15 years after the re-evaluations had initially got underway, MHLW published the complete results of its investigations of Kampo medicines, along with those for other pharmaceuticals.[33] This announcement was criticised for two reasons, the first being the unusually long period of time that it had taken regulators to complete their

---

32 Regulators should have disseminated their information to local governments, medical societies and industry representatives, to prevent any further drug-induced disasters.
33 The efficacy data report (http://www.fpmaj-saihyoka.com/efficacy/data/05/05_20140407-0407No1.pdf) and efficacy data are available via the Federation of Pharmaceutical Manufacturers' Association of Japan: http://www.fpmaj-saihyoka.com/efficacy/index.html

re-evaluations and provide their results to the public. The second criticism was that the announcement was issued without any explanation of the results of the individual drug evaluations, information that could have been beneficial to physicians and patients. Although one could argue that regulators were not required to provide any explanation in cases of positive re-evaluation results, the absence of any information following the announcement raised suspicion. Thus, since then, with the exception of *shoseiryuto* as a renal treatment, all the Kampo medicines subject to re-evaluations have remained on the market.

A stark difference can be seen between the repercussions of the post-evaluation for the biomedicines and the Kampo medicines industries. While there was no evidence to demonstrate that the Kampo medicines evaluated were ineffective for their assigned indications, such was not the case for certain categories of biomedicines, such as anti-cancer drugs, whose market size in Japan in the 1980s had surpassed even that of the United States. As shown in Umemura's study (2010), the re-evaluations of two top-selling anti-cancer biomedicines resulted in their removal from the market in 1989, a decision that had devastating economic effects on the companies marketing them in Japan and abroad.[34] In 1998, another category of biomedicines, cerebral circulation and metabolism-improving drugs, which had been approved for reimbursement under NHI since the mid-1980s, were also withdrawn following re-evaluation (MHW 1988). This not only resulted in tremendous financial losses for industry but also tarnished the image of the regulatory authorities that had granted NHI approval for the sale of drugs in this category to eleven manufacturers. On the other hand, for the Kampo medicines industry, the results of the re-evaluations were not unfavourable and had little if any negative impact on sales.

"New" GCP and their impact on the Kampo medicines industry

The re-evaluations took place at a time when Japanese regulators were engaged in negotiations designed to harmonise the clinical trial practices in the European Union, Japan, and the United States. This factor may have influenced their decision not to pursue the second series of re-evaluations, as this might have raised public suspicion regarding the validity of the re-evaluation results. Japan had introduced Good Laboratory Practices (GLP) in 1982, making the testing for toxicity, oncogenicity, and teratogenicity mandatory. However, the first GCP, designed to protect the safety

---

34 These Japanese drugs were used as cancer treatments. Amygdalin or Laetrile was thought to have similar cancer treating properties; however, the US FDA never approved it for that purpose. Also see, National Cancer Institute. https://www.cancer.gov/about-cancer/treatment/cam/hp/laetrile-pdq#_10

and human rights of trial Japanese participants, was not issued until 1989 (Tsutani 2013).[35]

Japanese standards for conducting trials differed significantly from those in Europe and the United States, the implications for which went beyond the realm of public health. By the mid-1980s, Japan's regulations for clinical trials had become the source of an international trade dispute, stemming mainly from Japanese regulators' refusal to accept foreign trial data in the approval of new drugs (Kuo 2008). Consequently, foreign firms hoping to market their products in Japan were required to perform costly new trials in Japan on Japanese subjects, which they perceived as a non-tariff barrier (Yongue 2008).

Bilateral talks began with US representatives in the mid-1980s.[36] However, by the mid-1990s, these talks evolved into the multilateral negotiations known as ICH (International Conference in Harmonisation of Technical Requirements for the Registration of Pharmaceuticals for Human Use) and involved government and industry representatives from the world's three major drug markets: the European Union, Japan, and the United States. The ICH negotiation process would eventually yield mutually agreed-upon standards for clinical trials that would be implemented in the three markets. The new regime would have a marked effect on the operations and strategies of Japanese pharmaceutical industry as a whole, including the Kampo medicines industry.

In 1998, the MHW implemented the new standards, which were initially called "ICH GCP" or "new GCP" to distinguish them from the previous, less rigorous domestic regulations. ICH GCP has affected the development of the Kampo medicines industry and is likely to continue to have a strong influence on its growth in the future. Under the ICH regime, trial data collected according to ICH standards is mandatory for all new drug approvals in Japan, including Kampo medicines. Since the introduction of ICH GCP, the cost of conducting clinical trials in Japan has risen considerably, encouraging large biomedicines firms to move their clinical development activities overseas (Yongue 2008). However, for Kampo medicines firms, which are much smaller in scale than their multinational biomedicine-producing counterparts, ICH GCP has further limited their opportunities to develop new Kampo medicines at home or abroad. Thus, while Japan became the

---

35 The introduction of J-GCP was prompted by a scandal in 1982 involving corporate data fabrication and misconduct in DB-RCTs. In response, the MHW established a working group to study clinical trial reliability issues in 1983. It was later decided to include ethical issues as well. To formulate the first GCP, Japanese regulators did not collaborate with international authorities or base their regulations on the principles of the Helsinki Declaration. See also the history of the World Medical Association: https://www.wma.net/who-we-are/history/
36 Trade disputes between the United States and Japan were discussed in the mid-1980s and early 1990s at a series of talks: the market-oriented, sector-specific talks (MOSS) and the Structural Impediments Initiative (SII).

first country in the world in 1969 to conduct RCTs on traditional medicines, specifically Kampo medicines, so far most of the clinical data generated from industry-sponsored or co-sponsored trials has only been used for the marketing of existing Kampo medicine products (Tsutani 1985).

Conclusions: The future of the Kampo medicines industry?

This chapter traced the historical background, introduction, and influence of GxP on the Kampo medicines industry's development as well as the changing regulatory environment within which it operated. The implementation of GxP can be characterised as having occurred more gradually for the Kampo medicines than for the biomedicines industry, since regulators needed to consider their distinctive features as medicines. Solutions for dealing with the differences were found, and today, GxP apply to the Kampo medicines industry in much the same way as for biomedicines. Moreover, in certain areas such as manufacturing (PIC/S) and clinical trials (ICH), it has been possible to integrate them into the same international regimes as biomedicines. Japan's measured approach to the implementation of GxP that began from an early date contrasts with the situations described by Chee in China and Kudlu in India (both this volume), where a different set of factors was in play. Whether state- (China) or market- (India) driven, the underlying force behind the introduction of GxP was in large part economic, given the perceived imperative to globalise the industry beyond national borders. The approach these countries took can be characterised as being far more outward-looking and export-oriented than the one seen in Japan, where maintaining domestic market share and ensuring continued NHI coverage were top of the industry's agenda.

In this study, two turning points specific to the Kampo medicines industry and its development stood out. The first was the 1976 reform, which boosted sales of both prescription and OTC Kampo medicines. This measure made Kampo medicines more affordable to patients and gave birth to the single system of NHI coverage for both biomedicines and Kampo medicines, which has emerged as a distinctive feature of Japan's medical system. The second turning point, occurring in the 1990s, was ADRs caused by what was then the top selling Kampo medicine, *shosaikoto*. For regulators, practitioners, and patients alike, these ADRs put an end to the "myth of Kampo medicine safety" and were followed by a sharp drop in demand for Kampo medicines. For the Kampo industry, this marked an abrupt end to a long period of uninterrupted economic growth. As shown in Figure 3.1, however, the Kampo industry witnessed a recovery since the early 2000s. Thanks to NHI coverage and steady demand for Kampo medicines, sales continue to rise despite the fact that not a single new prescription Kampo medicine has been launched since the 1970s. Some industry observers would characterise Kampo medicines as a maturing industry, an economist's term used to denote one that is neither pursuing new fields nor strategies of aggressive expansion into global markets. This is quite the opposite of other markets covered in this volume and elsewhere, whether desired or not (Chee, Kudlu, this volume; Craig 2011; Saxer 2013; Kloos et al. 2020) Yet this is not to say that the Kampo industry is stagnant, as the rising sales figures in Figure 3.1 clearly demonstrate. As shown in this chapter, particularly in the scientific and technological arenas the Kampo industry continues to be pioneering in the development of key technologies and methodologies that have aided regulators to integrate traditional medicines into the same global regulatory regimes as biomedicines.

What is on the horizon for the Kampo medicines industry? Although sales of Kampo medicines began to rise in the 2000s, the industry still faces major economic challenges. The first is higher production costs resulting from increased competition over limited raw materials, caused by rising demand from China's own growing domestic market for herbal medicines. As shown in other chapters, the ambitions of the Chinese state to make TCM a global industry places further pressure on Japan's domestic manufacturers and their efforts to secure sufficient raw materials. The growing cost of raw materials is a mounting financial burden for the industry, which could soon pose a threat to the affordability of Kampo medicines for the average Japanese patient.

The second challenge is the high cost of launching new medicines in the Japanese market since the implementation of ICH GCP. The combination of increasing raw material and clinical trial costs has had negative ramifications on the industry, which is comprised mainly of small- and medium-sized firms. This situation has further deterred them from investing in the launch of any new Kampo medicines or filing applications for additional indications. The high cost of launching a new medicine is also an issue in other Asian countries. As seen in Chee's chapter, however, this problem has been circumvented through the development of lesser regulated categories of health products and cosmetics. As prescription Kampo medicines are still more lucrative for manufacturers thanks to NHI coverage, the industry has yet to pursue the health products and cosmetics sector on a large scale.

Finally, given the negative impact of the ageing population, low birthrates, and rising healthcare costs on the national budget, the Japanese government might one day simply decide to eliminate or reduce NHI coverage of prescription Kampo medicines, in order to curtail overall healthcare expenditures. Since the 1980s, legislators have repeatedly tried to do away with NHI coverage and return to the pre-1976 situation, when patients covered the full cost of Kampo medicine use. However, despite bills put forth in 1983, 1993, 1997, 2009, and 2015, their attempts have failed. For more than two decades, legislative change has been averted thanks, at least in part, to the continued resistance of patients and lobbying organisations, one of the strongest being the JSOM. Thus for the time being, NHI coverage of prescription Kampo medicines through Japan's single medical system remains intact. In Japan as elsewhere in Asia, changes in regulatory policies have had a significant impact not only on the development of industry but also society's changing perceptions of Asian medicine.

Bibliography

Adams V (2002) Randomized Controlled Harm: Postcolonial Sciences in Alternative Medicine. *Social Studies of Science* 32(5–6): 659–690.

Agenosono H (2001) Kanpō ekisu seizai no rinshō hyōka (Current Status of Clinical Evaluation of Kampo Extract Products). *Rinsho Hyoka* 29(Suppl 16): 119–127.

Akazawa M, Yongue J, Ikeda S, et al. (2014) Considering Economic Analyses in the Revision of the Preventive Vaccine Law: A New Direction for Healthcare Policy Making in Japan? *Health Policy* 118(1): 128.

Akiba Y (2010) History of Kampo Extracts for Medical Use. *Tōyō Ishishi (Kampo Med)* 61(7): 881–888.

Akiba Y, Nakamura T, Nishikawa T, et al. (eds) (2012) *Iyakubungyō no rekishi (The History of Iyakubungyō)*. Tokyo: Yakujihō.

Arai I (2009) The Current Situation of Japanese Medicinal Plants Industry and Its Significance of the Pharmaceutical Industry, 5. Available at https://www.hdares.gov.tw/htmlarea_file/web_articles/hdais/1354/980108_1.pdf#search=%27The+Current+Situation+of+Japanese+Medicinal+Plants+Industry+and+its+Significance+of+the+Pharmaceutical+Industry%27 (accessed on 11 May 2018).

Arai I (2015) *Nihon no Kampōseizai sangyō no rekishi* (History of Kampo Medicines Manufacturers). *Yakushigaku Zasshi* 50(1): 1–6.

Asahi Newspaper (Japanese edition) (April 2, 1987) KM shōsaikotō: Effective in Prevention of Liver Cancer; Osaka City University testimony (Kanpō no shōsaikotō, kanzōgan yobō ni yūkō, Osaka-shidai de shōmei).

Asahi Newspaper (Japanese edition) (March 2, 1996) Side Effects Caused by KM shōsaikotō, 10 Deaths and Interstitial Hepatitis Since 1994 (Kanpōyaku shōsaikotō no fukusayōde shisha 10nin, 94nenikkō manshitsusei kaenmo).

Bowers J (1970) *Western Medical Pioneers in Feudal Japan*. Baltimore, MD: The Johns Hopkins Press.

Campbell J and Ikegami N (1998) *The Art of Balance in Health Policy Maintaining Japan's Low-Cost, Egalitarian System*. Cambridge: Cambridge University Press, pp. 107–108.

Craig S (2011) "Good" Manufacturing by Whose Standards? Remaking Concepts of Quality, Safety, and Value in the Production of Tibetan Medicines. *Anthropological Quarterly* 84(2): 331–378.

Hattori M (2006) Wakanyaku kenkyujo no kako, genzai, soshite mirai (The Past, Present, and Future of the Wakan-Yaku Institute), Annual report, Institute of Natural Medicine, University of Toyama (32), 6–12 (2006-03-01).

Howells J and Neary I (1995) *Intervention and Technological Innovation: Government and the Pharmaceutical Industry in the UK and Japan*. London: Macmillan, pp. 111–135.

Ishii K and Shibuya A (1985) Manseikanjya shippei nitaisuru shōsaikotō no chiryōkōka (Shosaikoto as a Treatment for Chronic Hepatitis Patients). *Yakuri to Chiryō* 2(10): 4807–4812.

JKMA, Japan Kampo Medicines Manufacturers Association (2011) Kanpō Yakushō Jittai Chōsa 2011 (Kampo Medicines Prescriptions Survey). Available at https://www.nikkankyo.org/serv/serv1.htm (accessed on 28 September 2021).

JKMA, Japan Kampo Medicines Manufacturers Association (2015) Chūgokusan genryōshōyaku kakaku chōsa (JKMA Survey of Prices of Crude Herb Raw Materials Produced in China). Available at: https://www.nikkankyo.org/serv/serv3.htm (accessed on 20 July 2020).

JKMA, Japan Kampo Medicines Manufacturers Association (2019) Kanpō seizaitō no seisan dōtai, heisei 30 nen yakuji kōgyō seisandōtai tōkei nenpō kara (Kampo Medicine Production from the Production Statistics of the 2018 Annual Report). JKMA, 20 September 2019. Available at: https://www.nikkankyo.org/serv/movement/h30/all.pdf (accessed on 21 July 2020).

JSHP, Japanese Society for the History of Pharmacy (1995) In: Gakkai NY (ed) *Nihon Iyakuhinsangyōshi (History of the Japanese Pharmaceutical Industry)*. Tokyo: Yakuji Nipposha.

Katahira K (1997) *Nōmoa yakugai: yakugai no rekishi ni manabi, sono konzetsuwo (No more Drug-induced Suffering: Learning from the History of Drug Induced Disasters so as to Eradicate Them)*. Tokyo: Kirishobō.

Kawaguchi T and Wada M (Oct 1985) Kanshikkan eno shosaikoto no kōka wo tsuikyū (Pursuing of Addition of Shosaikoto for Liver Disease). *Nikkei Medical* (0385-1699) 14(12): 7–11.

Kikutani T (2001) Watakushi no Kaimamita Kinsei Kampōshi no ichimen (A Glance at the Early Modern Period of the History of Kampo Medicine). *Nihon Ishigakushi* 47(4): 859–860.

Kitajima M (2017) *Kanpō no kagakuka (Kampo Science Visual Review)*. Tokyo: Raifu Saiensu, pp. 10–11.

Kloos S, Madhavan H, Tidwell T, et al. (2020) The Transnational Sowa Rigpa Industry in Asia: New Perspectives on an Emerging Economy. *Social Science & Medicine* 245: 112617.

Kosoto H (2014) *Kanpo no rekishi chūgoku nihon no dentōigaku (The History of Kampo Medicine Chinese and Japanese Traditional Medicines)*. Tokyo: Ajiashoten.

Kuo W-H (2008) The Voice on the Bridge: Taiwan's Regulatory Engagement in Global Pharmaceuticals. *East Asian Science, Technology, and Society* 3(1): 51–72.

He T, Ung COI, Hu H, et al. (2015) Good Manufacturing Practice (GMP) Regulation of Herbal Medicine in Comparative Research: China (GMP), cGMP, WHO-GMP, PIC/C and EU GMP. *European Journal of Integrative Medicine* 7(1): 55–66.

Hirayama C, Okumura M, Tanikawa K, et al. (1990) A Multi-Center Randomized Controlled Trial of Shosaiko-to in Chronic Active Hepatitis. *Kantansui* 20(4): 751–759.

Lock M (1980) *East Asian Medicine in Urban Japan*. Berkeley, CA: University of California Press.

MHW, Ministry of Health and Welfare (1985) Hyōjun tōzai tono hikakushiken ni kansuru shiryō (Data Related to Comparative Trials with Standard Decoctions), Attachment Table 1, Notification Number 120 of the Evaluation and Registration Division, Pharmaceutical Affairs Bureau, 31 May 1985.

MHW, Ministry of Health and Welfare Fifty-Year History Editing Committee (1988) *Kōseishō Gojūnen-shi (The Fifty-Year History of the Ministry of Health and Welfare)*. Tokyo: Kōseimondai Kenkyūkai, pp. 55–62.

MHW, Ministry of Health and Welfare (1998) Kōseishō kinkyūi iyakuhin jōhō saihyōka kekka ni motozuku nōjunkantaisha kaizenyaku 4 seibun ni kakawaru sōchi nitsuite (Emergency Drug Information: Measures for the Four Kinds of Drugs for Improving Cerebral Circulation and Metabolism Based on the Re-evaluation Results). Available at: https://www.mhlw.go.jp/www1/houdou/1005/h0519-1.html

MHLW, Ministry of Health, Labour, and Welfare (2008) Yakugai saihatsu bōshi no tameno iyakuhin gyōsei no minaoshi ni tsuite saishū teigen (Regarding the Review of Medicine Policies to Prevent the Reoccurrence of Drug-induced Disasters, Final Version) 28 April 2008, Available at: https://www.mhlw.go.jp/shingi/2010/04/dl/s0428-8a.pdf#search=%27http%3A%2F%2Fwww.mhlw.go.jp%2Fshingi%2F2010%2F04%2Fdl%2Fs04288a.pdf%27 (accessed on 22 July 2020).

Mizuta M, Matsuda A, Nawada H (Aug 1983) Manseikanenchiryō eno shōsaikotono hyōka(1) (Evaluation of Shosaikoto in Order to Treat Chronic Hepatitis Treatment). *Rinshō to Kenkyū (0021)* 60(8): 2592–2596.

Nishikawa T (2010) *Kusuri no Shakaishi (Social Accounts of Medicine)*. Tokyo: Yakujinipposha, pp. 25–43.

Oka H, Fujihara K, Hayashi S (1984) Manseikanjya niokeru shōsaikotō narabini keishibukuryōgan (Using shosaikoto and keishibukuryogan for Chronic Hepatitis Patients). *Kantansui* 9(5): 825–831.

Otsuka Y (1976) Chinese Traditional Medicine in Japan. In: Leslie C (ed) *Asian Medical Systems: A Comparative Study*. Berkeley, CA: University of California Press, pp. 332–333.

Sakuma A (1988) Past, Present, and Future of Clinical Trials in Japan in Biometry-Clinical trials and Related Topics. In: Okuno T (ed) *Proceedings of the ISI Satellite Meeting on Biometry, Excerpta Medica International Conference Series 787*. Osaka, Japan, 113–129.

Saxer M (2013) *Manufacturing Tibetan Medicine: The Creation of an Industry and the Moral Economy of Tibetaness*. New York, NY and Oxford: Berghahn Books.

Shim J-M (2015) The Relationship between the Use of Complementary and Alternative Medicine and the Use of Biomedical Services: Evidence from East Asian Medical Systems. *Asia-Pacific Journal of Public Health* 28(1): 51–60.

Shimazaki K (2009) Papers on the Local Governance Systems and Its Implementation in Selected Fields in Japan No. 13, The Development of Health Insurance Systems for the Elderly and Associated Problem Areas, Council of Local Authorities for International Relations, Institute for Comparative Studies in Local Governance, National Graduate Institute for Policy Studies.

Special Committee for Evidence-based Medicine (2002) The Japan Society for Oriental Medicine. EBM in Kampo 2002, Interim report [in Japanese]. *Nihon Toyo Igaku Zasshi* 2002(Suppl issue): 53.

Takeda Pharmaceutical Company (ed) (1984) *Takeda 200 nenshi (Two-Hundred-Year History of Takeda)*. Tokyo: Takeda Pharmaceutical Company.

Tanabe Pharmaceutical Company (ed) (1983) *Tanabe Seiyaku 300 shūnenshi (Three-Hundred-Year History of Tanabe Pharmaceutical Company)*. Tokyo: Tanabe Pharmaceutical Company.

Temin P (1980) *Taking Your Medicine Drug Regulation in the United States*. Cambridge, MA: Harvard University Press.

Terasawa K (2004) Evidenced-Based Reconstruction of Kampo Medicine: Part II – The Concept of Sho. *Evidence-Based Complementary and Alternative Medicine* 1(2): 119–123.

Tong D (2014) 17-19 Seiki chūnichi yakushu bōekishi genjyō to tenbō (The Research Actuality and Expectation of Traditional Herbal Medicinal Trades between Japan and China during the 17th and 19th Century). *Kyushu daigaku tōyōshi henshū* 42: 1–12, 2014 03.

Tsumura J (ed) (1964) *Tsumura Juntendō 70 nenshi (The Seventy-Year History of Tsumura Juntendō)*. Tokyo: Tsumura Company, pp. 5–6.

Tsumura J (1982) *Kanpō no hana juntendō jikki (The Blossoming of Kampo: The True Story of Juntendō)*. Tokyo: Tsumura Company, pp. 44–47.

Tsutani K (1985) Dentōyaku no hikakushiken no rekishi to genjyō (History and Current Status of Comparative Trials for Traditional Medicines). *Igakuno ayumi* 132(2): 103–106.

Tsutani K (1993) The Evaluation of Herbal Medicines: An East Asian Perspective. In Lewith G and Aldridge D (eds) *Clinical Research Methodology for Complementary Therapies*. London: Hodder and Stoughton, pp. 379–380.

Tsutani K (1998) Shūdan ni kiku koto to kojin ni kiku koto, kikime no komyunikeishon (Is it Effective on Group or Individual? Need for Effective Communication of Efficacy of Oriental Medicine). *Nihon Tōyō Igakuzasshi* 48(5): 569–598.

Tsutani K (2006) Ajia ni okeru dentō igaku no genjyō to mondaiten (Current Situation and Issues of Traditional Medicine in Asia), Minutes of International Symposium on Japan-China-Korea Traditional Medicines (Nichūkan de dentō igaku o kangaeru), Tokyo, 2 Feb 2006, 7.

Tsutani, K (2013) Gakujutsu Sōkaitokushū/Rinshō shinkenrinri daburu sutandaado no kaishō wa naruka. 1. Gakujutsu iinkai kenkyū rinri shoiinkai setsuritsu no haikei to katsudō (Special Issue on Clinical Trial Ethics: Will the Double Standard Issue be Resolved? 1. Background and Activities of the Ethics Task Force of the Academic Committee of the Japanese Society of Clinical Pharmacology and Therapeutics). *Rinsho Yakuri* 44(2): 127–130.

Tsutani K, Zhang X, Yamamoto N, et al. (1984) Shoyaku Kanpō Seizai no shikibetsu funōsei ni kansuru kannōshiken (Sensory Difference Tests of Pharmaceuticals of Herbs and Chinese Medical Prescriptions). *Rinsho Yakuri* 15(3): 469–472.

Tu Y and Tsutani K (2007) Chūigaku no genjyō shiriizu daiikkai, chūgoku ni ishimenkyoshō wa aruka? Chugoku no ishihōki to chūishi no genjyō (Is There a Physician's License in China? The Current Status of Chinese Doctors and Regulations Regarding Physicians and Doctors of Chinese Medicine). *Wakanyaku* 653: 2–6.

Umemura M (2010) Reconsidering Japan's Underperformance in Pharmaceuticals: Evidence from the Anticancer Drug Sector. *Oxford University* 11(3): 569–571.

Umemura M (2012) Reviving Tradition: Patients and the Shaping of Japan's Traditional Medicines Industry. In: Francks P and Hunter J (eds) *The Historical Consumer, Consumption and Everyday Life in Japan*. London: Palgrave Macmillan, p. 180.

Wada M (1997) *Iyaku Sangyōron (The Pharmaceutical Industry)*. Tokyo: Gyōsei, pp. 4–5.

Wakahara T, Kato N, Komori H (Nov. 1985) Mansei gankanjya nitaisuru shōsaikotō no chiryōkōka nitsuite (Regarding shosaikoto as a Treatment for Chronic Hepatitis Patients). *Gifu Municipal Hospital Annual Report* 4: 99–106.

WHO Western Pacific Region (2012) *The Regional Strategy for Traditional Medicines in the Western Pacific*. Geneva: WHO Publications, 47.

WHO Expert Committee on Specifications for Pharmaceutical Preparations (2014) Forty-eighth Report, Annex 2 WHO Good Pharmaceutical Practices for Pharmaceutical Products, WHO Technical Report Series, No. 986.

Yamada H (1995) Kōdoseichōki (The High Growth Period), in Nihon Iyakuhinsangyōshi (History of the Japanese Pharmaceutical Industry). *Japanese Society for the History of Pharmacy* (ed), Tokyo: Yakuji Nipposha, 21–33.

Yamada T (1996) The Tradition and Genealogy of Kampo Medicine (Yamada's English title). *Japan Society for Oriental Medicine* 46(4): 505–518.

Yamakawa K (1995) Kōdoseichōki (The High Growth Period), in Nihon Iyakuhinsangyōshi (History of the Japanese Pharmaceutical Industry). *Japanese Society for the History of Pharmacy* (ed), Tokyo: Yakuji Nipposha, 137.

Yamakawa K (2000) *Kokusai Yakugakushi higashi to nishi no iyaku bunmeishi (International Pharmacology History: The History of Eastern and Western Civilizations)*. Tokyo: Nakodo, pp. 6–7.

Yatsuhashi H (2016) Past, Present, Future of Viral Hepatitis C in Japan. *Eurasian Journal of Hepato-Gastroenterology* 6(1): 49–51.

Yongue J (2008) Shin'yaku Kaihatsu wo meguru kigyō to gyōsei (Corporate Development of New Drugs and Drug Policy). In: Kudō A and Ihara M (eds) *Kigyō to Gendai no Shihonshugi (Enterprises and Modern Capitalism)*. Kyoto: Minerva Shobo, pp. 166–191.

4 The pharmaceutical industry of Toyama prefecture, Japan

Haichi household medicines, intersectoral collaboration, and industrial clustering

Tomoko Futaya and Calum Blaikie

This chapter discusses the historical emergence and recent development of the pharmaceutical industry in Toyama prefecture, Japan. It shows how this region first became famous over 300 years ago for the production of *haichi* (配置) household medicines, a broad array of remedies primarily comprising *Wakanyaku* (和漢薬 Japanese and Chinese crude drugs)[1] and characterised by a specific mode of production, delivery, and payment-by-use (*sen'yōkōri* 先用後利). The chapter then shows how by successfully adapting to changing economic, political, and medical contexts over subsequent centuries, the region went on to become Japan's leading producer of both herbal and biomedical pharmaceuticals.

We examine three main factors that have shaped Toyama prefecture's pharmaceutical industry over this period. The first is the range of institutional and legislative changes that have influenced Japan's pharmaceutical industry in general (see also Arai et al., this volume). The second is the particular way that government bodies, academic institutions, and industry actors within Toyama prefecture cooperated to respond to these changes, especially from the early twentieth century onwards. The third concerns the clustering of a range of pharmaceutical producers and supporting industries in the prefecture over recent decades. The chapter argues that the interplay of these three factors enabled a unique industrial zone to develop in Toyama prefecture, comprising a mixture of traditional and biomedical pharmaceutical producers of various sizes and specialisations.

The Toyama case illustrates the wide range of contingent factors involved in the emergence of pharmaceutical industries, while highlighting the crucial role that intersectoral collaboration can play in their sustained success.

---

1 The term "*Wakanyaku*" literally translates as "Japanese and Chinese medicines" (see Arai et al., this volume), but actually denotes all the natural raw materials of plant or animal origin that are used in traditional medicines in Japan.

DOI: 10.4324/9781003218074-6

It also urges us to rethink relationships between "traditional" and biomedical pharmaceutical industries in Asia, which are often portrayed as entirely separate or indeed antagonistic. In Toyama, it was the historical success of the *haichi* household medicines industry that paved the way for biomedical manufacturers to flourish. Although the biomedical industry overtook its herbal counterpart during the twentieth century and is now far larger and more profitable, the two sectors coexist without apparent contradiction and both have benefitted greatly from collaborative institutional activities, local support systems, and industrial clustering. We further argue that *haichi* household medicine manufacturing took the form of a commercial patent medicine industry relatively early on in its history, incorporating medical knowledge and raw materials from several Eastern medical traditions as well as from the West to produce a broad range of classical, reformulated and hybrid medicines that became hugely popular throughout Japan. This opened up a distinct path to industrial growth that contrasts in instructive ways with that of Japanese Kampo (Arai et al., this volume; Umemura 2012) and other Asian "traditional" pharmaceutical industries (cf. Banerjee 2009; Bode 2008; Chee, this volume; Kloos, this volume; Lei 2014; Madhavan and Soman, this volume; Taylor 2005).

In the following sections, this chapter charts the changes that have taken place in pharmaceutical production in Toyama prefecture over the last three centuries. Firstly, it offers a historical overview of the origins and early development of the *haichi* household medicines industry between the seventeenth and nineteenth centuries. Secondly, it provides a detailed account of the expansion of the industry during the nineteenth and early twentieth centuries, including a succession of regulatory interventions and the industry's responses to them. Thirdly, it considers the evolving regulatory, industrial and market environment during the twentieth century. The fourth section discusses major institutional, organisational, and market-related developments in the twenty-first century, while the final section examines contemporary developments shaping this sector, including the spread of the *haichi* household medicine sales system beyond Japan.

Origins and early development of Toyama *haichi* household medicines

In order to understand why the pharmaceutical industry became so strongly rooted in Toyama prefecture from the late seventeenth century onwards, it is helpful to first consider several geographical features peculiar to the region, as well as the political, economic, and medical circumstances of the feudal era. Toyama prefecture is located in the central part of the Honshu side of the Japan Sea, within 270 kilometres of the three major metropolitan areas of Tokyo, Osaka, and Nagoya, giving it the excellent sea and land-based trade links. The prefecture has a rich and varied natural environment, with plentiful water of good quality. The Tateyama mountain range reaches an altitude of 3,000 metres, while the enormous Toyama Bay is more than 1,000 metres deep. Crucially, the "seven major rivers" flow in Toyama prefecture, forming a large alluvial plain. Aided by various irrigation projects, this area provided excellent paddy fields for seasonal rice cultivation, but was also vulnerable to severe flooding. In the Edo period, from the beginning of the seventeenth century until the middle of the nineteenth, the particular seasonal rhythms of Toyama forced people to engage in a range of economic activities in order to survive. Notable among these was seasonal migration, which enabled people to generate income while escaping the regular flood damage. As explained below, these factors played important roles in the birth of the region's pharmaceutical industry.

While there are various arguments concerning the earliest origins of the Toyama *haichi* medicines industry, the following reflects the existing consensus (Toyama Prefecture 1987: 9–14). In 1683, the Okayama clan's doctor, Mandai Jyokan, provided Toyama domain officials with information on how to manufacture a gastrointestinal medicine known as *Hangontan* (反魂丹), a locally adapted form of a classical *Kampo* formula. When Lord Maeda Masatoshi went to Edo Castle in 1690, one of the *Daimyō* (大名 feudal lords) present was suffering from severe abdominal pain. Lord Maeda provided the *Daimyō* with the Toyama-made *Hangontan* medicine he carried and the pain subsided. The other *Daimyō* who observed this event were impressed with the medicine's effects and asked Lord Maeda to sell the medicine to them. As the Toyama region suffered from severe river flooding at that time, the financial affairs of the Toyama clan were not good. To enable the inhabitants of the region to improve their incomes, Lord Maeda approved the peddling of *Hangontan* and other Toyama-produced medicines in other jurisdictions. Lord Maeda requested Matsui Gen'emon, who managed the medicine trade in Toyama castle town, to produce *Hangontan* and other medicines in large quantities, which he did, giving birth to a nationwide trade.

By the end of the eighteenth century, Toyama had become the centre of a network of medicine peddlers, known as *chōnushi* (帳主), who engaged in itinerant trade, in part inspired by the need to secure alternative sources of income during periods of flooding in their hometowns. This trade was based on the highly innovative *sen'yōkori* (pay-for-use) model, or "*haichi* medicine sales system." *Haichi* peddlers regularly deposited boxes containing many different kinds of household medicines at clients' houses, which the clients used as needed. The next time the peddlers visited each home, they collected the charge for the medicines that had been used and replaced them with new stock. Because medical services were not easily accessible for ordinary households during this period, many people found it highly convenient to have a wide variety of medicines ready in case of need and this system became widely accepted. The *chōnushi* and their clients established trusting relationships and the system had become highly popular by the mid-eighteenth century. Its popularity was such that the Toyama medicine peddlers were able to form a nationwide trade zone during the first half of the nineteenth century, which has continued into the present day (Toyama Prefecture 1987).

Several other important factors were involved in the early growth of the Toyama *haichi* medicine industry (Toyama Prefecture 1987: 9–12, 32–36). The first is that the *chōnushi* kept track of their accounts in a special kind of notebook called a *Kakebachō* (懸場帳). Each peddler recorded important data in their *Kakebachō*, such as clients' names and addresses, the types and quantities of medicines used, and the amounts of money paid. When borrowing funds, *Kakebachō* were used as collateral, as they represented the clientele and potential profits of the *chōnushi* possessing it. The *Kakebachō* could also be passed on to a new owner, allowing them to continue peddling medicines to a well-established network of clients. The use of *Kakebachō* was central to the development of the *haichi* medicine sales system, as it provided at once a detailed record of clients and their consumption patterns, a tool for planning future medicine production, and the basis upon which individual peddlers' business portfolios could be continued, expanded or sold on.

The second reason is that various efforts were made to improve the quality of the medicines, facilitated by trade networks that enabled good supplies of raw material to reach Toyama. Among the most important raw materials used in *haichi* medicines were Chinese items such as Chinese musk and Oriental bezoar. These were imported from China to Nagasaki, then sent to *Doshōmachi* (道修町), where the *kabunakama* (株仲間 guild of drugs) was established in the middle of the seventeenth century. This became a major distribution centre for drugs nationwide, to Osaka and onward to Toyama. Many of the medicinal ingredients collected in Japan also reached Toyama through wholesalers in Osaka. While some raw materials were also procured within the Toyama region, most were obtained through this nationwide economic distribution network.

From the latter part of the seventeenth century onwards, the major factor that enabled nationwide commerce to grow was the development of both land and sea trade routes, with the latter proving particularly crucial (Toyama Prefecture 1987: 69–90). The Tokugawa shogunate ordered Kawamura Zuiken to arrange westward maritime transport in 1671. It was a route from ports on the coast of the Japan Sea in both the Hokuriku and Tohoku regions to the West, descending southwards and entering the Seto Inland Sea via Shimonoseki, which enabled connection to Osaka. As this route opened, a system of maritime traffic centred on Osaka was formed, allowing a nationwide trading system to be established. The ships originally operating this route were called *Kitamaebune* (北前船). From the end of the seventeenth century, larger and more durable *Bezaisen* (弁財船) ships designed exclusively for trading began to appear, enabling bulk trade to progress. Boxes of finished medicines were sent from Toyama to Osaka and various areas of western and northern Japan by this westward shipping route, while raw materials came in the other direction.

Several other important changes took place in the way *haichi* medicines were produced and circulated between the late seventeenth century and the latter half of the eighteenth, when these medicines started to become popular on a large scale (Toyama Prefecture 1987: 180–191). During the Genroku period, at the end of the seventeenth century, the *haichi* peddlers mainly sold medicines formulated by a single pharmacist, Matsui Gen'emon (Mastuiya), who famously monopolised the production of *Hangontan*, the most popular *haichi* medicine. As the *haichi* medicine sales system developed, however, peddlers began setting up small pharmacies at their homes, producing several well-known *haichi* medicines as well as formulating their own prescriptions. In keeping with the mode of production prevalent during the Tokugawa period, the formulation of *haichi* medicines was a secretive matter, transmitted orally and largely within families. However, manufacturing processes were relatively simple and did not require elaborate pharmaceutical technology, making it quite easy for *chōnushi* to take up small-scale pharmacy.

It is unclear exactly when *chōnushi* began to make their own medicines in addition to selling them. However, as their number increased considerably during the early eighteenth century, it is reasonable to assume that some of the more successful among them were able to accumulate sufficient capital to invest in the production of household medicines during this period. By the late eighteenth century, it became clear that numerous *chōnushi* were recording high sales volumes, purchasing their own medicinal raw materials both in their home areas and along their peddling routes, and employing other peddlers to help them produce medicines at their homes. Thus, it gradually became customary that whenever employed peddlers returned to Toyama, they would engage in the medicine production process at their employer's house. As this cottage industry expanded, it became impossible for a single pharmacist to monopolise the production of *haichi* medicines, as had previously been the case.

As long-term trusting relationships became established between *chōnushi* and their clients, Toyama *haichi* medicines began to gain huge popularity from the mid-eighteenth century onwards. The *chōnushi* formed guilds for every region in which they conducted their itinerant trade (Toyama Prefecture 1987: 320). The number of guilds increased as the industry developed. By the mid-eighteenth century, the whole of Japan was divided into 18 travelling ranges, each with its own guild of licensed *haichi* peddlers. Three supervisors were elected for each guild, setting regulations that were observed voluntarily by the *chōnushi*. All the guilds helped each other mutually and banded together as a *Sōnakama* (惣仲間 general guild) to protect and further their commercial interests.

The Toyama clan managed the *haichi* peddlers through the general guild. They also monitored the distribution of medical raw materials, ensuring that *chōnushi* did not purchase poor-quality ingredients. The use of inferior raw materials and medicines had become a problem as medicine peddlers emerged in other domains. To prevent this from damaging their interests, the Toyama government ordered that only registered drug stores could deal with medicinal raw materials. In 1816, the Toyama government also established a monitoring agency for *Hangontan* (Toyama Prefecture 1987: 306–322). Since *haichi* medicine products became the most important trade items for the Toyama clan, many peddlers engaged in itinerant trade with other clans. The proceeds of their business not only contributed to the general economy of the region, but also their taxes became crucial to the Toyama clan's finances. By the mid-nineteenth century, a nationwide network involving more than 4,000 Toyama *haichi* medicine peddlers was well established. As they extended their networks across the nation, they developed a particular sales etiquette and other rules of the trade. Toyama's *Hangontan* agency also assisted in various negotiations between *chōnushi* and clients in other clans.

As the *haichi* medicine industry developed, organisational changes took place within the Toyama clan's government, including placing the Hangontan Agency under the control of the Toyama Clan Products Agency in 1844. Changes in administrative organisation showed the Toyama government attempting to control the distribution of medical ingredients and the *haichi* medicine sales business more strictly than before. For example, medicine packaging was produced displaying the symbol of the Toyama Clan Products Agency. The *chōnushi* were forced to use this packaging so that people could distinguish Toyama *haichi* medicine from similar patent medicines made elsewhere. The introduction of this early form of product branding proved successful and certainly strengthened the *haichi* medicine sales business. However, such measures did nothing to tighten government control over medicinal raw materials. To this end, a dedicated facility for medicinal ingredients was established in 1850, building on policies introduced in the early nineteenth century in order to strengthen control over the distribution of raw materials and to ensure the quality of the medicines produced by the Toyama clan.

Expansion, regulation, and transformation following the Meiji restoration

In the first half of the nineteenth century, Japan was still in the feudal era and governed by the Tokugawa regime. As we have seen, the political circumstances of the time meant that the *chōnushi* of the Toyama clan needed to exercise caution when entering regions ruled by other *Daimyō* families to sell their medicines (Uemura 1959), but were nevertheless able to extend their peddling activities right across Japan. At the same time, the Toyama clan strengthened distribution control of the raw materials used in their medicines. Feudal lords regulated the *chōnushi* and a government office was set up to collect transportation fees from them. This situation persisted until the Meiji Restoration of 1868, after which the entire system of government changed and strict medical regulations were introduced, strongly influenced by Western medical ideas and practices (Futaya 2000: 21–34). We shall now consider how the series of regulatory changes implemented during the Meiji period shaped the *haichi* medicines industry in important ways, while still allowing it to expand and develop its distinct identity and mode of operation. We also show how this growth built upon the governance system introduced during the earlier Edo period, but came increasingly to rely on close collaboration between industry, government and academic actors to help the industry adapt to the rapidly changing circumstances.

In 1868, the Tokugawa shogunate collapsed and the new Meiji government was established. In the early Meiji period, local administrative regions were reorganised. A part of the Kaga clan merged with the Toyama clan, resulting in the establishment of Toyama prefecture in 1883 (Toyama-ken Yakuzaishikai Sōkai Hyakujyūichinenshi Hensan Iinkai 2001: 28–29). The loss of the framework of feudal society presented the Toyama *haichi* medicines industry with new business opportunities and the industry prepared itself to take advantage of them. The new Meiji government, however, was much more enthusiastic about Western medicine and through legislation, regulation, and taxation, explicitly sought to modernise the Japanese pharmaceutical industry, in part by undermining its traditional medicine component.

The Meiji government put considerable effort into shaping and controlling the pharmaceutical industry, notably by heavily regulating the sale of *Wakanyaku* (Japanese and Chinese crude drugs) and encouraging the use of ingredients developed in the West (Futaya 2000: 21–22). However, herbs, minerals, and animal products from Japanese and Chinese medical traditions had long histories of use and were extremely popular among ordinary people. This made it very difficult for the Meiji government to rapidly alter the pharmaceutical market or the manufacturing industry that supplied it. New government policies introduced safety and efficacy as the most crucial parameters guiding the development of the pharmaceutical industry during this period. Because patent medicines were so widely consumed at the time, the government tried to eliminate those that they deemed harmful to the human body, while decreasing consumption of "cure-all" panaceas known as *manbyōyaku* (万病薬). In the early Meiji period, *haichi* household medicine manufacturers usually formulated and sold 40–100 kinds of patent medicine, including several kinds of *manbyōyaku*. Through the Patent Medicine Regulations of 1877, the government started to impose a two-yen business tax on each prescription of patent medicines, in the hope that this would bring about a general reduction in use and the disappearance of medicines they considered ineffective, non-essential, or indeed harmful.

In 1878, the Home Ministry ordered every prefecture in Japan to implement the Regulation of Patent Medicine Inspection. Although it was revised several times, this provided the basis for the regulation of patent medicines until World War II. These regulations categorised some oriental crude drugs and minerals as poisons or powerful drugs because the government decided that they were too strong for the human body, or that their effects were unclear. This meant that many *haichi* medicines could no longer be formulated as before.

Both the Patent Medicine Regulations and the Regulation of Patent Medicine Inspection acts had significant effects on the evolution of the *haichi* medicine industry in Toyama prefecture. Prior to this period, the *chōnushi* purchased crude drugs and formulated, packaged, and sold their medicines by themselves. When the Patent Medicine Regulation was implemented, the *chōnushi* established *dōgōsoshiki* (堂号組織 production groups for *haichi* medicines) in order to avoid having to personally shoulder the burden of expensive sales taxes. By joining together to form numerous small and medium-sized *dōgōsoshiki*, each with a nominal senior partner, the *chōnushi* played the role of both vendors and formulation clerks. This enabled them to continue producing *haichi* medicines in a similar manner to before, albeit with a smaller range of potential raw materials due to the regulations discussed above. In 1887, 22 *dōgōsoshiki* were registered in Toyama prefecture and many of these went on to formally become corporations in the early 1900s.

By the early twentieth century, the major players in the production of *haichi* medicines had transformed themselves from drug shops into patent medicine companies. Those *chōnushi* working for *haichi* medicine companies borrowed the trademark of their company and used the company's factory as their cooperative formulation place, but in fact continued to prepare medicines according to their own formulations and methods. This meant that the content, quality, and effectiveness of individual *haichi* medicines varied considerably, despite being made under the same name and ostensibly by the same patent medicine company. This lack of standardisation was one of the main targets of the Patent Medicine Affairs Law of 1914. Under this new law, patent medicine corporations were required to prepare their medicines according to standard formulations and under the control of qualified pharmacists.

The Toyama tax office was responsible for the next major change in the *haichi* medicines industry. In 1923, the government of Japan reformed the entire taxation system for medicines, abolishing specific patent medicine sales taxes and imposing general business tax on patent medicines instead. However, the Toyama tax office declared that it would continue to levy patent medicine sales tax on each *chōnushi* belonging to a *haichi* medicine company unless that company properly standardised the formulas for their medicines. This tax-driven regulatory development gave rise to significant changes in the formulation and production of *haichi* household medicines. Throughout the 1920s and 1930s, both the larger *haichi* medicine companies and the smaller pharmacies standardised the formulas for their household medicines. Within the rules of the Patent Medicine Affairs Law of 1914, there was room for manufacturers to independently create a "family medicine" with a personally devised recipe based on *Wakanyaku* or classical Kampo formulas. Many companies developed such formulations, utilising the traditional range of *Wakanyaku* but excluding those items banned under previous legislation. They also began to include raw materials used in Western medicine at the time, such as santonin and phenazone, thereby creating new hybrid drugs by combining elements of Eastern and Western pharmacologies. Many companies also started to produce the most popular *haichi* medicines in large quantities and to wholesale packaged medicines to their vendors, instead of various *chōnushi* making their own versions of them under the company name. These developments together led to the emergence of a particular form of patent medicine from merging classical with family-specific formulas and Eastern with Western raw materials, while setting *haichi* medicine producers firmly on the path to becoming industrial pharmaceutical manufacturing companies.

Toyama *haichi* medicines in the twentieth century

This section considers how a raft of new policies and regulations transformed the Toyama *haichi* medicine industry during the twentieth century, as well as how government and academic actors collaborated with the industry to help it adapt to the changes taking place (Futaya 2000). Major changes resulted from increased restrictions on patent medicines using raw materials derived from Japanese and Chinese medical traditions (*Wakanyaku*), from efforts to formalise and consolidate *haichi* manufacturers, from the advent of a national health insurance scheme, and from the introduction of good manufacturing practices (GMP). Whenever such institutional and regulatory changes occurred, the Toyama prefectural government, industry, and academia collaborated to respond flexibly and dynamically to them, thereby enabling the ongoing growth of this remarkable industry.

During the Edo period, *haichi* medicine peddlers purchased raw materials, formulated medicines, packaged them, and sold them on their own. In response to the Meiji government's introduction of various new pharmaceutical regulations, the *chōnushi* established *dōgōsoshiki* so they could produce their medicines at shared manufacturing facilities, as discussed above. The oldest patent medicine company in Toyama prefecture is Kokando Company Limited (henceforth Kokando), which was founded in 1876 as a *dōgōsoshiki* by 2,650 *chōnushi*. They made Murasawa Moriya, who was an old Samurai and a cashier of the Toyama clan, the company president, and became nominal vendors and pharmacists united under the Kokando name. The administrative expenses of the company were supported by the *chōnushi* according to the number of *Kakebachō* that they held. Although all medical packaging subsequently mentioned this manufacturing facility, the *chōnushi* continued producing many preparations individually. In the early 1900s, Kokando and many other *dōgōsoshiki* formally became *haichi* medicine companies, taking the industry into a new developmental phase.

Further evidence of this new phase came with the founding of the Kyōritu Toyama Pharmaceutical School in 1894, which was funded through subsidies from the *haichi* medicine companies, peddler associations, and Toyama City. It was upgraded to become Toyama Prefectural Vocational School for the Pharmaceutical Industry in April 1910. Students graduated after completing a three-year course and were given a licensed pharmacist's qualification.[2] In its early days, this school represented an important step in formalising the training and qualifications of pharmacists involved in the *haichi* medicines industry. It granted them greater official legitimacy and helped the *haichi* manufacturers adapt to the evolving legal and regulatory environment. The school went on to play a major role in the training of pharmacy students and the development of pharmaceutical science expertise within Toyama prefecture, while also facilitating collaboration between industry, state, and academic actors in the region.

However, as the Patent Medicine Affairs Law of 1914 came into force and the cost of raw materials imported from Europe increased during the interwar period, the prevailing methods of *haichi* medicine production could not continue. In 1916, this problem was discussed at a roundtable meeting attended by members of industry, government, and academia based in Toyama Prefecture. Several strategies were agreed upon for addressing the challenges the industry was facing, but it took time for the companies to adapt and for these strategies to bear fruit.

As discussed in the previous section, according to the Patent Medicine Affairs Law, each formulation was required to have the same standardised ingredients and to be produced under the supervision of a pharmacist at a registered pharmaceutical company. Many firms found it difficult to comply with this legislation. In 1923, the Toyama Taxation Authority put further pressure on firms to implement the "standardisation of formulas," in accordance with the amendments to the Patent Medicine Sales Tax Law. The government abolished the patent medicine tax and imposed general business tax on patent medicines instead.[3] To force compliance, the Toyama tax office declared that if *haichi* medicine companies did not implement standardised formulas for their medicines, it would levy patent medicine tax on each *chōnushi* belonging to that company. With such a change in the business environment, companies started producing popular *haichi* medicines in large quantities according to standardised formulas and

---

2   On these points, see *Toyama-ken Yakugyōshi, Tsūshi* (History of the Pharmaceutical Industry in Toyama Prefecture), Toyama Prefecture (1987: 567–574).
3   At this time, patent medicine tax originated from the patent medicine stamp duty tax established in 1882. The salesperson had to affix a stamp to the value of ten percent of the sale price on the wrapping of each patent medicine. If the *chōnushi* that belonged to *haichi* medicine companies did not follow the Toyama tax office's instructions exactly, their tax burden was significantly increased. Patent medicine tax was finally abolished in March 1926. See: Futaya (2000: 22–23).

wholesaling readymade medicines to their *chōnushi*. This enforced transition from *dōgōsoshiki* to *haichi* medicine manufacturing companies was a further step towards the formation of a true pharmaceutical industry.

According to a 1935 survey by Toyama City Hygiene Division, which studied 291 prescriptions for Toyama household medicines, 64 used only *Wakanyaku*, 68 contained mainly *Wakanyaku* with small quantities of Western ingredients added, 89 used mainly Western materials with a little *Wakanyaku* added, and 70 used only Western ingredients. Among the Eastern ingredients, *Oren* (黄連 *Coptis sp.*) and *Asen'yaku* (阿仙薬 *Acacia catechu*) were widely utilised, while Phenacetin and Acetanilide were commonly used Western ingredients. For reasons of convention, most preparations intended for children, women, and older people primarily used *Wakanyaku*, whereas those for general consumption used higher proportions of imported Western materials. While the *chōnushi* now bought many of their readymade medicines from wholesalers, they continued making the *Wakanyaku*-based preparations themselves and according to their own formulas, in so far as permitted under the medical sales law.

The government announced the Patent Medicine Operating Outline in February 1942, during World War II. In pursuit of higher productivity, its main aim was the consolidation of numerous patent medicine companies into fewer, larger companies for each prefecture (Hokuriku Ginkō Chōsabu Hyakunenshi Hensanhan 1978: 803–804). In Toyama prefecture, this meant that the former industrial array of two large factories, 150 smaller factories and 1500 un-mechanised *haichi* pharmacies and individual manufacturers were consolidated into 13 enterprises through integration or discontinuation. In August 1945, however, much of Toyama City was burned to the ground following intense firebombing. Almost all the *haichi* medicine manufacturers turned to ashes and 70 percent of the productivity in Toyama prefecture was lost.

After World War II, influenced by democratisation, the Pharmaceutical Affairs Law was fully revised and enacted on 29 July 1948 (Nishikawa 2004: 64). Under this new law, medicine manufacture and pharmacy operation came under a new system of registration. The *haichi* medicine sales system was recognised and registered as a legitimate pharmacy and drug sales business, and this registration has continued to be valid to the present day (Toyama Prefecture 1987: 823). Many factories resumed operations after 1946 and by 1947, productivity had recovered to the same level as before the war (Hokuriku Ginkō Chōsabu Hyakunenshi Hensanhan 1978: 804). By 1955, there were 210 pharmaceutical plants in Toyama prefecture and total production was valued at about 2.4 billion yen, of which *haichi* household medicine accounted for 84 percent, or roughly 2 billion yen. By 1968, the total pharmaceutical output of Toyama prefecture was 10.2 billion yen and *haichi* household medicine sales were worth 4.9 billion yen, showing an overall growth in sales volume but a reduction (to 43 percent) in terms of its share of the total output of the prefecture.

Part of the reason for the declining market share of Toyama *haichi* medicines compared to other pharmaceutical forms was the introduction of universal National Health Insurance coverage in 1961. Through this, the entire population of Japan gained access to state-sponsored, low-cost medical consultation and treatment by registered doctors. The nationwide demand for biomedical prescription pharmaceuticals grew exponentially as patient visits to clinics and hospitals increased rapidly and restrictions on the use of highly priced drugs such as antibiotics were relaxed (Futaya 2017: 168–170). Large pharmaceutical companies with access to investment capital, many of them based in Tokyo and Osaka, were the best placed to benefit from these new market opportunities. Biomedical manufacturers based in Toyama prefecture also took advantage of the increased demand for their products, but the producers of patent medicines were not able to grow at a comparable rate.

According to the *Annual Statistical Report on Production in Toyama Prefectural Pharmaceutical Industry, haichi* household medicines constituted about 80 percent of total production in the prefecture in 1960, but this had decreased to only 19 percent by 1975 (Toyama Prefecture 1983: 88–89). As many new kinds of medicine and vitamins were sold with the help of mass media advertisements from the mid-1970s onwards, the competition between household medicines and other types of pharmaceutical products intensified (Nihon Yakushi Gakkai 2016: 93). Indeed, it was from this period that the production of biomedical pharmaceuticals in Toyama prefecture began to increase sharply. In 1976, Toyama prefecture's pharmaceutical production accounted for 4.4 percent of Japan's total, ranking it in seventh place (Hokuriku Ginkō Chōsabu Hyakunenshi Hensanhan 1978: 806). However, in terms of the volume of household medicine produced for *haichi* sales, Toyama prefecture maintained its dominant position, accounting for 56.9 percent of the total nationwide production of 24 billion yen.

The introduction of GMP legislation in 1976 was a major factor in the increasing production of biomedical pharmaceuticals in Toyama prefecture in the second half of the 1970s, but it also held important implications for the *haichi* medicines industry (Toyama Prefecture 1987: 1002–1007, 1013). In 1968, the World Health Organization passed a resolution on the establishment of GMP, and legislation reflecting this was implemented in Japan in April 1976 (see Arai et al., this volume). The Toyama Prefectural Pharmaceutical Affairs Laboratory, pharmaceutical firms, government officials, and academics collaborated to respond to this regulatory change. In accordance with GMP guidelines, personnel were placed in all manufacturing facilities to monitor the production process, maintain quality and ensure hygiene standards. The infrastructure and equipment of pharmaceutical manufacturing facilities had to be upgraded at a substantial cost to include, for example, sterilisation rooms. Following consultations with manufacturers, Toyama's pharmaceutical promotion division established its own subsidy system to help firms meet GMP standards. At the same time, Toyama Prefectural Pharmaceutical Research Institute advised all pharmaceutical manufacturers on the technical aspects of GMP. This institute, formerly known as the Toyama Prefectural Drug Testing Laboratory, was established in 1929 by the Toyama Prefectural Patent Medicine Dealer Association. This pattern of institutional development clearly shows how the *haichi* industry paved the way for the biomedical industry to flourish.

In 1973, Toyama Prefecture Pharmaceutical Affairs Division worked with the pharmaceutical industry to establish the Pharmaceutical Quality Control Workshop. This workshop held lectures about quality management repeatedly until December 1975, the year before GMP was implemented, helping prefectural firms to attain GMP competence and certification. Adhering to GMP standards was particularly financially burdensome for the manufacturers of *haichi* medicines. It required a huge investment in facilities and quality control systems, especially for companies producing a wide variety of different formulations. Lacking the capital to invest in the equipment and procedures required to comply with GMP standards for the full range of products, most manufacturers were forced to reduce their portfolio of medicines, focus on those for which their formulation technology was superior, and explore new product forms for which regulations were less stringent, such as topical ointments. As a result, many *haichi* manufacturers became increasingly specialised in the manufacture and sale of a narrower range of medicinal products during the latter decades of the twentieth century.

The Toyama pharmaceutical industry in the twenty-first century

Among the many institutional changes that have shaped the Japanese pharmaceutical industry over recent years, there are three that have particularly affected Toyama prefecture. The first was the 2006 amendment to the Pharmaceutical Affairs Law, which allowed for contract manufacturing of pharmaceuticals. The second was the promotion of generic drugs, following the 2007 decision by the Ministry of Health, Labour and Welfare to increase the market share of generic drugs by 30 percent or more by 2012. The government subsequently raised these targets to an increase of 70 percent by 2017 and 80 percent or more by 2020 (Kōseirōdōshō 2016: 388–389). The third factor concerns the clustering of various kinds of pharmaceutical manufacturers and supporting industries in the region. Although forms of clustering started much earlier, arguably with the consolidation of the *haichi* industry in the eighteenth century, recent decades have seen considerable expansion of policies and incentives explicitly aiming to encourage industrial clustering. This section discusses how these changes contributed to variable growth rates across different sectors and thus shaped both *haichi* manufacture and the Toyama pharmaceutical industry as a whole.

Under earlier versions of the Pharmaceutical Affairs Law, contract pharmaceutical production was only permitted for certain parts of the manufacturing process. The 2006 amendment liberalised contract production by allowing all processes, including final product making, to be carried out under contract. Japan's major pharmaceutical manufacturers took this opportunity to reduce their costs by expanding contract manufacturing, which in turn allowed them to concentrate more resources on the development of new drugs. They commissioned other companies, which had small or medium-sized capital and excellent manufacturing technology, to make their products in order to reduce production costs. Many manufacturers with the appropriate technology and experience in formulation and quality management had been established in Toyama prefecture since the Meiji era and large numbers were selected for contract production, leading to significant increases in output[4]. The total production value of pharmaceuticals nationwide in 2005 was 6.3 trillion yen, of which Toyama prefecture accounted for 4.1 percent and was ranked in eighth place. By 2015, the total production figure reached 6.8 trillion yen, of which Toyama prefecture's share was 10.7 percent, raising it to the top rank. In the context of this impressive growth, the leap from 2005 to 2006 was particularly remarkable. In 2006, the value of Toyama's pharmaceutical production reached 441 billion yen, which was an increase of 167.5 percent over the previous year. This proved that the implementation of the amended Pharmaceutical Affairs Law was a key turning point for the Toyama pharmaceutical industry. According to *Annual Statistical Report on Production in Toyama Prefectural Pharmaceutical Industry*, the production value of prescription medicine was roughly 80 percent of the total amount of medicines produced in the prefecture in 2014 for both in-house and contract manufacturing. However, *haichi* medicine only constituted 5 percent of in-house production and 2 percent of contract manufacturing (Toyama-ken Kōseibu Kusuriseisakuka 1990–2016: 1–3). We return to consider the reasons for this below.

In 2014, there were 83 different pharmaceutical manufacturers active at 105 sites in the prefecture, ranging from producers of new drugs, generics, general-purpose OTC medicines, placebo materials, and drug substances, as well as *haichi* household medicines. Furthermore, a whole range of industries have become established in the prefecture to support the pharmaceutical industry by providing raw materials, pharmacy equipment and containers, packaging materials, and printing services. Many of these companies completely transferred their production bases to Toyama from other prefectures. A major reason cited for this relocation is the benefits gained from industrial clustering (Toyama-ken Iyakuhin Sangyō Kasseika Konwakai 2014: 7–9). The Toyama Prefectural Government's aggressive efforts to attract enterprises and promote pharmacies also influenced the

---

4 Noto Kazuhiro, *Kōkōgyōshisū to Toyama-ken ni okeru Iyakuhin no Dōkō* (Industrial Index and Trends in Pharmaceuticals in Toyama Prefecture): http://www.pref.toyama.jp/sections/1015/ecm/back/2009jun/tokushu/index2.html [accessed 27 June, 2018].

relocation of these companies. Although such clustering in recent times was mainly driven by the interests of those manufacturing biomedical pharmaceuticals, forms of clustering have much deeper origins in Toyama prefecture, as the above discussion of the early development of the *haichi* industry shows. Clustering has also proved beneficial for *haichi* companies over recent decades by improving access to inputs and services that supported their production, packaging, and marketing activities.

In order to respond to the changing institutional environment, the Drug Policy Division of Toyama Prefecture's Health and Welfare Department established the Toyama Prefectural Committee for the Revitalization of the Pharmaceutical Industry. Comprising representatives from industry, government, and academia, the committee convened in September 2009 and July 2013. This sentence has been changed: "It comprised representatives from industry, government, and academia and convened in September 2009 and July 2013." The new sentence reads as follows: "Comprising representatives from industry, government, and academia, the committee convened in September 2009 and July 2013." In their report of March 2010, the committee summarised their suggestions, outlined future policies, and proposed five concrete strategies, all of which the Toyama prefectural government subsequently implemented. First, pharmacists and engineers working in pharmaceutical companies were consulted about their working conditions and their views were subsequently reflected in operational plans and R&D activities, such as concerning the use of new technologies in the development of new drugs. Second, in order to make careers in the pharmaceutical industry more attractive, pharmaceutical companies held seminars and offered internships to pharmacy students. Third, Toyama Pharmaceutical Federation designated personnel to disseminate information and facilitate collaboration with related industries. Fourth, grants were offered and public relations activities were held to continue attracting new firms to the area. Fifth, a Japan External Trade Organisation (JETRO) project was launched in order to expand international exchange in the field of pharmaceuticals, in addition to the prefecture's ongoing exchanges with the Basel region of Switzerland.

The Toyama prefectural government's commitment to promoting the pharmaceutical industry was also reflected in the growth of the Toyama Prefectural Institute for Pharmaceutical Research from 2008 onwards. This institute focuses on drug formulation, pharmaceutical research and innovation in both biomedical and Wakanyaku-based medicines, on the quality evaluation of all pharmaceutical products, and on the provision of technical training for pharmaceutical company staff (Toyama Prefectural Government, Pharmaceutical Policy Division 2011: 5). They recruited a highly knowledgeable and experienced pharmaceutical technologist in 2008 and subsequently encouraged the use of specialised formulation machines in the prefecture. This notably included the expanded use of expensive tablet-making machines, for which subsidies were secured from the national economic stimulus scheme. As a result, new machines were used 200 times in 2013, compared to only six times in 2005 (Toyama–ken Yakuji Kenkyūkai 2015: 38, 102). Furthermore, a laboratory for innovation in pharmaceutical development and drug delivery was opened at the institute in 2015. In other words, from this period onwards, the Toyama government began seriously supporting pharmaceutical manufacturers to push forward into rapidly growing fields of innovation, while continuing to support the *haichi* industry, albeit at a reduced level.

In April 2018, the Toyama Prefectural Institute for Pharmaceutical Research was drastically reorganised into a three-centre system, with each centre pursuing a specific mission. The Research Centre for Drug Development and Quality Control focuses on strengthening research support for drug development and testing. The Centre for Innovation in Pharmaceutical Development and Drug Delivery aims to promote research and development of high value-added medicines such as biopharmaceuticals, utilising 25 of the most advanced analytical machines. It also supports cooperation in human resource development with universities and pharmaceutical companies in the prefecture (*Kateiyaku Shinbun* no. 3487). Thirdly, originally founded in 1967, the Centre for Medicinal Plants promotes the study, cultivation, and dissemination of medicinal plants and herbs. This centre tests cultivation, preparation, and processing methods for medicinal plants, as well as engaging in quality assurance (Toyama Prefectural Government, Pharmaceutical Policy Division 2011: 5). The current main research themes of this centre are promoting the branding project of *Toyama Shakuyaku* (富山芍薬 Toyama Peony), the development of medicines based on *Wakanyaku* so as to improve ease of consumption, and the development of medicines that affect the human immune system. Together, the activities of this institute symbolise the cooperation between industry, government, and academia, which has proved so crucial to the growth and adaptability of both the herbal and biomedical sectors of the prefecture's pharmaceutical industry.

It is clear that the Toyama government is fully committed to the slogan proposed by Toyama Prefecture Committee for the Revitalization of the Pharmaceutical Industry: "To realize Toyama as the medical capital of the world." As various pharmaceutical promotion schemes continued to be developed, capital investment by pharmaceutical companies in the prefecture exceeded 230 billion yen from 2005 to 2015, according to a survey conducted by Pharmaceutical Policy Division of Toyama Prefectural Government. This favourable environment also recently allowed Toyama prefecture to commission a major new drug manufacturer to increase generic drug production. As a result of these coordinated efforts, by 2015, the prefecture became the leader in pharmaceutical production within Japan, accounting for 10.7 percent of national production (*Kateiyaku Shinbun* no. 3442).

Meanwhile, however, nationwide production of *haichi* medicine decreased for 18 consecutive years, from 68.5 billion yen in 1997 to 18.9 billion yen in 2015 (*Kateiyaku Shinbun* no. 3442). In step with this general trend, the production volume of *haichi* medicine in Toyama prefecture also declined year after year. Following a peak of 31.2 billion yen in 1995, which represents almost half of total national production, it decreased to 20 billion yen in 2006 and then to 10 billion in 2013 (*Kateiyaku Shinbun* no. 3465). However, despite this general trend towards market contraction, Toyama prefecture remains Japan's most influential production area for *haichi* medicines. Looking at the breakdown of in-house manufactured *haichi* medicines in 2015, the leading treatments were cold medicines at 1.4 billion yen, followed by gastrointestinal agents at 1 billion yen, then antipyretic/analgesic/anti-inflammatory agents at 900 million yen. The fourth most popular was vitamins at 800 million yen, followed by Kampo preparations at 700 million yen.

The ranking of production value by types of *haichi* medicine did not change from 2010 to 2015. The Annual Statistical Report on Production in the Toyama Prefectural Pharmaceutical Industry (*Toyama-ken Yakuji Kōgyō Seisan Dōtai Tōkei Nenpō*) shows that, in 1999, Kampo preparations were ranked tenth in terms of the production value of *haichi* medicines, before moving up to fifth place by 2006.[5] Cardioprotective agents, which are traditional products of Toyama *haichi* medicine made from *Wakanyaku*, maintained annual production of about 2 billion yen in 1996 and were ranked in fifth place. However, the production volume of cardioprotective agents began to decline in 1997, dropping to tenth place, while Kampo medicine began to grow in 1999. In the 1990s, the production value of Kampo medicines was around 500 million yen, but its production value exceeded 1 billion in 1999 and kept fluctuating between 1 billion yen and 1.5 billion yen until 2007. In 2001, the ranking of cardioprotective agents and Kampo medicines was reversed, and two years later, the production of cardioprotective agents was further reduced to 1 billion yen. That is to say, the production value of conventional crude drug products, which had formerly been so representative of the Toyama brand of *haichi* medicine, has decreased, while on the contrary, the value of Kampo products has increased. According to Maki Umemura (2012), Japan revived traditional medicine in the latter half of the twentieth century by expanding the Kampo medicine market (see also Arai et al., this volume). Certainly, from the 1990s to the 2010s, the production trends for Kampo medicine in Toyama prefecture support this point. However, among the *haichi* medicines produced by pharmaceutical manufacturers in the prefecture, Kampo preparations still only accounted for about 8 percent in 2015. While roughly 50 percent of *haichi* medicines nationwide are produced in Toyama prefecture today, the changing structure and rhythms of Japanese life, the aging of *haichi* medicine vendors and

---

5   *Toyama-ken Kōseibu Kusuriseisakuka* (Pharmaceutical Policy Division, Health and Welfare Department, Toyama Prefectural Government) (1990–2016); *Toyama-ken Yakuji Kōgyō Seisan Dōtai Tōkei Nenpō* (Annual Statistical Report on Production in Toyama Prefectural Pharmaceutical Industry), Toyama: Toyama Prefecture.

the shortage of successors have become industrial problems, and consequently, the *haichi* medicine market continues to shrink (*Kateiyaku Shinbun* no. 3464).

Current situation of Toyama *haichi* medicine manufacturing and sales system

This section considers in more detail the current situation of the *haichi* medicine sales system in Toyama prefecture, the response of *haichi* manufacturers to the changing market conditions, and their prospects for the future. We begin by discussing the case of the Kokando Company, which is among Toyama prefecture's major *haichi* manufacturers with over 140 years of history, as mentioned above. Kokando is most famous today for producing and selling *Pana-Wan* (パナワン) and *Essen* (エッセン),[6] which are original, branded medicines developed through collaboration between the company, academic actors, and the Toyama Prefectural Institute. Although originally focused on *haichi* medicine manufacturing, the company has significantly developed Contract Manufacturing Organization (CMO) and over-the-counter (OTC) production activities over recent years. From 2009 onwards, the revised Pharmaceutical Affairs Law was fully enforced, allowing Kokando to engage in complete manufacturing processes and to establish a production system concentrated on tablets, pills, and liquid drugs.[7] As a result of continuing investment, the company's CMO business became the largest granule manufacturer in Japan. In 2018, the sales value of its CMO granule business was about 6.6 billion yen, while its healthcare business was worth 5.5 billion yen (*Kateiyaku Shinbun* no. 3486). At the same time, however, Kokando's *haichi* medicine sales value had dropped to 2.6 billion yen, down 7.1 percent from the previous year. This shows the continuation of a pattern of decline that had seen Kokando's wholesale *haichi* medicine sales decrease by half over the last 15 years, from a high of 5.3 billion yen in 2003.[8]

---

6 Developed in 2006, "Pana-wan" is a new type of pill-shaped gastrointestinal drug made from a mixture of 11 different animal and plant materials. In 2011, a second gastrointestinal medicine, "Essen", was released, consisting of six natural ingredients and produced in chewable form to make consumption easy for elderly people. See: Toyama Prefectural Government, *Pharmaceutical Industry in Toyama*, Toyama: Toyama Government, 2011: 6; Toyama Pharmaceutical Association, *Toyama's original medicine brand "PANA-WAN / ESSEN"* [Online]. Available from: http://www.toyama-kusuri.jp/en/aracalte/original/index.html [accessed 13 July, 2018].
7 Kokando Co., Ltd., *Heisei 15 nendo Eigyō Hōkokusho* (Business Report 2003) [Online]. Available from: http://www.koukandou.co.jp/wp-content/uplords/2015/02/H1504-1603ir.pdf [accessed 6 June, 2018].
8 Kokando Co., Ltd., *Heisei 15 nendo Eigyō Hōkokusho* (Business Report 2003) [Online]. Available from: http://www.koukandou.co.jp/wp-content/uplords/2015/02/H1504-1603ir.pdf [accessed 6 June, 2018].

Among the major reasons for this decline are the falling popularity of the household medicine delivery system, changes in the way people access medicines, and the declining number of *chōnushi*. The household medicine delivery system has weakened in part due to changes in the composition of Japanese households and to employment patterns. In former times, most households would contain at least a married couple and their children, and women largely stayed within the domestic sphere. Recent decades have seen the number of single-occupancy households increasing and larger numbers of women entering the labour market. It is now much less likely for *chōnushi* to find anyone at home when they come to call, and the *haichi* requirements for each household are much smaller than in former times, making peddling more challenging and less lucrative. Furthermore, with the 2006 revision of the Pharmaceutical Affairs Law, people can now purchase OTC medicines online or in convenience stores, further eroding the appeal of household medicine deliveries.

At its peak in 1934, *haichi* medicine sales in Toyama prefecture involved 13,360 people. After World War II, there were 9,810 registered *haichi* peddlers, but from 1963 onwards, the number declined year on year. By 2016, there were only 718 people involved, 60 percent of whom were over 60 years old (*Kateiyaku Shinbun* no. 3453). This environment, in which the peddlers were growing old but few successors were taking over from them, made it difficult for Kokando and other *haichi* medicine manufacturers to maintain their existing activities, let alone invest capital in new *haichi* medicine product development (*Kateiyaku Shinbun* no. 3466).

After struggling for some time to adapt to the changing regulatory and market environment, Kokando came to a major turning point in December 2017. In partnership with two other leading Toyama-based *haichi* manufacturers, namely Taikyo Phamaceutical Company and Naigai Yakuhin Company, they established a joint *haichi* medicine manufacturing and sales concern named Toyama Megumi Pharmaceutical Company Limited (*Kateiyaku Shinbun* no. 3479). Their aim was to promote project proposals and sales activities for the evolving needs of the *haichi* medicine market. This included consolidation of *haichi* medicine formulas and the creation of a new *haichi* medicine business model combining products and services. The new company manufactures and sells *haichi* medicines, medicated products, OTC medicines, health foods, and cosmetics (*Kateiyaku Shinbun* no. 3470). The most popular OTC medicine produced by Toyama Megumi Pharmaceutical Company is an antipyretic and analgesic agent called *Kerorin* (ケロリン). In continuous production since 1925, *Kerorin* still has a strong demand from consumers and sells well, despite the changes that have swept through the industry as a whole. Although the *haichi* medicine market continues to shrink, this new company is dedicated to making and supplying the best quality *haichi* medicines possible to cater to their remaining customers, while also branching out into new product forms.

It is clear that the Japanese *haichi* medicines market is in decline and that the 2006 revision of the Pharmaceutical Affairs Law played an important contributing role. Today, Toyama-based pharmaceutical manufacturers largely focus on CMO operations and OTC medicine production as the main core of their business. In 2018, the *haichi* medicine manufacturers jointly established a new company and began to explore business models that have advantages in *haichi* systems, with some early signs of success now becoming evident. In addition, actors from the Toyama pharmaceutical industry are involved in a project to transfer aspects of the *haichi* medicine system to other Asian countries, especially those with lower levels of economic development and poor access to medical facilities and other sources of medicine. The Institute of Natural Medicine of Toyama University has been engaged in a Japan International Cooperation Agency commissioned project "Primary Health Care Improvement Project through Quality Improvement of Traditional Drugs in Myanmar" since 2014, using their quality control expertise to help improve the standard and effectiveness of traditional medicines. The major *haichi* medicine companies of Toyama prefecture have also begun to expand into Mongolia, Myanmar, and other Association of Southeast Asian Nations (ASEAN) countries (*Kateiyaku Shinbun* no. 3453).

Conclusion

This chapter has traced the history of Toyama prefecture's pharmaceutical industry from its early beginnings, through the reforms of the Meiji era and the regulatory changes of the post-war period, into the present day. It has shown how the origins of this industry lie in the voluntary establishment of a general guild of *haichi* peddlers and the Toyama clan's efforts to control everything related to medicine production, using an organisational model from early modern times. It is clear that the historical success of this model laid the foundations upon which the entire Toyama pharmaceutical industry was subsequently constructed. Even though demand for *haichi* medicines has been in decline for several decades, and biomedical manufacturing has far superseded it in terms of scale and profitability, the *haichi* industry has remained vibrant and dynamic throughout. Furthermore, both sectors have benefitted greatly from the collaborative institutional activities, local support schemes, and industrial clustering peculiar to this region. Since the early twentieth century, an intersectoral collaboration between industry, government, and academia has been particularly crucial to sustaining the industry's remarkable trajectory. Such interactions meant that every time laws, regulations, business conditions, or demand patterns changed, pharmaceutical companies of all kinds were able to overcome the difficulties by altering their organisational structure, adapting their formulas, production methods, and technological inputs, or refocusing their activities onto new products and services.

The Toyama case challenges the popular image of "traditional medicine" as static and conservative, while also unsettling simplistic distinctions between "traditional" and "modern" pharmaceutical industries and their products. We have shown how the *haichi* medicines industry has always been dynamic, evolving in many ways over the years in response to a wide range of internal and external stimuli. Adapting to continuous waves of regulatory and legal changes during the nineteenth and twentieth centuries was highly problematic for *haichi* manufacturers, causing major upheavals, a great deal of unwelcome change to formulations and manufacturing methods, and the closure of many companies. However, it also proved productive by forcing the kinds of reorganisation and innovation necessary to maintain market footholds through periods of major socioeconomic and medical change. Standardised formulas, advanced production methods, and reliable quality control regimes are increasingly essential prerequisites to "pharmaceutical legitimacy" (Banerjee 2014) and thus to market success in contemporary Asia. Their adoption was crucial to the very survival of the *haichi* industry, let alone its continued vibrancy. Examples of the Toyama *haichi* industry's adaptability include the shift from dispersed to more centralised manufacture during the eighteenth and nineteenth centuries; the reformulation of medicines to include western ingredients and exclude banned substances during the nineteenth and twentieth centuries; and the standardisation of formulas, adoption of new product forms, and adaptation to GMP regulations during the twentieth century.

The latest phase of transformation has seen several of the larger *haichi* companies diversify their activities to include contract manufacturing of drug components and finished products for other pharmaceutical firms, as well as an increased focus on non-drug health and lifestyle products such as energy drinks and cosmetics. The latter development follows a pattern familiar in other Asian medical industries, where the diversification of product forms has allowed for new markets to be reached both at home and abroad, and considerable profits to be made while evading increasingly stringent regulations relating to drugs (Bode 2008; Banerjee 2009; Pordié 2015; Coderey and Pordié 2020; Chee, this volume; Kloos, this volume; Madhavan and Soman, this volume). What is less clear from the literature is the extent to which firms that started out producing herbal medicines in other parts of Asia have moved into CMO activities and the provision of specialised pharmaceutical services for the industry at large. Further research is required to establish why and how *haichi* manufacturing companies made these moves, and whether similar developments are taking place in other Asian medical industries.

We argue that as the *haichi* manufacturers negotiated the various phases of transformation described above, they carved out space for a new kind of industry to develop, for which labels such as "traditional" and "modern" hold little analytical value. In this context, such binary terms reflect essentialist notions of the purity, coherence, and boundedness of "medical systems," as well as implying inherent opposition and incompatibility between assumed modes of thought and practice. Such assumptions have very limited validity in the case of Toyama prefecture's pharmaceutical industry, hindering rather than helping efforts to understand its history and its current configuration. What actually occurred in Toyama is arguably better understood as the emergence of an evolving series of hybrid forms, perhaps constituting elements of an "alternative modernity" (Gaonkar 2001; Pordié and Gaudillière 2014: 4–5). The *haichi* companies did not simply adopt wholesale externally imposed ideas about how medicines should be formulated, produced, evaluated, or circulated, but rather engaged in ongoing dialectical processes involving a mixture of adaptation and resistance, alignment and divergence, continuity and innovation. This process did not result in a denuded, biomedicalised form of *haichi* medicine, but rather an inherently heterogeneous and innovative industry, drawing simultaneously upon its long history of herbal drug preparation and upon new technologies, methods, materials, and modes of organisation, albeit under varying degrees of choice and compulsion.

There is one key characteristic of the *haichi* industry that was crucial to this trajectory and sets it apart from the other Asian medical industries discussed in this volume. This is that the industry is founded in a particular mode of drug delivery and consumption, the *haichi* medicine sales system, rather than in a readily identifiable medical tradition with a specific set of texts, formularies, theories, and practitioners. Instead of being prescribed by practitioners following a textually delineated diagnostic process, as is usually the case in Kampo, Traditional Chinese Medicine, Ayurveda, or Sowa Rigpa, a broad selection of *haichi* medicines were delivered to homes and self-prescribed as needed, according to the symptomatic indications for each preparation. The medicines themselves have thus always been the core of the *haichi* system, with their prescription and consumption unmediated by physicians or clinical diagnostics. Furthermore, although many popular *haichi* medicines were based on well-known formulas with long histories, such as *Hangontan*, manufacturers did not use identical formulas to actually produce these medicines. Each manufacturer used their own version of these formulas and produced other medicines according to secret family recipes, as well as developing original formulations from time to time. These features arguably made the *haichi* industry more open to innovation at an earlier stage than its counterparts in India and Tibetan-speaking regions of Asia, where textually enshrined "classical" formulas were the mainstay of traditional pharmaceutical industries until the late twentieth century and remain crucial today (Bode 2008; Banerjee 2009; Craig 2012; Blaikie 2013; Pordié 2014; Kudlu, this volume; Madhavan and Soman, this volume).⁹ This openness is evident, for example, in the widespread development of new formulas by *haichi* companies during the nineteenth and twentieth centuries, and in the inclusion of components of Western origin in the majority of *haichi* medicines by 1935.

This latter practice of formulating entirely new hybrid medicines by combining *Wakanyaku* with Western chemicals is particularly striking, as we have not found any evidence of similar herbal-chemical combinations in other Asian medical industries. Further research into these practices would likely yield some very interesting results and is certainly required before any firm conclusions can be drawn concerning them. However, the available evidence allows us to posit the lack of singular bodies of medical theory, formulary texts, and practitioners in the *haichi* industry, the Meiji government's forceful preference for western medical knowledge and materials, as well as the centrality of the medicines themselves to the *haichi* sales system, as important contributing factors.

Taken together, the features described above support a view of *haichi* manufacturing as being a patent medicine industry from very early on, which contrasts in important ways with other Asian traditional medicine industries and opens up some interesting analytical perspectives. In particular, the process of pharmaceuticalisation appears to have been much less distinct and problematic than in other Asian cases. *Haichi* medicines did not have to be deracinated from a singular medical epistemology in order to be commercialised (cf. Banerjee 2009) because they were not deeply embedded to begin with and were understood as commercial products from the start. Pharmacy did not need to separate itself from the clinical realm of patient-healer dynamics in order to create a technologically, materially, and socially specific "reformulation regime" (Pordié and Gaudillière 2014) because there were no *haichi* physicians to begin with. There was no distinct, state-driven program of scientisation or integration with biomedicine to contend with either (cf. Chee, Kudlu, both in this volume), even though government policies were clearly shaped within this framework (Arai et al., this volume). Strictly speaking, *haichi* manufacture only became a patent medicine industry in the late nineteenth century with the introduction of official patents, but it had arguably adopted the form and approach of such

---

9 Stating that classical formulas remain central to the Ayurveda and Sowa Rigpa industries is not to suggest that they are produced in a uniform or standardised manner. Indeed, many of the references listed here mention considerable variation in the contents of classical formula-based medicines made by different manufacturers (see also Blaikie 2015, 2013; Kudlu 2016). Similarly, these references attest to a long history of innovation in the Indian "proprietary medicines" sector, while the contemporary "reformulation regime" in Ayurveda is highly dynamic (Pordié and Gaudillière 2014). We seek rather to underscore the absence of a core range of classical formulas identified with a single textual medical tradition in the *haichi* medicines industry, as well as the long history of broad product diversity and innovative formulation practices.

an industry from much earlier in its development. This meant there was no particularly stark or problematic shift from classical formulas to patent medicines, or from text-based and physician-led to pharmacy-based authority over formulation as seen elsewhere in Asia. The difficulties *haichi* companies faced mostly related to increasingly restrictive regulations, notably through successive changes to the Pharmaceutical Affairs Law and the introduction of GMP, as well as to falling market shares over recent decades. However, most companies found ways to adapt and continue their operations with help from state and academic collaborators. It is also remarkable that the distinctive *haichi* mode of drug delivery and consumption is currently being tested in Myanmar and Mongolia, and this key feature may end up having an enduring and beneficial impact beyond Japan, with or without the medicines themselves.

Bibliography

Banerjee M (2009) *Power, Knowledge, Medicine: Ayurvedic Pharmaceuticals at Home and in the World*. Hyderabad: Orient Blackswan.

Banerjee M (2014) "Contemporary Conversations between Ayurveda and Biomedicine: From Reformulating Drugs to Refashioning Parameters". *Asian Medicine* 9(1): 141–170.

Blaikie C (2013) "Currents of Tradition in Sowa Rigpa Pharmacy". *East Asian Science, Technology and Society* 7: 425–451.

Blaikie C (2015) "Wish-fulfilling Jewel Pills: Tibetan Medicines from Exclusivity to Ubiquity". *Anthropology & Medicine* 22(1): 7–22.

Bode M (2008) *Taking Traditional Knowledge to the Market: The Modern Image of the Ayurvedic and Unani Industry*. Hyderabad: Orient Blackswan.

Coderey C and Pordié L (eds) (2020) *Circulation and Governance of Asian Medicine*. London: Routledge.

Craig SR (2012) *Healing Elements: Efficacy and the Social Ecologies of Tibetan Medicine*. Berkeley: University of California Press.

Futaya T (2000) *Taishōki ni okeru Toyama Baiyakugyō no Seizaitōitsu to Seisankōzō no Hen'yō* (The Standardization of the Ingredients of a Medicine and the Change of the Structure of the Production of Medicines in Toyama in the Taisho Era). *Tochiseidoshigaku* 166: 19–36.

Futaya T (2017) *Kenkō to Iyaku* (Health and Medicine). In: Nakanishi S (ed) *Keizaishakai no Rekishi (History of Economic Society)*. Nagoya: Nagoya University Press, pp. 148–170.

Gaonkar D (ed) (2001) *Alternative Modernities*. Durham: Duke University Press.

Hokuriku Ginkō Chōsabu Hyakunenshi Hensanhan (1978) *Sōgyō Hyakunenshi (The Centenary History of Hokuriku Bank)*. Toyama: Hokuriku Bank.

Kateiyaku Shinbun no. 3442 (Household Medicine Newspaper) (2017a) Kateiyaku Shinbunsha (Household Medicine Newspaper Publisher), 5 April 2017.

Kateiyaku Shinbun no. 3453, (Household Medicine Newspaper) (2017b) Kateiyaku Shinbunsha (Household Medicine Newspaper Publisher), 25 July 2017.

Kateiyaku Shinbun no. 3464, (Household Medicine Newspaper) (2017c) Kateiyaku Shinbunsha (Household Medicine Newspaper Publisher), 5 Nov 2017.

Kateiyaku Shinbun no. 3465, (Household Medicine Newspaper) (2017d) Kateiyaku Shinbunsha (Household Medicine Newspaper Publisher), 15 Nov 2017.

Kateiyaku Shinbun no. 3466 (Household Medicine Newspaper) (2017e) Kateiyaku Shinbunsha (Household Medicine Newspaper Publisher), 25 Nov 2017.

Kateiyaku Shinbun no. 3470 (Household Medicine Newspaper) (2018a) Kateiyaku Shinbunsha (Household Medicine Newspaper Publisher), 1 Jan 2018.

Kateiyaku Shinbun no. 3479 (Household Medicine Newspaper) (2018b) Kateiyaku Shinbunsha (Household Medicine Newspaper Publisher), 25 Mar 2018.

Kateiyaku Shinbun no. 3486 (Household Medicine Newspaper) (2018c) Kateiyaku Shinbunsha (Household Medicine Newspaper Publisher), 5 Jun 2018.

Kateiyaku Shinbun no. 3487 (Household Medicine Newspaper) (2018d) Kateiyaku Shinbunsha (Household Medicine Newspaper Publisher), 15 Jun 2018.

Kokando Co., Ltd., *Heisei 15 nendo Eigyō Hōkokusho* (Business Report 2003) [Online]. Available at: http://www.Kokando.co.jp/wp-content/uplords/2015/02/H1504-1603ir.pdf

Kōseirōdōshō, Ministry of Health, Labour and Welfare (2016) *Koseirodohakusho* (White Paper on Health, Labour, and Welfare). Tokyo: Nikkei-Insatsu.

Kudlu C (2016) Keeping the Doctor in the Loop: Ayurvedic Pharmaceuticals in Kerala. *Anthropology and Medicine* 23(3): 275–294.

Lei SH-L (2014) *Neither Donkey nor Horse: Medicine in the Struggle over China's Modernity*. Chicago: University of Chicago Press.

Nihon Yakushi Gakkai (The Japanese Society for History Pharmacy) (2016) *Yakugakushijiten* (Encyclopaedia of Pharmaceutical History). Tokyo: Yakujinipposha.

Nishikawa T (2004) *Kusuri kara mita Nippon* (Japan from the Viewpoint of Medicine). Tokyo: Yakujinippōsha.

Noto K (2009) *Kōkōgyōshisū to Toyama-ken ni okeru Iyakuhin no Dōkō* (Industrial Index and Trends in Pharmaceuticals in Toyama Prefecture). Available from: http://www.pref.toyama.jp/sections/1015/ecm/back/2009jun/tokushu/index2.html

Pordié L (2014) Pervious Drugs: Making the Pharmaceutical Object in Techno-Ayurveda. *Asian Medicine* 9(1): 49–76.

Pordié L (2015) Hangover Free! The Social and Material Trajectories of PartySmart. *Anthropology & Medicine* 22(1): 34–48.

Pordié L and Gaudillière J-P (2014) Introduction: Industrial Ayurveda – Drug Discovery, Reformulation and the Market. *Asian Medicine* 9(1): 1–12.

Taylor K (2005) *Chinese Medicine in Early Communist China, 1945–63: A Medicine of Revolution*, London: Routledge.

Toyama-ken Iyakuhin Sangyō Kasseika Konwakai (Toyama Prefectural Committee for the Revitalisation of the Pharmaceutical Industry) (2014) *Kusuri no Toyama no saranaru Hiyaku ni mukete* (Steps toward Development of the Medicine Capital Toyama). Toyama: Toyama Prefecture.

Toyama-ken Kōseibu Kusuriseisakuka (Pharmaceutical Policy Division, Health and Welfare Department, Toyama Prefectural Government) (1990–2016) *Toyama-ken Yakuji Kōgyō Seisan Dōtai Tōkei Nenpō* (Annual Statistical Report on Production in Toyama Prefectural Pharmaceutical Industry). Toyama: Toyama Prefecture.

Toyama-ken Yakuji Kenkyūkai (Toyama Prefectural Pharmaceutical Affairs Research Society) (2015) *Toyama-ken Yakuji Kenkyūkai 60nen no Ayumi* (A 60 years History of Toyama Prefectural Pharmaceutical Affairs Research Society). Toyama: Toyama Prefectural Pharmaceutical Affairs Society.

Toyama-ken Yakuzaishikai Sōkai Hyakujyūichinenshi Hensan Iinkai (Editorial Committee for a 111 years History of Toyama Prefectural Pharmacist Society) (2001) *Toyama-ken Yakuzaishikai Sōkai Hyakujyūichinenshi* (111 years History of Toyama Prefectural Pharmacist Society). Toyama: Toyama Prefectural Pharmaceutical Society.

Toyama Prefecture (1983) *Toyama-ken Yakugyōshi, Shiryō Shūsei* (History of the Pharmaceutical Industry in Toyama Prefecture, Resource Collection). Toyama: Toyama Prefecture.

Toyama Prefecture (1987) *Toyama-ken Yakugyōshi, Tsūshi* (History of the Pharmaceutical Industry in Toyama Prefecture, Overall History). Toyama: Toyama Prefecture.

Toyama Prefectural Government (2011) Pharmaceutical Policy Division, Health and Welfare Department. *Pharmaceutical Industry in Toyama*. Toyama: Toyama Prefectural Government.

Uemura M (1959) *Gyōshōken to Ryōikikeizai* (Peddling Sphere and Economy of Feudal Lords). Kyoto: Minerubashobō.

Umemura M (2012) Reviving Tradition: Patients and the Shaping of Japan's Traditional Medicines Industry. In Penelope F and Hunter J (eds), *The Historical Consumer; Consumption and Everyday Life in Japan, 1850–2000*. London: Palgrave Macmillan, pp. 176–203.

Part II
South Asian medical industries

5 Globalising Ayurveda, branding India

Implications for the Ayurvedic pharmaceutical industry

Chithprabha Kudlu

Following the lead of Charles Leslie's pioneering work on Indian and other Asian medicines (Leslie 1969, 1976), studies of Asian medicine throughout the 1980s and 1990s focused on processes of modernisation in the context of medical pluralism, revealing a variety of configurations of national modernities. This approach soon came to be critiqued for treating heterogeneous medical systems as coherent epistemic systems, reifying their modern national identities (Langford 2002), and ignoring their fluid transnational histories (Alter 2005). It was only in the twentieth century that anti- and postcolonial nationalist movements throughout Asia redefined scholarly medical traditions as markers of national identity. Although these identities played a constitutive role in the modern biographies of Asian medicines, their symbolic power in constituting the modern nation gradually declined. While marginalisation within a biomedicine-dominated healthcare system was the cause for the decline in their political-economic power, their cultural symbolism appeared incongruent, and often antithetical to state regimes founded on scientific modernity.

Global attitudes towards traditional medicine began to change following the ethnobotanical discoveries of the 1970s. Fear of intellectual property appropriation from "big pharma" bioprospecting, combined with the emergence of a multi-billion-dollar global herbal supplement market, alerted newly liberalising Asian states to the revenue potential of traditional medicinal resources, knowledge, and practices (Pordié 2010), stimulating a revival of associated cultural nationalist symbolism. The emergence of the practice of nation branding in the late 1990s provided a legitimate global political and commercial space for the reinvention of the cultural nationalist identities of indigenous medicines.

The branded nation is qualitatively different from earlier forms of national imagining in that "the very idea of a viable nation" becomes "interlinked with the ability of the nation to enhance and realize its exchange value in the global circulation of capital" (Kaur and Wahlberg 2012: 577). The commercial practice of branding nations was an outcome of narratives of globalisation deployed at the end of the Cold War. It differs from other nationalist projects in that it is primarily "a commercial practice" which transforms

DOI: 10.4324/9781003218074-8

civic space into a calculative space dominated by marketing goals rather than social relations or governance. Consequently, it "selects, simplifies and deploys only those aspects of a nation's identity that enhances a nation's marketability" (Jansen 2008: 122).

Far from being unitary, national identities are forged through multi-layered and discrete representational practices. While marketability is a necessary criterion, anthropolgial and sociological analyses show that power acts as a key factor in determining which of the many representations get selected to constitute the nation brand (Dzenovska 2005; Kaneva 2011; Graan 2013). Given their symbolic value in constituting the national identity, cultural domains like cuisine, traditional medicine, and music came to be identified as soft-power resources to be exploited in the global market, in order to boost a nation's economic and political power. The ethnographic focus of nation branding studies has been largely limited to large-scale state-driven campaigns aimed at promoting the nation as a whole (e.g. Dzenovska 2005; Graan 2013). Studies of nation branding of specific culture-domains are few and far between, with the exception of cuisine. Less salient cultural domains like traditional medicine remain virtually unexplored.

The phenomenon of nation branding has also remained unexamined in Asian medicine literature, although attention has been paid to how national identities of Asian medicines are co-constituted by their transnational biographies (e.g. Zhan 2009; Pordié and Hardon 2015; Kloos 2017), Addressing the virtual absence of scholarly work on the relationship between Asian medicines and nation branding, this chapter explores Ayurveda's ongoing transformation into a global brand, with particular attention to implications for the Ayurvedic pharmaceutical industry. Besides calling attention to the emergence of Asian medical industries as one of the key domains for nation branding, I argue that nation branding has come to acquire a formative role in shaping the contemporary transnational identities of Asian medical industries. As Ayurveda increasingly perceives itself in global competition particularly with Chinese medicine, its case illustrates both the evolving relationship between Asian medicines and national identities, and the centrality of what Alter (2005) calls "transnational nationalisms" to the phenomenon of Asian medical industries more broadly.

Nation-branding efforts in the domain of Asian medicine are conceptualised and promoted by top-down, state-driven campaigns. The People's Republic of China (PRC) initiated an organised drive to promote traditional medicine in the late 1980s. China's thrust on scientisation as the means to promote the global expansion of Chinese medicine went on to influence policy and discourse of Indian medicine globalisation a decade later (Kudlu and Nichter 2019). Unlike Chinese medicine (Chee, this volume; Crozier 1970; Hsu 2008), indigenous medical traditions were sidelined in the healthcare policy of postcolonial India, until their global market potential was discovered in the mid-1990s (Islam 2017; Khalikova 2017b). A decade later, as national identity began to be recast as a global corporate

Globalising Ayurveda, branding India 141

brand identity to promote India as a tourist and investment destination (Kaur 2012), Ayurveda and yoga came to be officially designated as key soft-power resources to boost "Brand India" (Geary 2013; Edwards and Ramamurthy 2017).

While Ayurvedic globalisation has received some research attention (Banerjee 2004; Pordié 2010; Sujatha 2011; Bode and Payyapallimana 2013), the official marketing campaign and discourse surrounding Brand Ayurveda have gone unnoticed. Aiming to address this gap, this chapter begins by tracing Ayurveda's trajectory from a symbol of nationalism to a global brand, providing an overview of mainstream discourse – as circulating in media reports, academic publications, policy documents, and Ayurvedic conferences – surrounding Ayurvedic globalisation in India. In the second part of the chapter, this is complemented with ethnographic data on the commodification of Ayurveda in the southern Indian state of Kerala, collected between 2008 and 2012 (Kudlu 2013, 2016). Reviewing the historical role of national identity in Ayurveda's modernisation, I argue that the nation branding of Ayurveda in the global market constitutes a revival of cultural nationalist symbolism based on a Hindu national identity, with implications for the Indian system of medicines in general, and the Ayurvedic pharmaceutical industry in particular.

Besides expanding the understanding of the globalisation of Ayurvedic medicines in particular and Asian medicines in general, this analysis contributes to the emerging cross-disciplinary literature on nation branding. The emergence of nation-states as brand identities has been found to potentiate prevalent nationalist imaginations, enhancing their authority to subsume heterogeneous practices (Jansen 2008; Kaur and Wahlberg 2012; Graan 2013). I argue that by recasting Ayurveda as instrumental to promoting the nation as a brand, the state-mediated project of globalisation brings about a subtle but significant qualitative shift in the way the Ayurvedic pharmaceutical is imagined by its traditional stakeholders. Drawing insights from the literature on nation branding, I argue that the shift in the focus of Ayurvedic commodification from "nation building" to "nation branding" potentiates Ayurveda's cultural-nationalist identity at the cost of intrinsic lineage-based and regional variations.

Because the globalisation of Asian medicine has been driven largely by the global market for herbal supplements, standardisation pressures are higher on pharmaceuticals than on clinical protocols. Over the past decade, scholars studying Asian medicines have reported an increasing trend in pharmaceuticalisation (Adams 2002; Janes 2002; Hsu 2008; Pordié 2010; Pordié and Hardon 2015; Kloos 2017). However, Ayurveda had undergone significant pharmaceuticalisation prior to globalisation (Nichter 1989; Banerjee 2009). The industrialisation of Ayurvedic pharmaceuticals, initiated at a small scale from the late 1800s onwards, expanded fast and became well established by the 1970s. In the absence of state patronage, revenues from pharmaceutical sales had provided the founding capital for the modernisation and institutionalisation of Ayurveda (Leslie 1976, 1989). The Ayurvedic pharmaceutical sector today constitutes around 8667 registered manufacturers (Business Standard 2018) with an estimated turnover of 200 billion INR (3 billion USD), the vast bulk of which is generated through domestic sales. Despite the growing emphasis on the global market, exports actually account for only 15 percent of the total annual turnover (Economic Times 2018).

Besides intensifying the already prevalent trend of pharmaceuticalisation, globalisation also brought about significant qualitative changes. With Ayurveda being envisaged as a supplier to the global herbal supplements market, the entrepreneurial focus shifted from inward to outward. The pursuit of global marketability brought pressure to conform to global standards (Banerjee 2004; Pordié 2010). On this count, Ayurveda's experience is not different from that of other Asian medicines (see Arai et al.; Chee, this volume).[1] A more pronounced qualitative change arises from the policy push towards scientisation (Kudlu and Nichter 2019). Unlike Chinese medicine, which had undergone scientisation prior to globalisation, Ayurveda had preserved its distinct epistemological space, despite undergoing a certain degree of biomedicalisation (Banerjee 2004). The ideological shift in policy thus brought in expectations of standardisation that Ayurveda had hitherto never been subjected to (Banerjee 2004; Bode 2008, 2015; Madhavan 2009; Pordié 2010; Sujatha 2011; Kudlu and Nichter 2019).

Studies evaluating the impact of globalisation on Asian industrial medicines have largely approached the problem of standardisation as a product of scientisation, that is, prioritisation of a biomedicine-derived, evidence-based framework for evaluating safety and efficacy of pharmaceuticals (e.g. Adams 2002; Janes 2002; Craig and Adams 2008; Craig 2011; Banerjee 2013; Bode and Payyappallimana 2013). The centrality of this concern notwithstanding, I argue that the bulk of current pressures for standardisation on Ayurvedic medicines in the domestic sphere of practice and production emerge not from scientific modernity but rather from canonical Ayurveda. The imagination of Ayurveda as a single and coherent national medical system, with common canonical foundations, played a key role in providing the foundation for the professionalisation of Ayurveda in the 1970s. This imagination had its foundations in the Ayurvedic revivalist ideology that took shape in the early twentieth century, which valorised ancient texts over practices and effectively sidelined regional variations (Leslie 1969, 1976; Langford 2002). However, the goal of modernisation, of dissolving "multiple identities" to create "one Ayurveda" (Banerjee 2004: 89) had not been extended to discipline the manufacturing sector until the advent of globalisation.

---

1 The 2002 WHO Strategy for Traditional Medicine initiated the task of global harmonisation of regulatory regimes, carried forward by the 2014–2023 WHO Strategy for Traditional Medicine.

Public and policy discourse surrounding Ayurveda's globalisation today revolves around the issue of standardisation (or, more precisely, its lack), perceived to be the key stumbling block to Ayurveda's global future. Uniformity is imagined and valued as a natural virtue, a goal with origins in global market aspirations but increasingly internalised as a desirable end to achieve in the domestic market (Kudlu and Nichter 2019). This policy preoccupation with uniformity, I argue, is particularly inimical to classical medicines. Proprietary medicines being by definition distinct, standardisation demands would be restricted to batch-to-batch reliability in ingredient quality. Canon-based classical medicines,[2] on the other hand, can be theoretically expected to conform to uniform standards of drug composition and processing. In practice, products tend to vary widely, given inter-textual differences in drug composition, inter-regional variations in raw drug identities, processing methods, harvesting and pre-processing practices, and lineage-specific traditions (Blaikie 2015; Kudlu 2016).

Most ethnographic accounts of Asian industrial medicines, including Ayurveda, have focused on proprietary medicines (e.g. Nichter 1989; Banerjee 2009; Pordié and Gaudillière 2014; Pordié and Hardon 2015). Standardisation pressure on classical medicines has not been identified as a problem in itself. Although marginal in terms of profit share, the classical medicine industry is an integral part of the pan-Indian Ayurvedic therapy landscape. In an earlier paper (Kudlu 2016), I made a case for recognising the "alternative modernity" presented by industrially produced classical formulations. This alterity, I argue, is endangered by expectations to conform to standards of uniformity implicit in the imagination of Brand Ayurveda.

Providing a close examination of Indian medicine policy and the Ayurvedic pharmaceutical industry, this chapter reveals a gulf between policy discourses of standardisation and regulation on the one hand, and a ground reality of entrenched pluralism on the other. While the preoccupation with globalisation has expanded the state's role, as in the case of traditional medicine in China and Japan (see Chee; Arai et al., this volume), its regulatory power over the Ayurvedic industry has been limited owing to the historical dominance of the private sector. At the same time, increasing pressure towards rationalisation produced by the expansion of "regulatory globalization" (Kuo 2009) has enhanced the state's ideological power to set research and education agendas. This disjunction not only shapes the contemporary Ayurvedic industry in India but provides insights into some of the complexities of nation branding and transnational nationalisms in Asian medical industries more generally.

---

2 56 texts are officially approved as drug sources by the Indian Drugs and Cosmetics Act (DCA) 1940.

Revival of Ayurveda's cultural-nationalist symbolism

Ayurveda's "Indian" identity was forged during the early twentieth century as indigenous practitioners struggled to survive colonial delegitimisation. Leslie's (1969, 1976) pioneering studies showed how the evolution of modern Ayurveda was shaped by a medical revivalist ideology founded on European orientalism-inspired cultural nationalism. National leaders like Nehru and Gandhi were unreceptive to cultural nationalist ideologies, besides being sceptical of Ayurveda's scientific credentials. Nevertheless, they supported Ayurveda for its popularity and practical application, recognising it as culture rather than science (Langford 2002). Ayurveda's symbolic value that helped in forging a culturally unique, non-Western identity for the imagined Indian nation saw a sharp decline in post-independence India (Leslie 1989; Khan 2006). Practitioners' hopes of acquiring a better status failed to materialise, with the Nehruvian regime proving to be as unfriendly to traditional medicine (Khan 2006) as Republican China (Lei 2014). But unlike the latter, which attempted to ban Chinese medicine, India's federal democratic regime readily provided statutory legitimacy and relative autonomy to classical medical systems (Leslie 1969).

Organised practitioner resistance and the administrative constraints of healthcare were key factors that enabled the survival of both Chinese medicine (Lei 2014) and Ayurveda (Khan 2006). Chinese medicine practitioners had successfully used the economic nationalist cause to win allies in Republican China towards creating a "national medicine." Post-1950s, this plan was taken forward by the Maoist policy of healthcare integration, which combined the twin universalistic impulses of scientific modernity and cultural nationalism to formulate the "Project of Scientizing Chinese Medicine" towards the goal of creating a unified "Chinese medicine" (Lei 2014: 262–276). In India, on the other hand, biomedical professionals' vested interest in guarding their professional boundaries, combined with traditional medicine practitioners' resistance to an integrated healthcare model, led to the development of parallel spheres of practice and production (Langford 2002). Although Indian medical systems were granted legitimacy, with the ideology of science taking centre-stage in building "modern India," colonial healthcare policies favouring biomedicine continued.

Poor state patronage[3] eroded Ayurveda's public support base, turning into a backdoor for the practice of biomedicine (Leslie 1989). Although integral to the making of urban middle-class identity in parts of North India (Berger 2013), institutionalised Ayurveda had been largely inaccessible to the masses (Nichter 1989; Hardiman 2009), evident from poor popular knowledge of Ayurvedic concepts and products (Langford 2002;

---

3 Indian medical systems along with Homeopathy received less than 4 percent of the central health budget (Banerjee 2009).

Nisula 2006). A recent national survey of utilisation of Ayurvedic healthcare pegs the usage at a low of 6.9 percent (Rudra et al. 2017). Observing its marginal status in the daily lives of average Indians, Khalikova (2017a: 43) states that "Ayurveda simply did not exist as a constituent of Indian identity." The image of Ayurveda projected from India to the rest of the world was "often one more of shame than pride," observes American Ayurvedic practitioner-scholar Robert Svoboda. Unlike the Chinese diaspora, who patronised Chinese medicine, Indian immigrants were acutely embarrassed to associate themselves with Ayurveda, which was widely perceived as an obsolete field of endeavour (Svoboda 2008: 123).

The lost symbolic value of Ayurveda was rediscovered in the late 1990s, when the Indian state discovered the global market potential of traditional medicine. In 1995, a separate Department for Indian medicines was set up within the Central Health Ministry (later renamed AYUSH).[4] In 1999, the Planning Commission set up a Task Force to devise strategies to promote trade and conservation of medicinal plants. Underscoring India's potential to become a major player in the global herbal market, the Task Force Report observed that controlling the quality of raw materials, finished products, and processes is an "absolute necessity if one is to produce goods for world market" (Planning Commission 2000: 23). The first step towards regulating the Indian medicine industry came with the Good Manufacturing Practices (GMP) Guidelines in 2000. The first independent national policy on Indian medicine was formulated in the same year (see Banerjee 2004). The regulation of medicinal plants and manufacturing processes were primarily aimed at disciplining unruly pharmaceuticals to reduce "product variability," considered the key impediment to the global future of Ayurvedic pharmaceuticals.

Meanwhile, the broader project of economic globalisation was fast-unfolding in newly liberalising India. The 1990s, celebrated as a "decade of tourism" had opened India to new ideas of marketing, leading to the "Incredible India" campaign of 2002. An attempt to transform India into a globally competitive corporate brand was initiated in the mid-1990s by the Congress-led coalition government, with the establishment of the India Brand Equity Foundation in 1996. But the project sat on the back-burner until it was revived in 2002 by the new, right-wing Bharatiya Janata Party (BJP)-led coalition government. The idea of "Brand India" crystallised by 2004 and was primarily aimed at marketing India as an attractive destination for Foreign Direct Investment and tourism (Kaur 2012). Drawing on the orientalist symbolism of India as a spiritual destination, Ayurveda and yoga were designated as key soft-power resources to promote wellness

---

4 Ayurveda, Yoga and Naturopathy, Unani, Siddha, and Homeopathy, with Sowa Rigpa added in 2010.

tourism and to provide "credible competition" to China's hold over "the alternative lifestyle in the West" (Bagchi 2004).

Producing Brand India through Brand Ayurveda

Just as the global gaze accentuates the imagination of a universal "Indianness," it reinvigorates Ayurveda's cultural-nationalist symbolism in constituting the nation. "National identity, formulated as a brand, becomes a resource to be managed and developed by state and commercial projects alike," observes Graan (2013: 166). The symbolic power of cultural nationalist imaginaries formerly used for constructing a national solidarity vis-à-vis the colonial other is now used to bolster a commercial brand identity in the global market, which can then compete with other nation brands. Designated as "national heritage" to be exploited to serve India's global ambitions, Ayurveda has once again become a salient constitutive element in forging a national identity, albeit with the context shifted from a domestic healthcare space to transnational market space. Articles on Ayurveda in Indian science journals tend to follow a formulaic narrative beginning with a eulogy on Ayurveda's golden age, followed by a lament on its decline during Persian and colonial regimes, then ending with a hope of recovering Ayurveda's lost glory through globalisation (e.g. Dubey et al. 2004; Raj et al. 2011). The dream is not just to earn substantial revenues on the market but to be a "global leader." What is at stake is not just Ayurveda, but "Brand India." An undercurrent of anxious urgency pervades this narrative, with India being seen as having "a long way to catch up" with a highly successful China.

The shift in focus from nation building to nation branding has made the global market a key site for the construction of a "global Indianness" (Kaur 2012: 610). The emergence of nation states as brand identities potentiates prevalent nationalist imaginations (Jansen 2008; Kaur and Wahlberg 2012; Graan 2013), with cultural nationalistic ideologies playing a key role in the modernisation of Asian medicines across countries (Hsu and Barrett 2008). The nation branding of Ayurvedic medicines in western markets is particularly conducive to a revival of cultural nationalism, as Ayurveda's western career takes place within a predominantly medico-religious milieu, combined with meditation and yoga. Ayurveda's authenticity in the West is rooted in the European orientalist imagination of an ancient Hindu India, harking back to a mythical Aryan Vedic past (Reddy 2002; Smith and Wujastyk 2008). This makes Ayurveda a useful resource for resurgent right-wing cultural nationalist attempts of constructing a Hindu national identity as part of the project of promoting Brand India.

Although directed at a global audience, nation branding opens up a new space for politics in the domestic arena. The symbolic power derived from its global status is used to consolidate established structures of dominance and to counter internal challenges to state authority and national authenticity

(Graan 2013). As Ayurvedic stakeholders seek global markets for financial profits and legitimacy (Banerjee 2004), and policy goals of globalisation overtake domestic healthcare priorities (Sujatha 2011), the global market emerges as a key site for the construction of Ayurveda's identity.

In late 2014, signalling a marked policy change in favour of Indian medicine, the newly elected BJP-led government upgraded the AYUSH Department to the status of an independent ministry. For the Hindu nationalist ruling regime, the symbolism of yoga and Ayurveda serves its cultural nationalist agendas back home. Promoting Brand Ayurveda in the global market furthers the goal of constructing a Hindu identity for India. Official discourse on Ayurveda in the domestic context had long ignored other medical systems (i.e. Unani, Siddha, and Sowa Rigpa), while "appropriating heterogeneous herbal therapies under the umbrella of Ayurveda" in order to establish a link between "Ayurveda and Indian identity, constructing Ayurveda as a symbol of Indian civilization" (Khalikova 2017b).

Kaur and Wahlberg (2012: 576) argue that both Indian and Chinese nation branding projects strive to subordinate the unruly "internal other" using three languages of difference: subscribing to a global hierarchy of standardised indices; the commodification of essentialised national-cultural differences; and employing emotive assertions of alterity. While the branded nation strengthens already-dominant identities, it is considered qualitatively different from earlier nationalist imaginations as it strives to create a competitive market identity rather than a collective community (Jansen 2008). By packing political agendas of cultural nationalism within "forward looking" economic ventures, it provides a veneer of modernist glamour and respectability to projects hitherto deemed communal or parochial. While the yoga popularisation drive is ostensibly aimed at boosting India's soft power abroad, it has also been used to push the *hindutwa* (Hindu nationalist) agenda back home (Hindustan Times 2015), and standardising yoga protocols is considered a part of this strategy (Indian Express 2016).

Nation branding is a "monologic, hierarchical, reductive form of communication" (Jansen 2008: 134) intended to privilege one message and marginalise dissenting voices. At the same time, nation brand images also emerge as sites of popular contestation with the potential to be used for constructing alternative identities (Graan 2013). To counter yoga's *hindutwa* symbolism, Kerala's Marxist party staged a massive public yoga demonstration to promote a "non-religious, de-Hinduized, pure yoga" to develop "resistance to lifestyle diseases" (Basheer 2016). Realising the futility of opposing a globally reputed brand, it chose instead to emphasise yoga's secular credentials. In the Ayurvedic arena too, Kerala has been able to maintain its historic regional distinctiveness by establishing Kerala Ayurveda as a niche brand in the global market, capitalising on western tourist demand for Kerala-specific wellness therapies (see Abraham 2013; Madhavan 2013; Kudlu 2013, 2016). Kerala has also presented an alternatively modern model of Ayurvedic industrialisation, centred on supplying classical medicines to the clinic (Kudlu 2016; Madhavan and Soman, this volume).

Although nationalist attention to Ayurveda falls far short of yoga, its symbolic value as a representative of the "nation" is well recognised. In early 2016, the Minister for AYUSH made headlines for adding two categories to the growing list of "anti-national" activities: "Ayurvedic doctors who prescribe non-Ayurvedic medicines" and "biomedical doctors who advise patients not to take Ayurvedic medicines." Citing Ayurveda's global legitimacy, he asked, "how can anyone oppose a medical system that the world is showing interest [in]?" (Times of India 2016).

Ayurveda's value at home is clearly seen as derivative of its global value, while its global reputation is deployed to bolster its weak public image back home. However, Brand Ayurveda in the global market continues to be predominantly shaped by its transnational history, independent of Indian Ayurvedic policies and practices. Primarily reproduced as "Indian ethnomedicine" for western audiences (Reddy 2002), "Global Ayurveda" is constituted by plural practitioner-led paradigms dominated by a spiritualised approach to healthcare (Smith and Wujastyk 2008), in stark contrast with modern Ayurveda in India, which has embraced centralised standardisation emulating the biomedical template (Warrier 2008).

Pressures of scientific modernity

Inevitably, the lure of global markets comes with fears of intellectual property loss, resource scarcity, and delegitimisation. In the mid-1990s, western patents on neem and turmeric brought home the importance of guarding "national wealth" from "western bio-pirates" (Gaudillière 2014). The Planning Commission (2000) recommended the setting up of a National Medicinal Plant Board (NMPB) for conservation and cultivation of medicinal plants, and a Traditional Knowledge digital database (TKDL) as a defensive tool against patenting. Both plans were implemented in 2001, a year that turned out to be eventful for Ayurveda as it also saw the drafting of the first national policy on Indian medicine and a bill on intellectual property (see Banerjee 2004, 2009).

In the same year, Ayurveda also appeared in the UK's list of "unscientific traditional medicines," which triggered the birth of the "World Ayurveda Congress" (WAC). The WAC was conceptualised as an advocacy forum meant to "to unite all concerned parties ... to offer robust scientific support" to defend Ayurveda in anticipation of "impending European legislation to bar Ayurveda from the continent" (WAC n.d.). Another major blow to Ayurveda's global reputation was dealt by reports of heavy metal residues in exported medicines (Saper et al. 2004), leading to the tightening of regulatory regimes across western countries (Banerjee 2004). Though sections of the Ayurvedic community alleged conspiracy (e.g. AMAM 2005), in the collective national introspection that followed, the finger of blame pointed firmly inward.

The perceived urgency to safeguard Ayurveda from biopiracy and delegitimisation catapulted the project of scientific translation to the centre stage, with ethnopharmacology emerging as the focal discipline (see Pordié 2010). Paradoxically, institutionalised modern Indian Ayurveda has been found unwilling to cater to western expectations of spiritual-holistic Ayurveda (Warrier 2008).[5] Despite its centrality to the Indian cultural nationalist agenda both at home and abroad, the policy approach to Ayurvedic globalisation is centred on scientisation (Bode 2008; Banerjee 2009; Sujatha 2011; Madhavan 2013). Ethnobotanists, ethnopharmacologists, and allied scientists who advocate a science-based approach have become influential in shaping official and public discourse on Ayurveda, as well as in setting policy agendas. Poor standardisation is considered the primary culprit for Ayurveda's poor global performance. The responsibility of making Ayurveda globally respectable and saleable is placed squarely on the shoulders of Ayurvedic pharmaceutical companies. More precisely, the blame for poor global performance is attributed to the failure of these companies to adapt to modern standards of production (Kudlu and Nichter 2019; Madhavan and Soman, this volume).

Several forums like the WAC have come up since mid-2000s, forging a motley community of stakeholders who periodically come together to organise grand Ayurvedic conferences, aptly dubbed "epistemic carnivals" by Cohen (1995). There are few conferences on Ayurveda today that do not carry the prefix "global" or "world." Globalisation was the primary focus of six of the seven conferences I participated in between 2008 and 2016. The division of labour observed by Cohen (1995) between "big rooms" and "small rooms" persists, but on a different axis. "Big rooms" feature high-profile speakers, including modern scientists, pharmaceutical and herbal industry proprietors, "progressive" Ayurvedic manufacturers, and western CAM practitioners. Besides setting the tone of the conference, "big room" talks help in conveying Ayurveda's "global value" to home audiences. Scientific presentations by Ayurvedic professionals are relegated to "small rooms," where individual career aspirations combine with "big room" agendas, steering the research focus steadily towards scientific validation, particularly concerning Ayurvedic pharmaceuticals (see Pordié 2010: 57–58).

Over the past decade, speakers gathering together in these conference carnivals have produced a collective discourse aimed at integrating Ayurveda in the global market. Furthermore, the refrain of "poor standardization hindering Ayurveda's global potential" has entered public discourse via media reports of such conferences. Ayurvedic manufacturers' conservative attitudes, inadequate standardisation, poor investment in scientific research, or poor quality of production are commonly identified hurdles in Ayurveda's

---

5 A similar conflict between Western spiritualised forms and scientised mainland practice has been observed in the context of Chinese medicine in the United States (Furth 2011).

global career (Kudlu 2013; Kudlu and Nichter 2019). Feature articles and op-eds in business and pharma sections of reputed periodicals air public statements and solicited opinions of scientists heading state research institutions, stakeholders from biomedical and herbal product industries, R&D scientists, and marketing managers from large Ayurveda companies.

These new stakeholders, who were formerly not associated with Ayurveda, have become default spokespersons of Ayurveda's progress (e.g., Dogra 2006; Jagdale 2007; Sharma 2008). Their opinions and assessments regularly feed into public discourse through the media. Take, for example, an article on the Ayurvedic industry in the pharma section of a leading national daily (Sharma 2008). Based on the opinions of modern herbal industry stalwarts and Ayurvedic marketing professionals, the article identifies the lack of standardisation of products as the root cause for Ayurveda's poor global success. The respondents pin the blame of low-quality drugs on the "high level of fragmentation in the market" and the presence of "too many small and localized players [who] damage the reputation of the entire industry as a whole." Advocating standardisation, quality control mechanisms and investment in modern research, they locate the "lack of adequate scientific data" as a key hindrance to the progress of the industry.

Ayurveda's experience with globalisation and the discourse that followed foreshadows the developments the nation as a whole would confront a decade later. Kaur's (2012) insightful analysis of Brand India campaigns shows how in the late 2000s, resistance to farm land acquisition and corruption scandals had similarly created an "anxiety of negative publicity" to Brand India. The "public and collective introspection" blamed India's failure to realise its global potential on an "old India" out of sync with times (615). Kaur invokes the trope of "two nations" to capture the "tension between a nation that is in harmony with the markets, and its other, which continues to resist the same" (619). The "sense of urgency" to salvage the image of Brand India that motivated corporate activists to join forces with the anti-corruption mobilisation (617) was, in the context of Ayurveda, directed towards standardisation and scientisation.

The current BJP-led government's professed Hindutwa ideology has not led to an approach more sympathetic to Ayurvedic ethos and epistemology. Six conferences after the founding of WAC, there has been little change in policy rhetoric surrounding Ayurveda's globalisation. The title of the government's press release on the proceedings of the 6th WAC reads, "Government to push for standardisation in Ayurvedic drug production: AYUSH to lead Brand India thrust in global Pharma." Expressing regret for "missing the bus," the Health Minister states, "It is a pity that China has captured such a huge share of the world market whereas India's presence is nonexistent. We are determined to develop Brand India through Ayurveda" (PIB 2014).

In early 2016, inaugurating the "Vision Conclave" of the Global Ayurveda Festival in Kerala, Prime Minister Narendra Modi urged the Ayurvedic community to focus on translation research. "The truth is bitter," he said, "The fault is not Ayurveda's, but of the *ayurvedawallahs* who have failed to translate their science into modern language." The blame for the failure to replicate the Chinese model was squarely laid at the door of the Ayurvedic community, ignoring vast differences between them in state patronage. Hailing the Prime Minister as an inspiration for an "Ayurveda revolution," the Minister of Science and Technology proclaimed with pride, "Now Ayurveda has been recognised by the WHO... We have the protocols ready to propagate Ayurveda globally... We are pretty sure we can show the way to rest of the world."

The constant presence of "the world" as a patronising and legitimising authority in the everyday imagination of Ayurveda carries with it an implicit and invisible rationalising power. This process is best captured by the concept of "worlding" formulated by Mei Zhan (2009) to describe the transnational processes by which TCM is constituted. Not only are actors, ingredients, knowledge, and technologies assembled from different places, the very identities of Asian medicines are produced through translocal encounters and entanglements, as they strive to comply with international quality standards, biodiversity protocols, and consumer demands.

The policy rhetoric's failure to acknowledge Ayurveda's epistemological distinctiveness suggests an internalisation of global hierarchy of value associated with scientific modernity (Kudlu and Nichter 2019: 125–128). I argue that global market demand for scientific modernity combined with its ability to reinvigorate the cultural nationalist symbolism of Ayurveda in western markets creates an ideal climate for the coming together of two opposing ideologies, comparable to the emergence of Maoist healthcare integration policy in the PRC (Lei 2014). The conflict between the two ideologies, manifest in the struggle between *misra* Ayurvedists (integrationists) and *shuddha* Ayurvedists (purists) has shaped the evolution of Ayurveda in independent India. However, as Langford (2002: 111) points out, both had been united in their desire to adapt the modern institutional structure to create a uniform national identity for Ayurveda: "both are national signs, the first relying on the ideological seductiveness of cultural authenticity and the second on the ideological seductiveness of modernity."

The purist worldview (advocating Ayurvedic exclusivity) that had dominated Ayurvedic policy up to the 1970s was officially marginalised in 1977,[6] after the centralisation of the Ayurvedic curriculum under the Central Medical Council of India. Although biomedical instruction was included in the Ayurvedic curriculum, rather than leading to an integrated system of healthcare, it has produced a system best described as "medical parallelism" (Wolfgram 2009), characterised by "conceptual bilingualism" (Naraindas

---

6 By this time, student protests had already forced the inclusion of introductory biomedical instruction in many Ayurvedic colleges (Langford 2002).

2006: 2659). While scientific modernist ideology has dominated healthcare policy and state research approach to Indian medicine, its organising influence on Ayurvedic clinical practice and industry has been limited. As mentioned earlier, Ayurvedic practice and production flourished in the private sector relatively free of the universalising pressures of both cultural nationalist and scientific modernist ideologies, leading to the proliferation of multiple/alternative/vernacular modernities (Hardiman and Mukharji 2012; Pordié and Gaudillière 2014; Kudlu 2016).

The discovery of Ayurveda's global economic value, I argue, creates conditions similar to the colonial era, as it brings Ayurveda once again face to face with the "western other." In the colonial context, Ayurvedic practitioners had struggled to meet western standards for escaping delegitimisation. In the postcolonial context, the influential and lucrative western medical markets are actively sought by Ayurvedic industrial stakeholders as a source of legitimacy (Banerjee 2004). The encounter with "cultural others" and the need to build a unique brand identity revived a cultural nationalist symbolism of Ayurveda, while at the same time subjecting it to pressures of scientific modernity. As in the colonial context, Ayurveda's economic value to the state is primarily derivative of its extractive value. If the colonial state's interest was to extract useful botanical substitutes to reduce the cost of European medicine exports (Mukharji 2009), today Ayurveda is seen as a supplier of pharmaceuticals to the global market (Banerjee 2004).

Noteworthy to both the contexts is also the survival of an alternative discourse of economic nationalism. In the colonial era, despite nationalist leaders' allegiance to biomedicine and distrust in Ayurveda's scientific credentials (see Langford 2002: 108–109), practitioners had exploited cultural nationalist sentiments to promote the consumption of Ayurvedic medicines in opposition to western medicine, riding on the bandwagon of the *swadeshi* movement. Such nationalist tropes continued to be part of Ayurvedic marketing strategies post-independence (Langford 2002; Bode 2008). The global context provides for a reinvention of *swadeshi* "firmly embedded in neoliberal modernity, nationalism and the-more-the-better consumerism" and "invoking the principles of self-reliance and self-sufficiency" (Khalikova 2017b: 110–114). This development has to be understood in the context of the structural transition in the global medical landscape. The shift in the global health order towards a neoliberal ideology of self-care, Hsu (2008) points out, is increasingly shaping the landscape of Asian medicine, driving it towards consumerist pharmaceutical-centric commercialisation.

National uniformity for a global future

The perceived necessity to create a standard Indian Ayurveda for the global market has led to discourses that privilege uniformity over diversity. Goals of global marketability have generated a slew of standardisation programs, creating templates of "Good Practices" to cover the entire gamut of traditional medicine practice and production, including manufacturing, clinical practice, collection, and cultivation practices (Arai et al., this volume). Standard setting in these domains tends to be based on Ayurvedic classical text-based templates that are correlated, validated, or aligned with bio-scientific measures.

In the early twentieth-century struggle to portray Ayurveda as secular and scientific, medical revivalists adopted the orientalist narrative of an ancient scientism, followed by a medieval process of "sacrilization," to be corrected by a project of "secularization" (Leslie 1976). As ancient Sanskrit texts were valorised, intervening centuries of practice, regional variations, innovations, and fruitful exchanges with other healing practices were overlooked (Langford 2002). Founded on this reinvented classical framework, the centralised professionalisation of Ayurveda in the late 1970s led to the sidelining of non-mainstream textual and non-textual traditions (Cleetus 2007; Hardiman 2009). But as noted earlier, in the absence of state patronage, Ayurvedic modernisation was largely driven by bottom-up forces of marketisation (Crozier 1970; Leslie 1989), leading to a heterogeneous landscape of pharmaceutical production dominated by an unorganised sector, inhabited by a variety of stakeholders including large corporates, physician-owned companies and physician co-operatives (Bode 2008: 49; Abraham 2013; Kudlu 2013, 2016).

As mentioned earlier, classical Ayurvedic medicines vary in composition from text to text and also due to regional variations in raw drug identities, variations in methods of pre-processing and processing (Kudlu 2013). In the mainstream discourses on Indian Ayurveda, such diversity in pharmaceutical products and practices is seen as the primary stumbling block to the global success of Ayurveda (Kudlu and Nichter, 2019). According to the Planning Commission (2000: 107), "the single most important factor which is standing in the way of wider acceptance of drugs based on medicinal plants is non-availability or inadequacy of standards to check or test the quality by modern instrumental methods." This report underscored the need to speed up the development of pharmacopeia standards because "countries like China have gone ahead and have captured a major share of global export market. India cannot wait" (108). Poor quality of production was attributed to irregularities in medicinal plant trade and to industries "managed on traditional ethos and practices" (17).

This condescending attitude towards collectors underlies official discourse and regulatory approaches towards the quality control of medicinal plants. As studies of raw drug supply chains in this volume show, such approaches are mired in misconceptions that are incongruent with the complex social and material reality of collection, trade, and production. The top-down perspective assumes a linear flow, failing to grasp the diversity of horizontal flows and the intricate webs of social relationships that facilitate them (see Dejouhanet and Sreelakshmy; van der Valk, this volume;

cf. Kudlu 2013). Combined with a failure to comprehend the needs of the small-scale Ayurvedic industry, this led to the failure of India's first Ayurvedic industrial cluster (Madhavan and Soman, this volume).

In mainstream Ayurvedic discourse today, achieving national uniformity of medicines and clinical protocols is presented as an obvious and inevitable goal. A brief vignette from a panel discussion I observed at the Global Ayurvedic Festival held in Calicut, Kerala in 2016, will illustrate the point. The session entitled "Pan-Indian Clinical Practices" was the first of its kind I had come across in my eight years of field experience. Presentations in conference sessions tend to be dominated by academic presentations on clinical trials, pharmacognostic studies, pharmacological standards, and other such translational research; little room is provided to doctors to present clinical case studies. This session, featuring four doctors hailing from different parts of the country, was chaired by the Director of Kerala's Ayurvedic Medical Education, a former State Ayurvedic Drug Controller I had interviewed multiple times during the period of my fieldwork. Disregarding the theme of the session, each of them went on to present an experience-based account of clinical practices. The first presented a detailed account of Bengal-specific Ayurvedic practices; the second presented an elaborate typology of inter-practitioner differences in southern Karnataka; and the third described diagnostic protocols developed by state-run medical colleges of Andhra Pradesh.

This joyous celebration of regional particularism was interrupted by the last speaker, a young doctor from Kerala, who began his speech by lamenting the "lack of standards" in Ayurvedic practice. After extolling at length on the distinctness of Kerala Ayurveda and the heterogeneity of Keralan medicines, clinical protocols, and therapies, he called attention to the need to bring "unity in diversity." Sharing his experiences as a member of a national working group on harmonising clinical protocols, he stated it was a Herculean task to undertake, but it was the "need of the times." While he clarified that standardised protocols were not expected to replace classical practice, he said it was to be mandatorily included in the Ayurvedic curriculum and instituted in primary health clinics. Interestingly, however, while belabouring the need and urgency of standardisation, his speech was peppered with repeated references to the superiority of Ayurveda's individualistic epistemology, betraying an underlying anxiety about contravening Ayurvedic principles by imposing uniform standards.

This ambivalence found its culmination in the concluding remarks by the chair. A visibly moved Dr. T. Sivadasan said it was the first time he had encountered such a vibrant inter-state exchange on clinical practices, which he hoped would become a norm in future conferences. Contrasting Ayurveda's variability with biomedicine's uniformity, he stated, "uniqueness is the beauty of Ayurveda, that is *my* belief." Making it doubly clear it was his "personal view," he stated apologetically that he could not elaborate

Globalising Ayurveda, branding India

on standardisation as it was a "sophisticated concept" and he had not "studied it well enough." While such standards could be theoretically conceptualised, it was difficult to implement them on the ground, he said. For that matter, even standardisation of drugs was incomplete and "even Kerala's educated class" was reluctant to take Ayurvedic medicines, he said, owing to a perception of them being "not at all standard." He concluded by ambiguously stating that he agreed with his junior colleague that they had "miles to travel" before "educating the rest of the world."

Although uncomfortable with the idea of disciplining Ayurveda's natural diversity, Dr. Sivadasan found it difficult to disagree with what was presented as the zeitgeist. Outsider orientation has evidently caused a subtle shift in the way Ayurveda is being imagined. Constantly fed by the globalising discourse, the average Ayurvedic practitioner is beginning to become conscious of the mismatch between neat imaginations of Ayurveda as a cohesive "medical system" and its messy lived practices. In a recent workshop on standardising Ayurvedic medicines, the vice president of Kerala's largest practitioner body stated that while it was important to create standards to export, "having a common standard in the country would help the industry at least in its domestic market" (Nambudiri 2016).

What had begun as a response to the global market has clearly attained a life of its own: the construction of a uniform Ayurveda that had begun as a program to meet an imagined global future had gradually evolved to be an implicit goal for domestic practice. With the global hierarchy of value associated with scientific modernity becoming internalised in the Ayurvedic discourse, uniformity and universality were beginning to be considered naturally superior to heterogeneity and localness.

Discourse vs market realities

Policy and public discourse on Ayurvedic globalisation have been preoccupied with standardisation for over a decade and a half now, but it is important to note that little of this talk has translated into regulatory action. The only significant regulatory step thus far, GMP, was implemented in a highly relaxed fashion, in contrast to the rushed and stringent implementation in China (Saxer 2012). Though mandatory since 2003, it took over a decade to bring two-thirds of Indian medicine manufacturers into the GMP compliance net. Interactions with drug control department officials revealed that considerable flexibility was shown to accommodate the constraints faced by small manufacturers. As of 2015, around 80–85 percent of manufacturing units were reportedly GMP compliant, but no step has been taken to close non-complying units.[7]

---

7 "AYUSH in India Reports" of the AYUSH Department (2004–2005 to 2014–2015).

Moreover, Ayurveda's path to GMP has been relatively free of the epistemological conflicts described elsewhere (e.g. Craig 2011). The focus has been mainly on creating hygienic storage and processing environments and instituting batch-wise documentation and quality testing. Manufacturers continue to follow in-house production protocols, while state pharmacopeia and formularies are not considered binding. As Banerjee (2002) notes, GMP have also been sensitive to system-specific requirements. In fact, a recent AYUSH-commissioned report recommends that the exemption given to Ayurvedic doctors and hospitals be extended to artisanal units focused exclusively on supplying medicines to Ayurvedic doctors (Chandra 2011: 246–247). Moreover, inter-country variability in standards is common, given that GMP guidelines provide for flexibility in adaptation. Even in countries such as China and Japan, which are stringent in enforcing GMP, regulations have been tuned to meet the needs and constraints of the industry in the domestic market (see Chee; Arai et al., this volume). Observing the wide variation between GMP standards in different countries, Saxer (2012: 499) points out that "although GMP bears all the marks of a global form, it is important to stress that it is neither Western nor an international standard."

Heavy metal testing was made mandatory for exports in 2006, but no attempt has been made to extend this to domestic products, implicitly acknowledging cost constraints (in the case of herbal products) and epistemological incompatibility with the biomedical concept of safety (in the case of herbo-mineral products, Banerjee 2013). During the course of this study, I witnessed two important regulatory policies shelved: the Clinical Trials Draft Bill 2008 and Kerala Ayurveda Health Centres Ordinance 2007. Both met with fierce resistance, the former from Indian medicine manufacturers across the country and the latter from Ayurvedic hospital owners in Kerala. Interviews with stakeholders revealed that in both cases, apprehensions boiled down to two issues: cost concerns for small manufacturers and hospital owners, and problems arising from the imposition of biomedical regulatory templates. Stakeholders argue that such regulatory policies create a double whammy: while laying obstacles in the path of genuine Ayurvedic professionals, they ease access to unscrupulous profiteers backed by big capital.

In implicit acknowledgement of the irrelevance of imposing blanket global standards on domestic players, the policy regime has gradually shifted towards voluntary certification schemes. In 2009, accreditation schemes were announced for AYUSH products[8] and services in collaboration with the Quality Council of India and the National Accreditation Board for Hospitals, respectively. In 2011, standards for Good Agricultural Practices (GAP) and Good Field Collection Practices (GFCP) were announced. After years of soft-pedalling the clinical trial bill, in 2013, the AYUSH department

---

8   AYUSH Standard for Indian market; premium mark for international markets.

came up with Good Clinical Practice guidelines (Shankar 2013). None of these standards are mandatory as yet.

The national pharmacopeia and formularies produced by the state are not binding on the industry, which continues to rely on in-house standards. Even among standard setters, there is an unspoken deference to traditional variability. Banerjee (2009: 98–99) observes "the translation project" of the Ayurvedic Formulary as embodying "a struggle between the sheer diversity in manufacturing practices of the old and the new," with constant references to "age-old practices faithfully reproduced from the texts and a reference to variations in large-scale manufacture." The lack of clarity and silences on critical aspects like efficacy and quality control inadvertently end up "demonstrating the reality of the existence of diversity and ambiguity in manufacturing methods."

In 2010, the AYUSH ministry published a draft gazette notification adding three new categories of proprietary medicines: Ayurvedic supplements, Ayurvedic cosmetics, and Ayurvedic extracts. An amendment was made to drug licensing conditions for proprietary medicines, making it mandatory to supply evidence of safety and efficacy based on clinical trials, but only if the medicines claimed to treat new indications or were presented in forms absent in classical texts. While a section of the industry welcomed this as a progressive move, including the manufacturers association from the State of Karnataka (Kudlu 2013), the Ayurvedic Drug Manufacturers of India questioned the rationale of including extracts and supplements under AYUSH regulations, ruing the failure of policymakers to follow a consultative process when formulating drug regulatory policies (Shirodkar 2010). In early 2018, giving in to pressure from a section of the industry, the government issued clarification withdrawing the clinical trial requirement. The policy change was justified as a move to facilitate the growth of the industry, citing inordinate delays in issuing drug licenses owing to the lack of adequate facilities for conducting clinical trials. Nevertheless, the move received considerable bad press for rescinding on its earlier commitment to strengthening the regulatory framework in order to improve the global competitiveness of the Indian medicine industry (e.g. Chandna 2018; Smitha 2019).

Thus, while the mainstream discourse on Ayurvedic globalisation continues to be preoccupied with standardisation, the state has followed a soft path to regulation. Another regulatory move that the government attempted to push hard, the Access and Benefit Sharing Notification of 2014, has also met with stiff opposition from Indian medicine practitioners and industry bodies, who have taken the government to court contesting its legality (Nautiyal 2016). Clearly, the state's approach to regulation falls far short of the totalising narrative projected by the policy discourse.

Meanwhile, some stakeholders have begun to grumble about "talk not translating into action." While genuine acknowledgment of sector-specific cost and epistemological constraints is one of the factors behind this inaction, another factor is the state's inability to impose unilateral policies on a powerful private sector – for better or for worse, depending on the perspective of each stakeholder. AYUSH insiders who demand better regulation see the state's unwillingness "to put money where the mouth is" as the primary constraint. Some interviewed manufacturers pointed out that the state's commitment to regulatory infrastructure falls far short of its interest in selling Ayurveda to outsiders. A recent investigative report by a national media group provides substantiation to their claims. Over 60 percent of officially recognised Ayurveda and Unani colleges and hospitals were found to be running in abysmal conditions, without meeting basic regulatory stipulations with regard to infrastructure and trained faculty. Many colleges had no functional hospitals and were graduating doctors without any clinical exposure (Pandey 2018).

While the BJP-led regime's nationalistic enthusiasm has generated a mood of hopeful optimism, there are already serious misgivings arising about the conspicuous mismatch between promised and actual budgetary allocations for the National AYUSH Mission (Ghosh 2015); the absence of Indian medicines in the 2015–2020 Foreign Trade Policy (Sharma 2015); and the government's reluctance to implement the Central Quality Control Scheme designed to strengthen regulatory frameworks and facilitate AYUSH exports (Shirodkar 2015). The chairman of the Kerala Ayurvedic industrial cluster complained that none of their suggestions were considered and "no proactive step was taken by the minister despite repeated representations" (Kunnathoor 2015).

Media reports of project announcements and budgetary promises by the state tend to be little more than political announcements intended to create media hype. After every budget announcement, reports flood the media creating a gung-ho narrative, highlighting percentage increases over previous years, while the proportion of the total health budget allocated to all the six AYUSH systems together has remained stagnant at around three percent. Inadequacy of funding has been flagged as a matter of prime concern by none other than the central minister for AYUSH (The Hindu Business Line 2019), and this issue was also raised in a parliamentary debate in July 2019 (TOI 2019).

It is common for projects to remain on paper or even be dropped mid-way due to inadequate budgetary allocation (Bode and Shankar 2017). The BJP-led government, re-elected for a second term in May 2019, continues to reassert its Hindu identity and to keep its core electoral constituency pleased with periodic announcements of schemes on Ayurveda. Its defaulting on these schemes often remains unreported or unnoticed, given the marginality of the Indian medicine sector.

State bureaucracy and the established Ayurvedic pharmaceutical industry

Early market trends indicate that the difference between global and local market logic is implicitly or explicitly recognised by entrepreneurs, who use the strategy of diversification to balance their global ambitions with domestic market stakes. In terms of their attitude towards globalisation, Ayurvedic manufacturers lie at various points on the continuum between "progressives" advocating aggressive modernisation, and "conservatives" who adhere to traditional practices (e.g. Kamath 2008). Of the leading Ayurvedic companies, manufacturers like Dabur and Charak advocate a progressive approach, whereas most of the large Kerala-based manufacturers tend towards conservatism (Abraham 2013; Kudlu 2013, 2016).

Classical-focused manufacturers desirous of exploiting global opportunities follow the tried and tested strategy of product diversification. Not only are separate product portfolios diligently maintained, production facilities too are segregated to prevent the traditional and the modern impinging on each other, both literally and figuratively. Traditional kitchen-factories continue to coexist with ultra-modern WHO-GMP factories (see Bode 2008: 123). Coimbatore-based Arya Vaidya Pharmacy makes this distinction clear on its website.

> In Kanjikode factory we are manufacturing traditional Kerala type medicines in the traditional way of processing (all classical forms including new forms). In our second factory at Thennalipuram we are manufacturing only proprietary medicines (syrup, hard gelatine capsules, granules, hair oil, cream, ointments and Ayurvedic transparent soap). Now we have started …a new factory as per WHO-GMP specifications …
>
> (AVP, n.d.)

Given vast differences in global and domestic consumption contexts, pragmatic-minded manufacturers find little reason to apply the standards of one market to the other. The distinction between the two markets is well expressed by Mr. Jayesh Chaudhary, the MD of Mumbai-based Vedic Life Sciences, a leading contract research organisation for nutraceuticals and herbal medicines:

> The West does not understand Ayurveda but we keep harping on Ayurvedic medicines. These classes of goods do not exist in the West… Indian marketers would be better off first getting a presence in the existing segments of dietary supplements, functional foods and herbal personal care products and then build a new segment like Ayurveda… Leading Ayurvedic houses must either shed their traditional ideologies or be content with a domestic market… India's indigenous medicine manufacturers have to cater to the price-sensitive domestic healthcare needs, whereas for global compliance, we need to follow international guidelines. With no compromises, we can formulate a separate set of regulations to accommodate the realities of overseas and domestic markets. This way exports can develop without blocking access of the Indian consumer to affordable traditional medicine.
>
> (Chaudhary 2008)

Mr. Chaudhary sees no contradiction between domestic and global market standards. Recognising them to be mutually irrelevant, he advises the industry to diversify its product strategies. Policies that seek to streamline the domestic Ayurvedic market to meet an imagined future in the global market appear to be uninformed by this pragmatic market knowledge. The recent AYUSH Department Task Force notes, "While international standards for GMP have been prescribed by WHO for herbal medicines, the AYUSH regulation is still short of international standards like GMP...therefore AYUSH products are not globally competitive" (AYUSH 2015: 17).

Thus, the Ayurvedic pharmaceutical market displays increasing heterogeneity in forms, formulations, and trajectories, in line with the findings of recent studies of Asian industrial medicines (Blaikie 2015; Bode 2015; Pordié 2015; Pordié and Hardon 2015). A quick glance at Ayurvedic entrepreneurial strategies indicates a dissonance between pragmatic logics of practice and the ideals that dominate policy discourse. The imagined conflict between domestic and global standards that dominates Ayurvedic discourse comes across as being starkly incongruous with the ground reality. Inadequate standardisation of production in the domestic market, widely held responsible for Ayurveda's lacklustre global career, appears to have little bearing on their global ventures.

Although the Chinese medicine industry appears to be no less heterogeneous than India's (Zhan 2009), since the 1980s it has been subjected to significant centralised standardisation, reducing regional diversity (Wang et al. 2016). For socialist countries like China, the transformative change in the era of globalisation was brought about by marketisation. Traditional medicines hitherto well-patronised by the state were forced to undergo a fast-paced market expansion to meet global demands (Janes 2002; Hsu 2008). The differential impact of State patronage and regulatory policies on the modernisation paths of Asian medical industries is illustrated by several contributions to this volume (Arai et al.; Blaikie and Craig; Futaya and Blaikie; Kloos). Of particular relevance is the study by Blaikie and Craig, which shows that while lack of state recognition and support adversely affects Nepal's Sowa Rigpa cottage industry, it also grants pharmacists a large degree of freedom over the scale, mode, and orientation of medicine production.

In the case of Ayurveda, an increase in state intervention was the most noteworthy of globalisation's impacts. As observed earlier, in the absence of state patronage, Ayurveda had to rely on the pharmaceutical market for survival. Ayurvedic modernisation was largely led by practitioner-entrepreneurs who had ventured into the modern marketplace by scaling up and adapting their own family/lineage traditions to meet the demands of mass production (Bode 2008; Banerjee 2009; Madhavan 2013; Kudlu 2016). As a result, the Indian state's bureaucratic power over the industry was limited. By the time state pharmacopeia standards began to emerge, in-house production protocols had become far too entrenched (see Bode 2008: 49).

Ayurveda's combative attitude towards biomedicine, in contrast to the biomedicine-friendly path followed by Chinese medicine during modernisation (Banerjee 2004), made it less vulnerable to biomedicalisation (Pordié and Gaudilliere 2014). When the winds of globalisation began to blow, Ayurveda already had a robust private sector that was anxious to preserve its established stakes in the domestic market, even as it dreamed of a global future. The state's interest in regulating the Ayurvedic industry to serve its global market ambitions had to contend with a century-old private sector industry whose "market logic" (Bode 2008) was strongly tied to the domestic market. Despite the hype surrounding the global market, the share of exports in the turnover of Indian medicine has remained stagnant at 10 percent over a decade and a half (cf. Kamboj 2000; Sharma 2008, 2015). From a modern business perspective, the "conservative and fragmented" nature of this market is one of the biggest hurdles to Ayurveda's globalisation (see Sharma 2008, 2015).

In appraising state power, it is important to make a distinction between "state as a bureaucratic apparatus" and "the state as producer of ideology" (Janes 2002: 274). In contrast to state-patronised Asian medicines like Chinese medicine (Crozier 1970), Ayurveda has sustained itself without state support for over a century. Dependence on the pharmaceutical market for sustenance created a robust private sector not easily amenable to bureaucratisation. As of today, state ideology on Ayurvedic standardisation is slow to translate to reality, given its limited bureaucratic power. But with the spread of "regulatory globalization" (Kuo 2015), informal channels of medicine flow are increasingly restricted and centralised regulatory barriers tend to augment the role of nation states as mediators (e.g. Meier zu Biesen 2017).

Consequently, India's policy on Ayurveda, with its skewed focus on globalisation (Sujatha 2011), has visibly expanded the state's influence as a producer of ideology. This power is not always directly visible in regulatory policy, but it acts unobtrusively through research and training policies which play an important role in shaping collective imagination. With the power to set research and education agendas, the state wields significant influence in shaping the collective imagination. There are some indications that the state's relentless focus on globalisation has led to the internalisation of the "global hierarchy of value" (Herzfeld 2004) of scientific modernity. Ayurvedic commodities and services circulating within Ayurveda's traditional sociotechnical networks are subject to top-down pressures of rationalisation, even when no deliberate attempt is made to target the global market. Such processes are less likely to be visible as they may not show overt signs of globalisation or scientisation.

At the same time, Ayurveda, like other Asian medicines in the global market, is split by a Cartesian mind-body dichotomy between "physiologized" and "spiritualized" markets (Hsu 2008). The discussion in this chapter has been limited to the state-driven discourse of scientisation, as the focus of the analysis was the Ayurvedic pharmaceutical industry. A study of Ayurveda in transnational locations would have to pay attention to "the nationalness," that is, "the symbolic, nonterritorial linkage between a product and its nation in the context of commodities disconnected from the country of origin" (Ng and Skotnicky 2016), as well as to the various interactions and conflicts between the dominant spiritualised model of transnational Brand Ayurveda and the state-driven project of scientisation centred on the global pharmaceutical market.

Conclusion: Discourse, reality, and imagined global futures

Besides shaping the global destinies of medical traditions, nation branding has the potential to reinvigorate cultural-national identities of Asian medicines in their countries of origin. By potentiating Ayurveda's cultural-national identity, the global gaze creates a climate conducive to the realisation of one of the central but incomplete projects of Ayurvedic modernisation, namely the construction of "Indian Ayurveda." Nation-branding Ayurveda does not entail concrete processes distinguishable from the economic objective of the state's globalisation project, but by reinvigorating the cultural nationalist identity central to the construction of modern Ayurveda, it enhances its ideological power to subjugate heterogeneous practices. This is visible in an increased emphasis on standard-setting both in Ayurveda's domestic and global policies, which I argue owes to the coming together of two hitherto divergent universalising discourses of cultural nationalism and scientific modernity.

In the mainstream discourse surrounding Ayurvedic globalisation, there is an increasing concern with inadequate standardisation. In the domestic sphere, the Indianness of Ayurvedic medicines and services circulating within their customary sociotechnical networks was taken for granted; an imagined collective national identity had been superimposed on Ayurveda's pluralistic milieu without generating any perceptible contradiction. Nation-labeling for the global market engenders a self-conscious cross-examination of domestic Ayurvedic practices and products with the benchmark of nation-based uniformity, laying a fertile ground for discordance between idealistic imaginations of a classical text-based Indian Ayurveda and the disorderly habitus of practiced Ayurveda. In other words, discrepancies between multiple versions of Ayurveda that had remained inconspicuous in its domestic commodity life are rendered explicit and problematic in the context of its imagined global future.

However, a review of Indian medicine policies and trends in the Ayurvedic pharmaceutical industry indicates that the totalising specter projected by the state-driven mainstream discourse on globalisation is not borne out by developments on the ground. Presenting an overview of Ayurvedic regulatory regimes and entrepreneurial strategies, I have called attention to the dissonance between global imaginations and ground realities. The commodity career of Ayurveda has evolved over a century catering to domestic clientele, making it resistant to radical shifts in product strategies. The amenability of Asian medical traditions to top-down processes of globalisation is differently shaped by their particular histories of modernisation. If the most transformative of globalisation's impacts for state-driven Chinese medicine was privatisation and pharmaceuticalisation (Farquhar 1996; Hsu 2008), for a market-driven system like Ayurveda, it was expansion in state power (see Banerjee 2004).

There is a possibility that the policy makers' inability to differentiate between domestic and global market demands and constraints could lead to the restructuring of domestic Ayurvedic production to meet global standards, with far-reaching consequences to Ayurveda's traditional stakeholders (Madhavan and Soman, this volume). Theoretically, it is possible to envisage a pragmatic policy that promotes the globalisation agenda without losing sight of Ayurveda's practical and epistemological particularities. In other words, the local and global futures of Ayurvedic pharmaceuticals may not necessarily be at odds today, but imagining them to be so can actually produce the contradiction. Whether and to what extent nation branding impacts Ayurveda's domestic market trajectory depends on the extent of control state-generated processes are able to garner over an Ayurvedic milieu hitherto largely built by bottom-up processes. This in turn would be partly contingent on regulatory regimes in the global market and partly on the relative strength of global and domestic market forces.

Bibliography

Abraham L (2013) From Vaidyam to Kerala Ayurveda. *IIAS Newsletter* 65: 32–33.
Adams V (2002) Randomized Controlled Crime Postcolonial Sciences in Alternative Medicine Research. *Social Studies of Science* 32(5–6): 659–690.
Alter J (ed) (2005) *Asian Medicine and Globalization*. Philadephia: University of Pennsylvania Press.
AMAM (2005) President's Message. *Ayurvedic Heritage* 1(3): 1.
Appadurai A (1996) *Modernity at Large: Cultural Dimensions of Globalization*. Minneapolis: University of Minnesota Press.
AVP (n.d.) www.avpAyurveda.com
AYUSH (2015) *Final Report of the AYUSH Department Task Force*. New Delhi: Govt. of India.
Bagchi I (2004) Minting cultural currency. *India Today*. http://indiatoday.intoday.in/story/mea-mandarins-repackage-brand-india-promote-indian-food-music-films-yoga-tourism-it/1/196143.html
Banerjee M (2002) Power, Culture and Medicine: Ayurvedic Pharmaceuticals in the Modern Market. *Contributions to Indian Sociology* 36(3): 435–467.
Banerjee M (2004) Local Knowledge for World Market: Globalizing Ayurveda. *Economic and Political Weekly* XXXIX(I): 89–93.
Banerjee M (2009) *Power, Knowledge, Medicine: Ayurvedic Pharmaceuticals at Home and in the World*. New Delhi: Orient Blackswan.

Banerjee M (2013) Politics of Knowledge in the Debates on Toxicity in Ayurvedic Medicines. *Asian Medicine* 8(1): 153–179.

Basheer, K (2016). A "Marxist" version to counter "Hindutva" yoga? *The Hindu Business Line*. http://www.thehindubusinessline.com/news/national/a-marxist-version-to-counter-hindutva-yoga/article8065364.ece

Berger R (2013) *Ayurveda Made Modern: Political Histories of Indigenous Medicine in North India, 1900–1955*. London: Palgrave Macmillan.

Blaikie C (2015) Wish-fulfilling Jewel Pills: Tibetan Medicines from Exclusivity to Ubiquity. *Anthropology and Medicine* 22(1): 7–22.

Bode M (2008) *Taking Traditional Knowledge to the Market*. New Delhi: Orient Longman.

Bode M (2015) Assembling Cyavanaprash, Ayurveda's Best-Selling Medicine. *Anthropology and Medicine* 22(1): 23–33.

Bode M and Payyapallimana U (2013) Evidence-based Traditional Medicine: For Whom and to What End? *eJournal of Indian Medicine* 6(1): 1–20.

Bode M and Shankar P (2017) Ayurvedic College Education, Reifying Biomedicine and the Need for Reflexivity. *Anthropology and Medicine*. DOI:10.1080/13648470. 2017.1287258

Business Standard (2018) 8667 licensed pharmacies and 55 licensed laboratories in private and cooperative sectors in the country for providing quality AYUSH drugs, https://www.business-standard.com/article/news-cm/8667-licensed-pharmacies-and-55-licensed-laboratories-in-private-and-cooperative-sectors-in-the-country-for-providing-quality-aysuh-drugs-118010100277_1.html

Chandna H (2018) Modi govt's love for Ayurveda may be undermining ancient medicinal system. *The Print*, 14 Dec 2018.

Chandra S (2011) *Report on the Status of Indian Medicine*. New Delhi: Department of AYUSH.

Chaudhary J (2008) Running the Export Marathon. *Express Pharma* Feb: 16–29.

Cleetus B (2007) Subaltern Medicine and Social Mobility: The Experience of the Ezhava in Kerala. *Indian Anthropologist* 37(1): 147–172.

Cohen L (1995) The Epistemological Carnival. In: Bates D (ed) *Knowledge and the Scholarly Medical Traditions*. Cambridge: Cambridge University Press, pp. 320–343.

Craig SR (2011) "Good" Manufacturing by Whose Standards? Remaking Concepts of Quality, Safety, and Value in the Production of Tibetan Medicines. *Anthropological Quarterly* 84(2): 331–378.

Crozier R (1970) Medicine, Modernization, and Cultural Crisis in China and India. *Comparative Studies in Society and History* 12(3): 275–291.

Dogra S (2006) Breaking barriers. *Express Pharma*. http://www.expresspharmaonline.co m/20080831/market01.shtml

Dubey NK, Kumar R and Tripathi P (2004) Global Promotion of Herbal Medicine: India's Opportunity. *Current Science* 86(1): 37–41.

Dzenovska D (2005) Remaking the Nation of Latvia: Anthropological Perspectives on Nation Branding. *Place Branding* 1: 173–186.

Economic Times (2018) AYUSH Ministry aims to triple market share of its medicines and services. https://economictimes.indiatimes.com/industry/healthcare/biotech/healthcare/ayush-ministry-aims-to-triple-market-share-of-its-medicines-services/articleshow/66476239.cms?from=mdr

Edwards L and Ramamurthy A (2017) (In)credible India? A Critical Analysis of India's Nation Branding. *Communication, Culture and Critique* 10: 322–343.

Farquhar J (1996) Market Magic: Getting Rich and Getting Personal in Medicine after Mao. *American Ethnologist* 23(2): 239–257.

Furth C (2011) The AMS/Paterson Lecture: Becoming Alternative? Modern Transformations of Chinese Medicine in China and in the United States. *Canadian Bulletin of Medical History* 28(1): 5–41.

Gaudillière J-P (2014) An Indian Path to Biocapital? The Traditional Knowledge Digital Library, Drug Patents, and the Reformulation Regime of Contemporary Ayurveda. *East Asian Science, Technology and Society* 8(4): 391–415.

Geary D (2013) Incredible India in a Global Age: The Cultural Politics of Image Branding in Tourism. *Tourist Studies* 13(1): 36–61.

Ghosh A (2015) AYUSH department in a fix as government squeezes fund. *Indian Express*, 21 April.

Graan A (2013) Counterfeiting the Nation? Skopje 2014 and the Politics of Nation Branding in Macedonia. *Cultural Anthropology* 28(1): 161–179.

Hardiman D (2009) Indian Medical Indigeneity: From Nationalist Assertion to the Global Market. *Social History* 34(3): 263–283.

Hardiman D and Mukharji PB (2012) Introduction. In: Hardiman D and Mukharji PB (ed) *Medical Marginality in South Asia: Situating Subaltern Therapeutics*. London: Routledge, pp. 2–35.

Herzfeld M (2004) *The Body Impolitic: Artisans and Artifice in the Global Hierarchy of Value*. Chicago: University of Chicago Press.

Hindustan Times (2015) India's soft power? Cultural nationalism? Or Hindutva push? The many views on Yoga day. http://www.hindustantimes.com/india/india-s-soft-power-cultural-nationalism-or-hindutva-push-the-many-views-on-yoga-day/story-eqtlR1hJT6mLKJBFrtIZhM.html

Hsu E (2002) The Medicine from China has Rapid Effects: Chinese Medicine Patients in Tanzania. *Anthropology and Medicine* 93: 291–313.

Hsu E (2008) The History of Chinese Medicine in the Peoples Republic of China and its Globalization. *East Asian Science, Technology and Society* 2(4): 465–484.

Hsu E and Barrett RL (2008) Traditional Asian Medical Systems. *International Encyclopedia of Public Health* 6: 349–357.

Indian Express (2016) UGC writes to varsities: Govt's "yoga protocol" says chant "om", opposition protests. http://indianexpress.com/article/india/india-news-india/ugc-writes-to-varsities-on-yoga-day-govts-yoga-protocol-says-chant-om-opposition-protests-2806086/

Islam N (2017) *Chinese and Indian Medicine Today: Branding Asia*. Singapore: Springer.

Jagdale S (2007) Call for a Change. *Express Pharma*. http://www.expresspharmaonline.co m/20080831/market01.shtml

Janes C (2002) Buddhism, Science, and Market: The Globalization of Tibetan Medicine. *Anthropology and Medicine* 9(3): 267–289.

Jansen SC (2008) Designer nations: Neo-liberal Nation Branding – Brand Estonia. *Social Identities* 14(1): 121–142.

Kamath G (2008) Trouble brewing: Ayurveda is caught between the purist and the experimenter. *Businessworld*. http://www.businessworld.in/index.php/Miscellaneous/Trouble-Brewing

Kamboj VP (2000) Herbal Medicine. *Current Science* 78(1): 5–39.

Kaneva N (2011) Nation Branding: Toward an Agenda for Critical Research. *International Journal of Communication* 5: 25.

Kaur R (2012) Nations Two Bodies: Rethinking the Idea of "New" India and its Other. *Third World Quarterly* 33(4): 603–621.

Kaur R and Wahlberg A (2012) Governing Difference in India and China: An Introduction. *Third World Quarterly* 33(4): 573–580.

Khalikova V (2017a) *Institutionalized Alternative Medicine in North India: Plurality, Legitimacy and Nationalist Discourses.* PhD Dissertation, University of Pittsburgh.

Khalikova V (2017b) The Ayurveda of Baba Ramdev: Biomoral Consumerism, National Duty and the Biopolitics of "Homegrown" Medicine in India. *South Asia: Journal of South Asian Studies* 40(1): 105–122.

Khan S (2006) Systems of Medicine and Nationalist Discourse in India: Towards "New Horizons" in Medical Anthropology and History. *Social Science and Medicine* 62(11): 2786–2797.

Kloos S (2017) The Pharmaceutical Assemblage: Rethinking Sowa Rigpa and the Herbal Pharmaceutical Industry in Asia. *Current Anthropology* 58(6): 693–717.

Kudlu C (2013) *Brand Kerala: Commodification of Open Source Ayurveda.* PhD Dissertation, Washington University in St. Louis.

Kudlu C (2016) Keeping the Doctor in the Loop: Ayurvedic Pharmaceuticals in Kerala. *Anthropology and Medicine* 23(3): 275–294.

Kudlu C and Nichter M (2019) Indian Imaginaries of Chinese Success in the Global Herbal Medicine Market: A Critical Assessment. *Asian Medicine* 14: 104–144.

Kunnathoor P (2015) Displeasure growing among Ayurveda community in Kerala over delay in considering their demands by AYUSH Ministry. www.pharmabiz.com

Kuo W-H (2009) The Voice on the Bridge: Taiwan's Regulatory Engagement with Global Pharmaceuticals. *East Asian Science, Technology and Society* 3(1): 51–72.

Kuo W-H (2015) Promoting Chinese Herbal Drugs Through Regulatory Globalization. *Asian Medicine* 10(2): 316–339.

Langford J (2002) *Fluent Bodies: Ayurvedic Remedies for Postcolonial Imbalance.* Durham: Duke University Press.

Langwick S (2010) From Non-aligned Medicines to Market-based Herbals: China's Relationship to the Shifting Politics of Traditional Medicine in Tanzania. *Medical Anthropology* 29(1): 15–43.

Lei SH-L (2014) *Neither Donkey nor Horse: Medicine in the Struggle over China's Modernity.* Chicago: University of Chicago Press.

Leslie C (1969) Modern India's Ancient Medicine. *Society* 6(8): 46–55.

Leslie C (ed) (1976) *Asian Medical Systems: A Comparative Study.* Berkeley: University of California Press.

Leslie C (1989) Indigenous Pharmaceuticals, the Capitalist World System and Civilization. *Kroeber Anthropological Society Papers* 69–70: 23–31.

Madhavan H (2009) Commercializing Traditional Medicine: Ayurvedic Manufacturing in Kerala. *Economic and Political Weekly* 44(16): 44–51.

Madhavan H (2013) Revisiting the Kerala Ayurvedic Sector: Towards a Pharmaceutical Vicious Circle? *IASTAM Newsletter* 65: 32–34.

Meier zu Biesen C (2017) From Coastal to Global: The Transnational Flow of Ayurveda and its Relevance or Indo-African Linkages. *Global Public Health.* //dx.doi.org/10.1080/17441692.2017.1281328

Mukharji PB (2009) Pharmacology, "Indigenous Knowledge", Nationalism: A Few Words from the Epitaph of Subaltern Science. In: Pati B and Harrison M (ed) *The Social History of Health and Medicine in Colonial India.* New York: Routledge, pp. 195–212.

Nambudiri S (2016) Efforts on to standardize Ayurveda. *Times of India*. http://timesofindia.indiatimes.com/life-style/health-fitness/health-news/Efforts-on-to-standardize-Ayurveda/articleshow/51087837.cms

Naraindas H (2006) Of Spineless Babies and Folic Acid: Evidence and Efficacy in Biomedicine and Ayurvedic Medicine. *Social Science and Medicine* 62(11): 2658–2669.

Nautiyal S. (2016) Case related to ABS non-compliance to come up for hearing soon at Nagpur bench of Bombay HC. www.pharmabiz.com

Ng KH and Skotnicky T (2016) "That British Sound": Talk of Nationalness in Global Capitalism. *Signs and Society* 4(1): 1–29.

Nichter M (1989) Pharmaceuticals, Health Commodification and Social Relations: Ramifications for Primary Health Care. In: Nichter M (ed) *Anthropology and International Health: South Asian Case Studies*. Dordrecht: Kluwer Academic Publishers, pp. 233–277.

Nisula T (2006) In the Presence of Biomedicine: Ayurveda, Medical Integration and Health Seeking in Mysore, South India. *Anthropology and Medicine* 13(3): 207–224.

Pande T (2018) The Big Debate: Time to fix alternative medicine mess via operation Ayurveda, CNN-IBN, April 20. https://www.news18.com/videos/india/the-big-debate-time-to-fix-alternative-medicine-mess-via-operation-ayurveda-1724833.html

PIB (2014) Government to push for standardization in Ayurvedic drug production. pib.nic.in/newsite/PrintRelease.aspx?relid=111136

Planning Commission (2000) *Report of the Task Force on Conservation and Sustainable Use of Medicinal Plants*. New Delhi: Planning Commission of India.

Pordié L (2010) The Politics of Therapeutic Evaluation in Asian Medicine. *Economic and Political Weekly*, 45(18): 57–64.

Pordié L (2015) Hangover Free! The Social and Material Trajectories of Party-Smart. *Anthropology and Medicine* 22(1): 34–48.

Pordié L and Gaudillière J-P (2014) The Reformulation Regime in Drug Discovery. *East Asian Science, Technology and Society* 8(1): 57–79.

Pordié L and Hardon A (2015) Drugs' Stories and Itineraries: On the Making of Asian Industrial Medicines. *Anthropology and Medicine* 22(1): 1–6.

Raj S, Karthikeyan S and Gothandam KM (2011) Ayurveda – A Glance. *Research in Plant Biology* 1(1): 1–14.

Reddy S (2002) Asian Medicine in America: The Ayurvedic Case. *The Annals of the American Academy of Political and Social Science* 583(1): 97–121.

Rudra S, Kalra A, Kumar A and Joe W (2017) Utilization of Alternative Systems of Medicine as Health Care Services in India: Evidence on AYUSH Care from NSS 2014. *PloS One* 12(5): e0176916.

Saper RB, Kales SN, Paquin J, et al. (2004) Heavy Metal Content of Ayurvedic Herbal Medicine Products. *Journal of the American Medical Association* 292(23): 2868–2873.

Saxer M (2012) A Goat's Head on a Sheep's Body? Manufacturing Good Practices for Tibetan Medicine. *Medical Anthropology* 31(6): 497–513.

Shankar R (2013) AYUSH Dept. issues good clinical practice guidelines. www.pharmabiz.com

Sharma U (2008) Transforming Ayurveda. *Express Pharma*. www.expresspharmaonline.co m/20080831/market01.shtml

Sharma U (2015) Reviving AYUSH. *Financial Express*. http://www.financialexpress.com/pharma/cover-story/reviving-ayush/88919/

Shirodkar SN (2010) ADMA seeks clarification on Rule 158 (B) treating herbal extracts as Ayurvedic drugs. www.pharmabiz.com, Oct. 5.

Shirodkar SN (2015) AYUSH sector concerned over delay in implementing central scheme for quality control of drugs. www.pharmabiz.com

Smith F and Wujastyk D (2008) Introduction. In: Wujastyk D and Smith F (ed) *Modern and Global Ayurveda: Pluralism and Paradigms.* New York: SUNY Press, pp. 1–28.

Smitha N (2019) A disservice to Ayurveda. *Deccan Chronicle*, 19 July.

Sujatha V (2011) What could Integrative Medicine Mean? *JAIM* 2(3): 115.

Svoboda R (2008) The Ayurvedic Disapora: A Personal Account. In: Wujastyk D and Smith F (ed) *Modern and Global Ayurveda: Pluralism and Paradigms.* New York: SUNY Press, pp. 117–128.

The Hindu Business Line (2019) AYUSH Ministry rues inadequate funding, 18 July.

Times of India (2016) Doctors prescribing non-ayurvedic medicines are anti-national. http://timesofindia.indiatimes.com/city/kolhapur/Doctors-prescribing-non-Ayurvedic-medicines-are-anti-national/articleshow/52058067.cms

Times of India (2019) Rajya Sabha members ask for more fund allocation for AYUSH, 15 July.

WAC (n.d.) www.ayurworld.org/wac

Wang J, Guo Y, and Li GL (2016) Current Status of Standardization of Traditional Chinese Medicine in China. *Evidence-Based Complementary and Alternative Medicine* http://dx.doi.org/10.1155/2016/9123103

Warrier M (2008) Seekership, Spirituality and Self-discovery: Ayurveda Trainees in Britain. *Asian Medicine* 4(2): 423–451.

Wolfgram M (2009) *Ayurveda in the Age of Biomedicine: Discursive Asymmetries and Counter-Strategies.* PhD Dissertation, University of Michigan.

Zhan M (2009) *Other-worldly: Making Chinese Medicine through Transnational Frames.* Durham: Duke University Press.

6 Industry dynamics and clustering in Ayurvedic pharmaceutical production in South India
The case of CARe Keralam

Harilal Madhavan and Sajitha Soman

Amidst optimistic projections of continuous growth and development for the Indian Ayurveda industry, debates over processes of institutionalisation, pharmaceuticalisation, and public health mainstreaming remain widespread and contentious. A good amount of research exists today on the transformation of Indian indigenous medicines into modern health products for the middle class and the reshaping of pharmaceutical practices under the banner of globalisation. Studies on topics such as the anti-colonial struggle and the beginnings of commercialisation (Bala 1992; Panikkar 1992; Kumar 1998, 2001; Madhavan 2008), the emergence of the Ayurveda industry and its increasing prominence in policy frameworks (Abraham 2009; Banerjee 2009), regional growth and dynamics (Bode 2008; Islam 2008; Madhavan 2009; Kudlu 2016), and processes of standardisation, biomedicalisation, and customisation (Naraindas 2006; Banerjee 2008; Pordié 2010; Sujatha and Abraham 2012) have informed us in great detail about Ayurveda's historical trajectory, its contemporary status and the challenges it is facing. Further studies have explored Ayurveda's changing form and content in the global market (Reddy 2002), the factors influencing its degree of commercialisation (Patwardhan et al. 2005), and the government's responses to Ayurvedic mass production (Banerjee 2009). One insight all these studies have in common is that it is impossible to fully understand the Ayurveda industry without considering the various manifestations of raw material sourcing activities, production processes, and marketing practices at both state and local levels.

Taking the case of Kerala, the South Indian state most associated with Ayurveda and its industry, this chapter examines the Confederation of Ayurvedic Renaissance – Keralam Limited (henceforth CARe Keralam), a recently initiated industrial cluster for promoting the mass production and export of Ayurvedic medicines. This public-private partnership was developed within a nationwide context of mainstreaming indigenous medicines into public health delivery, aiming to provide common-use facilities for cooperative learning, collaborative technological upgradation and joint capacity building to small and medium enterprises (SME). It highlights the global trajectory of the Ayurveda industry, which, in common with the wider

DOI: 10.4324/9781003218074-9

Asian medicine industry, increasingly seeks to cater to a larger demand outside its original geographical area. The idea behind CARe Keralam was closely aligned with the cluster concept, which refers to geographic concentrations of interconnected companies, specialised suppliers, service providers, related industries, and associated institutions (like standards agencies and trade associations) in a particular field, which compete but also cooperate with one another while benefitting from location-specific externalities (Belleflamme et al. 2000: 159; Porter 2000: 15). Clusters have been widely promoted at the policy level in developing countries to help SME overcome growth constraints and compete with larger or more advanced players, mainly by facilitating innovation, generating regional networks, fostering collective efficiency, and generally upgrading the value chain (Humphrey 1995; Schmitz 1997; Gereffi 1999; Schmitz and Nadvi 1999; Humphrey and Schmitz 2000; Bair and Gereffi 2001; Guerrieri and Pietrobelli 2004; Giuliani et al. 2005).

Despite the indubitable benefits of clusters in general and the promising beginnings of CARe Keralam in particular, this cluster failed to make a significant impact on Kerala's Ayurveda industry. Documenting CARe Keralam's trajectory as an illustrative case of the complexities of mass production in Ayurveda, with implications that extend far beyond its immediate context, this chapter argues that the cluster's underperformance can be explained by two main factors. The first lies in the structure of the Ayurveda industry itself, particularly the parallel reliance of small firms on the low-profit classical medicines sector and large companies on more profitable non-classical flagship products, as well as its dependence on long-established, trust-based raw material sourcing mechanisms. The second factor concerns rigidities in the institutional political economy, including financial sourcing patterns in related sectors like medicinal plants and tourism. By not adequately taking these two factors into account, a critical minimum push in terms of the cluster's coverage and growth could not be achieved and the scheme failed to reach its stated goals.

While this case offers important policy lessons in the context of Ayurveda and India more broadly, particularly by demonstrating the need for regionally customised promotion strategies, it also provides critical insights into the social, political, and economic factors shaping the development of other Asian medical industries. The story of CARe Keralam reflects many pertinent characteristics of Asian medical industries today, including localised pharmaceutical development efforts, the role of governance structures, and the incompatibilities raised by nation-branding exercises (see Arai et al.; Campinas; Chee; Futaya and Blaikie; Kudlu, this volume). It also highlights some interesting specificities concerning this particular industrial regime, such as the role of complex cooperative raw material collection systems, public-private relations at multiple levels of production and questions of sustained public funding in Ayurvedic drug research, among other issues. By forcing us to grapple with the often messy details of how local, regional, national, and transnational elements of pharmaceutical assemblages articulate with one another (Kloos 2017), this example enriches discussions concerning the major challenges that Asian medical industries are confronting in their contemporary phases of emergence and development.

The policy framework: Markets and clusters

The development of CARe Keralam's cluster strategy took place in the context of – and partly contributed to – two major paradigm shifts in India: the changing national policy framework regarding Indian medicines and a general industrial context of increasing corporatisation. The Eleventh (2007–2012) and Twelfth (2012–2017) Five Year Plans (FYP) of India contained extensive policy strategies that aimed for the mainstreaming of Indian medical systems in order to improve public healthcare delivery, health promotion, and disease prevention. Mainstreaming was to be accomplished at the primary level by providing training to AYUSH (Ayurveda, Yoga and Naturopathy, Unani, Siddha, and Homeopathy)[1] practitioners in primary care and national health programs; at the secondary level by establishing AYUSH departments in district hospitals; and at the tertiary level by establishing AYUSH "Centres of Excellence" for referral, research, development, and supervision. This initiative significantly increased the budget outlay for AYUSH. The original outlay in the Tenth FYP (2002–2007) was 12.14 billion INR (203 million USD), which subsequently tripled to 35.26 billion INR (588 million USD) in the Eleventh FYP, before jumping further to 100.44 billion INR (1.67 billion USD) in the Twelfth FYP. This final figure constituted around 3.75 percent of the total budget of the Ministry of Health and Family Welfare (MoHFW). In the Eleventh FYP allocation, the development of the AYUSH industry was given high priority, as evidenced by a direct budget allocation of 5.05 billion INR (84 million USD), rivalled only by outlays for research and development (R&D) and medicinal plant research. The report of the Working Group on AYUSH for the Twelfth FYP sought an allocation of 10.11 billion INR (168 million USD) for supporting the development of at least one industry cluster in each state, which constituted a major share of the industry allocation. This "Scheme for Development of AYUSH Clusters" was a central sector scheme and co-terminus with the Twelfth FYP.

In addition to funding for core AYUSH areas like education, research, and medicinal plant conservation, four important dimensions were added to the rationale of funding in the Eleventh FYP: (1) mainstreaming of AYUSH

---

1 AYUSH has replaced the older terminology of "Indian Systems of Medicine and Homeopathy" or ISM-H. The acronym is also used for the Department (since 2014, Ministry) of AYUSH, which has additionally included Sowa Rigpa (Tibetan medicine) since 2010.

in public healthcare, (2) technological upgradation of the AYUSH industry, (3) assistance to Centres of Excellence, and (4) revitalisation and validation of community-based local health traditions. All these dimensions were expected to enhance AYUSH's social and community outreach, as well as expand its domestic and global markets. Since previous financial support for individual projects had failed to make much impact, financial flows were channelled into tied composite funding, in which similarly funded projects were bundled together. In the Eleventh FYP, ongoing schemes concerning the strengthening of the Department of AYUSH, statutory institutions, hospitals, dispensaries, and laboratories were merged into a core strategy of "systems strengthening" and furnished with adequate budgetary provisions. Many of the earlier funding channels were thus integrated into the main agenda of mainstreaming AYUSH into public healthcare delivery. The cluster approach was considered as a multi-faceted project with outcomes not only for the industry (which was identified as a domain of growth), but also for the mainstreaming of AYUSH pharmaceuticals through the National Health Mission (NHM),[2] the MoHFW's flagship programme in the Twelfth FYP period.

Against the background of the long-standing marginalisation of Indian medicines in public healthcare delivery, this mainstreaming initiative was certainly laudable. Although it has an annual turnover of approximately 300 billion INR, or 4.4 billion USD (CII 2018),[3] the Indian Ayurveda industry remains dominated by SME and even smaller micro-enterprises, of which more than 80 percent are located in identifiable geographical clusters (ibid.).[4] Two key dimensions of cluster development, then, are to enable these SME and micro-enterprises to deliver quality products that are competitive in the market, and to facilitate their transition towards large-scale production. Another dimension consists in the AYUSH sector's upgradation of the value chain, or more specifically the transformation of the industry's global image as a raw material supplier into that of a major knowledge products exporter. This is particularly pertinent considering that the export of raw herbs and value-added extracts of medicinal herbs are gradually increasing over the years. India exported 330.18 million USD worth of herbs during 2017–2018, with a growth rate of 14.22 percent over the previous year.

---

2 The National Health Mission is India's flagship health sector programme for revitalising rural and urban health sectors by providing flexible finances to State Governments. It comprises four components, namely the National Rural Health Mission, the National Urban Health Mission, Tertiary Care Programmes and Human Resources for Health and Medical Education.
3 Data concerning the overall turnover of the Ayurvedic industry in India remains inconclusive. While the above study claims that the turnover surpasses 4.4 billion USD, the Ministry of AYUSH reported it as 2 billion USD in 2015.
4 According to the Ministry of AYUSH, there are 8667 licensed AYUSH drug manufacturers in the country, out of which 1179 (13.60 percent) are reported as not being compliant with the prescribed GMP (as answered by Minister of State for AYUSH Shripad Yesso Naik in a written reply in the Lok Sabha on 19th December, 2017)

The export of value-added extracts of medicinal herbs/herbal products during 2017–2018 stood at 456.12 million USD, recording a growth rate of 12.23 percent over the previous year (GoI 2019).[5] These two items – herbs and value-added products – constituted 70 percent of the total exports, with only the remainder of around 30 percent consisting of finished products. At present, Indian AYUSH exports continue to be led by a trader's vision rather than one inspired by value-added knowledge products and it is this vision that current policies seek to change.

The second paradigm shift that clustering initiatives like CARe Keralam sought to address is the increasing corporatisation of the Indian medicine sector. In such a context, the survival of SME and micro-scale manufacturers calls for cooperation rather than competition, and the state of Kerala provides a good example of this. There exists an increasing demand for Ayurvedic medicines in Kerala, not only from the mainstream hospitals or over-the-counter (OTC) drug outlets but also from a thriving tourism industry. At the southwestern tip of India and bordered by the Arabian Sea to the west, Kerala is the country's main destination for Ayurvedic health tourism. The government-supported Ayurvedic tourism industry generated about 40 percent of the state's total tourism revenue of almost 4 billion USD in 2012, which increased to 5.1 billion USD in 2018 (Ramesh and Joseph 2012; Cyransky 2016; GoK 2019). In the course of the tourism sector's rapid growth in Kerala, Ayurvedic clinics, spas, and wellness centres mushroomed in the 1990s and early 2000s. To date, the government of Kerala has officially accredited roughly 130 such facilities, but an even higher number of non-recognised institutions continue to operate as well (GoK 2019).

According to the President of the Ayurvedic Manufacturers Association of India (personal communication 2017), Kerala is also home to the second-largest number of Ayurvedic manufacturers in India after Uttar Pradesh, with over 700 SME engaged in the industrial manufacture and distribution of traditional Ayurvedic and herbal products. As described in earlier studies (Madhavan 2009; Kudlu 2016), around ten leading firms constitute the largest share of the total output (50–60 percent), while numerous SME constitute the other 40 percent. Although 10–12 percent of India's Ayurvedic manufacturing units are located in Kerala, their share in terms of value addition is only 5 percent or less. If the latest large entrant Patanjali Ayurved Ltd with its 80–100 billion INR turnover is taken into account, this share is even less. The leading Ayurvedic firms in Kerala have their outlets all over the state, but their spread clearly establishes a pattern of regional monopolies: Kottakkal Arya Vaidya Sala (AVS) in North Kerala, Sitaram, Oushadhi, and Vaidya Ratnam (Thrissur) in Central Kerala, and Nagarjuna Herbal Concentrates

---

5 Press Information Bureau, Government of India. This information was given by the Minister of State of Commerce and Industry, in a written reply in the Lok Sabha (Lower House of India's bicameral Parliament) on January 07, 2019.

and SD Pharmacy in the South. Pankajakasthuri essentially caters to all regions of Kerala. The largest concentration of Ayurvedic producers is centred in Thrissur and Palakkad (North Kerala), and if we also include the northern parts of Ernakulam, Malappuram, and Kozhikode, the number of units engaged in the manufacture of Ayurvedic medicines is around 400 in that region of North Kerala, forming the largest cluster of units in the state.

Kerala's Ayurveda industry is unique in that a large number of traditional Ayurvedic houses have merged or collaborated with multinational corporations interested in the brand name "Kerala Ayurveda," which is associated with claims to ancient traditions and authentic practices. This trend was initiated by firms like Reliance Retail through its Reliance Wellness Unit, Hindustan Unilever Ltd's Ayush Spa Clinics, and Pantaloons Retail (India) Ltd's Tulsi brand of Ayurveda drugs and health centres. Recently, the Aluva-Kochi-based company Kerala Ayurveda Ltd (KAL) announced a merger with Coimbatore Arya Vaidya Pharmacy (AVP). KAL was formerly a public limited company but is now listed on the stock market and owned by Ramesh Vangal, the former head of PepsiCo India, while AVP is the second-largest Ayurvedic company in South India after Kottakkal AVS. The main aim of their merger was to compete more aggressively in the Indian wellness market, which has an annual sales value of some 9 billion USD. Yash Birla, an industrial group worth 40 billion INR (0.7 billion USD) in 2015, is currently looking for more acquisitions within the state, including negotiations with two major Kerala Ayurvedic companies with large chains of treatment centres and drug outlets. The group recently acquired a majority stake in Kochi-based Kerala Vaidyasala (part of KAL) to form Birla Kerala Vaidyasala (BKV), which is now involved in negotiations to acquire the Nagarjuna Group. Three companies, namely Kerala Ayurveda, Nagarjuna, and AVP, were the leading pharmacies claiming to offer authentic "Kerala brand" Ayurveda. This brand is rapidly growing in value and is becoming increasingly attractive to massive corporate firms such as Birla.

This new corporatisation strategy is based on the agglomeration of large industrial firms with highly respected, tradition-oriented Ayurvedic family companies. Its main aim is to capitalise on the huge recent growth in Ayurvedic health tourism. Many of the Ayurvedic firms mentioned above are connected to the oldest lineage of Ayurveda in Kerala, the Ashtavaidyas,[6] whose "brand name" and time-tested authenticity was seen as having the

---

6 Between the thirteenth and seventeenth centuries, with generous royal and individual patronage, a fertile intellectual milieu developed around temples in Kerala, especially in the Malabar region, where scholarship and scientific research on medicine, mathematics and astronomy made significant progress. The *Ashtavaidya* culture evolved in this environment, blending the Ayurveda of *Ashtangahridayam* with the knowledge and practices of local healers, and *Ashtavaidyas* represent the Brahmin scholar physicians who were masters of the eight branches (Ashtanga) of Ayurveda mentioned in classical texts. For more details, see Menon and Spudich (2010).

potential to create "new demand." A large number of tourists visit Kerala primarily to receive Ayurvedic treatments and the state has increasingly realised the huge potential in this fast-growing market (Basi 2012; Kannan and Frenz 2017; Kudlu 2016). For example, BKV invested around 500 million INR (8 million USD) to open more than 200 new resorts in various cities across India. The company operates spa centres across Kerala and Goa, as well as in cities like Mumbai, Bangalore, Kolkata, and Chennai. Concurrently, AVP initiated a collaboration with Hindustan Lever for establishing 48 "Ayush" spa clinics in Chennai, Bangalore, Maharashtra, Delhi, Hyderabad, and Kochi.

Given this context, cluster promotion seems to be pertinent for many SME in order to facilitate upgradation to large-scale production, process evaluation, and brand promotion so that they may survive alongside, or even compete with, the large corporate entities that increasingly dominate the field. Another way clustering aims to support this is by establishing strong links between these small units and credit facilities. More importantly, however, clusters are expected to work as a single window source for good quality raw materials (collected from various parts of the country) for both SME and large firms with more than one billion INR turnover. As envisaged by the Government of India, the development of AYUSH clusters is assumed to be both participatory and cost effective, while providing critical mass for the customisation of enterprises according to the "collaborating while competing" principle. The scheme also envisioned the identification of reputed AYUSH knowledge institutions in the non-governmental and private sectors and their attachment to these clusters as Centres of Excellence through an upgrading of their functions and facilities. Overall, it aimed to support innovative proposals of the state governments and private organisations to promote AYUSH interventions for community healthcare, encouraging the inclusion of both AYUSH practitioners and medicines in public health programmes. According to a public health professional in Thiruvananthapuram:

> AYUSH drugs have proved potential to tackle community health problems resulting from nutritional deficiencies, epidemics and vector-borne diseases. Tropical infections cause significant morbidity and mortality especially in this region of India and re-emerging infectious diseases […] create troubles in the community. Ayurveda drugs turned out to be very effective in the recent Chikungunya and Dengue outbreaks in Kerala. Easily accessible medicines of this sort can play a very important role in maintaining Kerala's credentials on the public health front.

By 2018, ten such cluster projects had been accepted across India (Table 6.1), with four already in place and functioning. They are implemented through a Special Purpose Vehicle (SPV), a corporate body registered as a company, in which AYUSH enterprises control a minimum of 51 percent with the

Table 6.1 Approved Ayurveda clusters in India in 2016

No.	Name of the cluster	Location	Status
1	CARe Keralam Limited	Thrissur, Kerala	Functioning
2	Maharashtra AYUSH Centre Pvt Ltd	Pune, Maharashtra	Near completion
3	Herbal Health Research Consortium Pvt Ltd	Amritsar, Punjab	Functioning
4	Konkan Ayurpharma Private Ltd	Sangameshwar, Maharashtra	Near completion
5	AYURPARK Healthcare Limited	Bengaluru, Karnataka	Functioning
6	Traditional AYUSH Cluster of Tamil Nadu Pvt Ltd	Chennai, Tamil Nadu	Ongoing
7	Rushikulya Ayurvedic Cluster Pvt Ltd	Ganjam, Orissa	Ongoing
8	Lepakshi AYUR Park Pvt Ltd	Anantpur, Andhra Pradesh	Court case
9	Sanskar Ayush Medicare Pvt Ltd	Haridwar, Uttarakhand	Near completion
10	M/s Ayushraj Enterprises Pvt Ltd	Jaipur, Rajasthan	Functioning

Source: Q&A, Question No. 438, Lok Sabha, Indian Parliament, 2016.

remainder held by government agencies, banks, or other strategic partners. State governments must play proactive roles in these schemes, participating actively in terms of land procurement, external infrastructure development, the gaining of necessary project-related clearances, and dovetailing with other relevant schemes. Due to a lack of independent research data concerning the other clusters, it is not possible to compare them directly with CARe Keralam, making this case study all the more crucial.

Cluster development carries significant implications for the structure and growth of the Ayurveda industry. As the Managing Director of AVP, Coimbatore pointed out:

> Since the Ayurveda industry in India has a large number of small and medium units, the clusters in Ayurveda should aim for a holistic growth model where three major challenges should be addressed: supply chain management, common infrastructure, and capacity development. In the case of supply chain management, the standardization of quality and supply of raw materials, as well as common facilitation centres for testing are important. Skill upgradation and new cluster parks with tax subsidies are pertinent for common infrastructure, while social capital creation, access to technology, access to institutional credits, certification facilities, quality and complaints awareness are necessary for capacity development.

The cluster approach was thus expected to provide solutions to a whole range of important problems. In this light, the next section discusses in detail the genesis of the CARe Keralam cluster, its performance, and the main challenges it faced.

Towards a "Kerala brand": The CARe Keralam Ayurveda industry cluster project

The idea of cluster promotion in Kerala started even before the Department of AYUSH initiated it. The annual combined turnover of Ayurvedic industrial units in the state was estimated at 8–10 billion INR (120–150 million USD) in 2016, according to the Ayurvedic Drug Manufacturers Association of India (ADMA). Although the industry grew by 10–11 percent in the first decade of this century (Madhavan 2009), a non-conventional approach was considered necessary to sustain this growth momentum. The ADMA and the Kerala Industrial Infrastructure Development Corporation (KINFRA), a governmental organisation, initiated efforts to bring Ayurvedic product manufacturers together on a common platform in order to improve their collective efficiency. A series of meetings was held under the auspices of KINFRA and the Kerala State Industrial Development Corporation (KSIDC) with the aim of reaching sufficient consensus among manufacturers to form a consortium. Once convened, this consortium set itself the objective of jointly promoting Kerala as a global destination for sourcing Ayurvedic products and services of internationally acceptable standards. The state government then formed a public-private partnership in the form of a SPV – a legal entity created for a limited business acquisition or transaction, which can also be used as a funding structure – including all types of Ayurvedic medicine manufacturers (small, medium and large) and with the participation of KINFRA and KSIDC.

Most of the leading Ayurvedic manufacturers in Kerala joined this cluster, with the exception of Kottakkal AVS, whose official status as a charitable trust rather than a company did not allow for its inclusion, despite its position as the largest Ayurvedic firm in the state. Beside the leading firms, around 240 smaller companies located all over Kerala also joined the campaign, with a considerable combined share equity (see Table 6.2).

The cluster compiled a feasibility report that identified the industry's constraints at various stages (nodes), with the intention of addressing and finding solutions for each issue, as outlined in Table 6.3.

Table 6.2 Initial costs of the CARe Keralam project

Contributor	Share (million INR)
AYUSH Cluster Scheme	100.0
Ayurvedic Manufacturing Units (240 members)	68.8
KINFRA and KSIDC	10.0
Total cost	178.8

Source: Interview with CARe Managing Director, November 2014.

Table 6.3 Constraints of the industry at various nodes

Node	Constraints
Cultivation	• Sourcing of raw drugs from the wild or from traders • Farmers don't get adequate value for their produce; hence they hesitate to cultivate medicinal plants • Lack of awareness of pre- and post-harvest activities (Good Agricultural Practices) on the part of cultivators
Manufacturing	• Testing requirements at raw material, work-in-progress and final product stages • Technology constraints • Poor documentation of processes, products, and benefits • IPR related issues
Marketing	• Integration with mainstream markets • New market access • New product development • Visibility and branding
Policy level	• Regulations/tax implications on value-added processes outside manufacturers' premises • Restricted use of animal sources for some generic drugs

Source: Author interviews with Ayurvedic manufacturers in Kerala, December 2015–March 2016.

The main objectives mentioned in the cluster's project framework were:

1 To upgrade the process technology of Ayurvedic drug manufacture to enable competition in the global market.
2 To promote the export of Ayurvedic products and reduce export bottlenecks.
3 To develop a Centre of Excellence for Research in Ayurveda, approved by international and national organisations such as the WHO and Government of India.
4 To establish a Kerala brand of Ayurvedic products.
5 To provide training for Ayurvedic manufacturers on the importance of safety, quality, and efficacy of medicinal plants.
6 To protect Ayurveda from adulteration in both manufacturing and treatment and to protect the intellectual property rights (IPR) of Ayurvedic manufacturers.
7 To provide plantation facilities for farmers by supplying free or subsidised seedlings in order to reduce threats to medicinal plant resources and the local communities that depend on them.

These objectives highlight many of the key issues that Asian medical industries have been grappling with over recent decades.[7] When the consortium

---

7 Many chapters in this volume address these issues, notably: Arai et al.; Campinas; Dejouhanet and Sreelakshmy; Futaya and Blaikie; Kudlu; and van der Valk.

submitted its project proposal to the Department of AYUSH, based upon the above objectives, it was not only approved but also led to the initiation of a new nationwide scheme for cluster promotion.

The components of the cluster development scheme

Once officially established, the consortium set to work commissioning and constructing common facilities with the aim of raising the quality, safety, and marketability of Kerala-made Ayurvedic pharmaceutical products. These common facilities were fairly comprehensive and of a very high standard. One of the cluster's main objectives was to facilitate the labelling of Ayurvedic products, which is a core prerequisite for the marketing of such products as drugs in foreign markets. In order to achieve this and other goals, the project launched a fully-fledged laboratory for herbal and Ayurvedic products, with three sections: a quality control (QC) and R&D laboratory, a Toxicity Study Centre (TSC), and a Process Validation Laboratory (PVL) to assist with scaling-up operations. It further established a raw material store and mini-lab, IT and marketing infrastructure, a Common Facility Centre (CFC) for production and packaging, and a medicinal plant nursery. The cluster proposal notes that:

> Lack of information about toxicity makes it difficult to compare the benefit-risk profile of herbal medicines. Even if no adverse drug reaction is reported, long-term toxicity, mutagenicity and genotoxicity studies need to be conducted, as these things are not clinically evident. Many herbs can have direct toxic effects, allergic reactions, effects from contaminants and/or interactions with drugs and other herbs. The Toxicity Study Centre is expected to examine the side effects considering the interaction with other herbs and modern drugs.

The main purpose of the PVL was to provide R&D facilities to SME, thus contributing to innovation and continuous regeneration of the Ayurveda industry beyond the market-leading firms. Because the PVL can perform around 25 process validations at a time, its services could also be offered for a fee to a range of industry clients, potentially providing an important source of income.

A major share of basic raw materials for the consortium's production of Ayurvedic medicines (as well as that of many other companies) was planned to be procured and supplied directly by CARe Keralam in order to avoid the low-value but high-cost additions of middlemen (cf. Dejouhanet and Sreelakshmy, this volume). The raw material store could contain around 500 items at a time and was equipped with all necessary amenities to improve their shelf life, including specially built pallets separating each item. The quality of all raw materials acquired by the consortium was tested in an attached mini lab, with only those that passed the quality tests admitted to the store.

A total of 20 acres of land was identified in different regions across the state, including Wayanad, Thrissur, Idukki, and Trivandrum districts, which had one acre of land each allocated for cultivation. Interested and capable farmers were mobilised and trained in the techniques and technology of medicinal plant cultivation required for growing high-quality materials. In order to provide the necessary incentives for reliable medicinal plant cultivation and thus to ensure sufficient material availability, CARe Keralam offered a buy-back guarantee to the cultivators. In turn, cultivation was expected to reduce pressure on wild resources while ensuring that only high-quality raw materials were used in the production of Ayurvedic medicines.

CARe Keralam's CFC ensured the production and packaging of Ayurvedic products according to standardised norms. It contained expensive equipment for testing, measurement, quality and safety certification, and other key processes too large to be affordable by individual small manufacturers (e.g. machines for soft gelatin capsule filling, coating, and carbon dioxide extraction). The packaging section concentrated on incorporating specialised packing materials and features such as resalable spouts and openings, as well as developing unique bottle designs that would address growing environmental and safety concerns in the field of medicinal product packaging.

The expectation was that by making such state-of-the-art facilities available to SME at an early stage of their industrial development, small firms would benefit greatly while improving collective efficiency across the entire industry. While competing on some levels, individual firms could thus also reap benefits through multilateral horizontal collaboration, including product upgradation, participation in international trade fairs, access to information about global demand, and connections to international buyers.

CARe Keralam made an excellent start towards achieving these aims. It generated revenue of 190 million INR in 2013, mostly through medicinal plant sales to Ayurvedic manufacturers in Kerala and income from tests conducted at the toxicology lab. In addition to enabling small firms to develop new drugs, CARe Keralam was involved in setting up 50 innovation centres in colleges across Kerala. Within three years of its establishment, the CFC completed a scientific validation study on the efficacy of *Nizhakathakadi Kashaayam*, an Ayurvedic anti-diabetes formulation, and had submitted its drug master file dossier to the (by then) Ministry of AYUSH. The dossier contained quality control parameters for the drug's ingredients, a product profile, details of the manufacturing process, toxicity studies and data on its anti-diabetic activity in rats with streptozotocin-induced diabetes. It also included formats for regulatory submission, drug licensing, and GMP certification, besides identifying 20 other popular formulations for scientific validation with a view to ensuring wider acceptability for Ayurvedic medicines, which are mostly marketed as food supplements outside of India.

Collaboration with various government departments and leading firms also generated some leverage for the consortium. For example, the National Innovation Council supported CARe Keralam to prepare dossiers for 20 formulations, as well as funding the efficacy studies. CARe Keralam also signed collaboration agreements worth 50 million INR with large Ayurvedic manufacturing firms like Kochi-based Dhathri group for manufacturing tablets, conducting clinical trials, process validations, and new product development. This ongoing collaboration currently focuses on developing remedies for diabetes, cardiovascular diseases, arthritis, and spondylitis and has already made some important advances.

Despite such early successes and a comfortable start-up capital, the cluster's performance did not live up to expectations after its first five years of operation. In 2018, the company reportedly had a debt of 120 million INR (2 million USD). With a new set of directors and support from the Ministry of AYUSH, CARe Keralam now strives hard to come up with better connections, selective collaborations, and informed investments. One problem was that the cluster was under-utilised, as explained by Deputy Drug Controller of Ayurveda, Dr Smart P. John: despite bringing together a large number of SMEs and supporting numerous medicinal plants cultivators, the cluster's facilities were only actually used by a few companies. In order to manufacture formulations at CARe Keralam, producers needed a "25E license" from the Kerala State Drug Controller, which had up to that point issued only ten such licenses for soft gel capsules to SMEs. These licenses ensure that SMEs continue to avail themselves of the services offered by CARe Keralam, but also mean that a failure to do so may result in their manufacturing license being suspended. Many small private firms (unless funded by government schemes) were unwilling to adhere to this, as it creates numerous complications without offering many benefits. Such a situation further illustrates the lack of coordinated planning and the resulting poor linkage between the cluster and the various concerned government departments.

The consortium had taken a 70 million INR loan to invest in the trading of plants and production of finished goods but instead spent it mostly on infrastructure and working capital, which later turned into a liability. While the failure in terms of financial management is quite evident in the recent past and its implications are analysed in the following sections, the initiative did also produce some positive early outcomes, albeit inadvertently. For example, it spurred better connections between a range of stakeholders in terms of raw material sharing, networks for adaptable techniques of production, as well as research into medicinal plants and new formula development, as mentioned above. This reflects the continued potential that collaborative work in this field holds, so long as due diligence is exercised in order to effectively understand the heterogeneity within the sector, to follow up efficiently on positive leads and to avoid costly wrong turns.

Conflicting structures: Profitable nutraceuticals and surviving pharmaceuticals

In order to understand what went wrong and to establish the extent to which the general objectives of the cluster could or could not be achieved, it is useful to juxtapose CARe Keralam's initial performance with the larger structure of Kerala's Ayurveda industry. Most medicine producers in Kerala belong to various traditional lineages. While moving from small pharmacies attached to clinics or home-based medicine production to large-scale commercial operations, most tended to confine their innovations to the category of classical drugs. As Kudlu (2016: 3) describes it, Kerala's Ayurvedic industry was a "classical drug-centric pharmaceutical regime" dominated by physician manufacturers. When opportunities arose for commercial production, practitioners across castes and communities came forward to make their "unique" family medical recipes commercially available, largely marketing them under their family name (Abraham 2013). Along with medicines from classical texts, formulations from local texts were also produced and marketed as Ayurvedic medicines, catering mainly to a local clientele. According to a State Drug Control Department official, around 70 percent of entrepreneurs in this field are Ayurvedic doctors, despite a post-1990s influx of non-traditional entrepreneurs. The predominance of physician-manufacturers in Kerala's Ayurveda industry partly explains the dominance of the classical drug-centric business strategy. Even in the case of the leading manufacturers such as AVS, AVP, SNA Oushadhasala, and Nagarjuna, industrial production follows strong family traditions of classical practice. One further explanation for this pattern is that the current market structure for Ayurvedic medicines was initially shaped by the public health requirements of the state towards the end of the nineteenth century (Madhavan 2008).

Another characteristic of the contemporary Ayurveda industry in Kerala is that a large number of firms concentrate on the domestic market, with very few companies seriously catering to external demand (see Kudlu, this volume). While even the domestic market is divided between medicines, health supplements, beauty care products, and so on, according to Dr Joy Varghese, the Additional Director of CARe Keralam, "around 75–80 percent of the production in Kerala (in terms of volume, less in terms of value) falls in the 'classical medicine' category." Despite spectacular growth rates across the rest of the country, the Ayurvedic nutraceuticals and cosmetics market is still underdeveloped in Kerala. Many larger firms like Pankajakasthuri, Dhathri, Anoop Pharma, and Nagarjuna make most of their profits from only one or two flagship nutraceutical/cosmetic products. According to the MD of Pankajakasthuri, the profit margins of OTC nutraceuticals are over 30 percent, while those of classical products are below five percent of the total production cost. Dhathri herbal hair oils, Pankajakasthuri granules for respiratory issues, Nagarjuna tooth powder and Kamilari liver capsules are among the OTC products that have made a big impact on Kerala's Ayurvedic nutraceutical market, resulting in significant vertical growth for their respective companies. In this context, market access becomes an important issue, especially for larger firms with over 100 million INR turnover. This has resulted in an expanded focus beyond state boundaries, as evidenced in the idea of "Kerala brand promotion." Given this larger picture, if CARe Keralam is seen as an attempt to encourage mass production and modernisation with a global market vision, its failure partially reflects the predominantly conservative and classically oriented approach of its stakeholders.

At the firm level, competition is virtually absent in both classical and non-classical categories. The larger firms have very different types of products, making product substitution impossible at the consumer level. Many producers have established their own niche through a non-classical flagship product, while in the classical category, lineage-derived authenticity defines the demand, as epitomised by Kottakkal AVS. Most of the smaller producers operate only in the classical category, some of them with up to 400 classical products in their portfolio. R&D is mostly confined to public laboratories and leading private manufacturing labs, making overall R&D investments appear low. The value chain is mostly supplier-driven in the case of classical medicines and buyer-driven in the case of food supplements. Most innovations in the nutraceutical market derive from consumer choices and partially take the form of "experiments in the market." The reformulation has thus become the norm for innovation in this category (Pordié and Gaudillière 2014). The proprietary drugs developed through this reformulation regime have become the major drivers of reconfiguration in the Ayurveda industry and this is possibly influencing other Asian medical industries also. Attractive labelling, marketing, and advertising also push demand for reformulated drugs. In the classical drug category, on the other hand, the market has long followed a price-leadership model, in which AVS played the lead role by setting the prices. Over the last decade or so, the public firm Oushadhi has also acquired a leadership role, with a more diversified product profile and increasing government reinvestment in its expansion.

Ayurveda's industrial structure in Kerala clearly played an important role in shaping and determining the utilisation patterns of CARe Keralam's facilities. Most of the leading private pharmacies have their own R&D labs and thus have no need to depend on the public facilities available at the consortium. At the other end of the spectrum, most of the SME (accounting for 30–40 percent of total production volume) are mainly confined to the classical medicines category, which does not require strict biomedically derived QCs, toxicity tests, or process validations. The large firms, furthermore, have little interest in exporting their products to Europe or the USA due to their strict quality and toxicity standards, and therefore tend to target "easier" destinations with a large Indian diaspora, such as the United Arab

Emirates or countries like Hungary (which has more relaxed import regulations for food supplements), instead of investing in costly process or product innovations. Indeed, companies with flagship products spend much more on advertisement (over 15 percent of the turnover) than on basic research (1–2 percent), while technological innovations are relatively insignificant or even non-existent (Madhavan 2014). Their lack of active participation in the cluster and under-utilisation of its technological facilities consequently had negative impacts on the expected technology transfer to SME. In fact, the only place where any substantive learning or knowledge exchange took place was in the workshops and trade fairs organised by the cluster. In the words of one CARe Keralam official:

> Over time, even the larger firms who took initiative in creating the consortium hardly contracted their work to the consortium. But their holding the key positions of its governance body kept the small firms away from actively participating with the consortium, as they only had a small role to play in both share-holding and the governance structure.

The business and development strategies of a few large companies targeting the global market, mainly through proprietary medicines produced according to international standards, thus came together under a single roof with many SME, who were aiming to supply local and domestic markets with affordable classical formulas. This inevitably created conflicting priorities, which were exacerbated by differential access to finance and managerial influence. The inadequate representation of SME in the internal power structure of the organisation also had negative consequences for its envisioned horizontal linkage with sectors like tourism and medicinal plants. Few leading firms in the Ayurvedic tourism industry approached CARe Keralam for any kind of medicines, despite the high quality of its drugs. The two dimensions of the "joint actions" of a typical cluster – sharing large equipment and horizontal interactions for knowledge transfer – led to a number of interactive workshops and joint cultivation schemes in the initial years, but these were not followed up with any systematic vision.

In Kerala, an institutionalised cooperative system has long been in place specifically for the collection and marketing of non-timber forest products. Since 1978, it has relied on a network of public cooperative societies under a State Federation, with medicinal plant collection rights exclusively given to members of scheduled tribes (Dejouhanet 2014; Dejouhanet and Sreelakshmy, this volume). Since 1981, the Federation led the collection and sale of plants, supplying them first to Oushadhi, the main publicly owned company in the state, and selling leftover materials through auctions to private companies, traders, or wholesalers. This system gave a monopoly to tribal collectors and marketing preference to public companies, thereby relegating important stakeholders to the margins: non-tribal collectors, former traders of medicinal plants, small private companies not able to pay the required advance for participating in auctions, and so on. However, Dejouhanet (2014) reports that between 1995 and 2005, an estimated 67 to 90 percent of forest goods were traded outside this cooperative system. This is hugely significant given that 91 percent of the plants used in Ayurvedic manufacturing comes from the wild. Of this, 43 percent are "cultivated in the wild," meaning that manufacturing firms engage in *in situ* cultivation with the help of various tribal groups, ensuring ready availability of raw materials in addition to those collected directly from truly wild sources (Sasidharan and Muraleedharan 2009). According to Oushadhi's managing director, the company purchases around 500 plant varieties with a total value of around 400 million INR annually. About 25 percent of these raw materials are sourced directly from farmers, while the rest is procured from the Scheduled Caste/Scheduled Tribe (SC/ST) Federation (except for sandalwood, which is purchased from the Gujarat State Forest Development Corporation). This long-standing arrangement between the public company and SC/ST federation led many other producers to continue with their own diverse networks of collectors and traders, as described in detail by Dejouhanet and Sreelakshmy in this volume.

One of CARe Keralam's major objectives was to upgrade the industry through an effective rearrangement of these complicated raw material supply networks while simultaneously introducing better quality standards. Even though in the first year of its operation, CARe Keralam successfully entered the medicinal plant supply market with a 150 million INR turnover, ineffective management saw it gradually succumb to the supply rigidities of the former market structure. By the end of its third year of operation, the prices quoted by CARe Keralam for most plant categories were 30–40 percent higher than the firms' traditional sources.[8] Although the better quality was assured by the consortium, most of the producers stayed with their traditional supply sources, which were much cheaper and based on mutual trust. While most leading companies like Kottakkal AVS and Vaidyaratnam had long-standing informal networks that they were unwilling to give up, the main problem for SME were the high auction advances, especially in the context of market and regulatory fluctuations. Despite some successes,[9] the consortium thus failed to incentivise a formal channel of raw material supply by developing effective linkage with the farmers and the SC/ST Federation.

A second important set of objectives for the cluster was to help firms to upgrade their manufacturing processes and to help the SME obtain GMP

---

8 Source: Interview with the managing director of a leading manufacturing firm in Thrissur.
9 One important achievement was the facilitation of new models of cooperative cultivation partnership. CARe Keralam arranged a number of interactive sessions on cooperative medicinal plant ventures and their dissemination. This facilitated the establishment of the successful Mattathur Labour Cooperative Society in Thrissur, which cultivates medicinal plants (including plumbago, bitter gourd and sida) in all 23 wards of the Mattathur Panchayat throughout the Kudumbashree program.

certification and training that would enable them to reach out to external markets. At present, around 50 percent of Ayurvedic producers in Kerala have GMP accreditation, some of which have been facilitated by CARe Keralam. Although no major impact of the cluster's initiatives is visible in this field as yet, its potential remains, provided the firms are cautious in marketing and branding their products with both an AYUSH stamp and a Kerala brand name. However, a major criticism was voiced by a prominent manufacturer from North Kerala:

> The government is only interested in promoting public firms like Oushadhi, while other manufacturers are harassed in terms of excise raids, tax revisions[10] and so on. The policy is one of curtailing the competitive spirit in the sector, and it's not for good. The government is trying to brand only the public firms' products, which is against the promise made by the consortium.

Against this background, the larger hope behind India's Ayurvedic cluster schemes of capturing a larger share of the global market (see Kudlu, this volume) appear far-fetched in the context of Kerala. Several of the core stated objectives of the cluster had this orientation, notably GMP training, technology transfer, and the development of an international marketing centre for Ayurvedic medicines. The cluster's former managing director, Mr Raman Karimpuzha, confirmed these intentions when he emphasised that the business plans in the second year of the consortium expected a 3 billion INR (50 million USD) turnover in the fifth year. This was visualised as taking place through export promotion and the branding of Ayurvedic products in the global market, with improved market facilitation provided by the consortium. For companies deliberately targeting only local markets, any push into the global market diverged from the reality of the industry. For them, any upgradation in the value chain was confined to the logic of local demand and minor innovations in the classical drug category. If the industry was able to facilitate the production of better quality products at affordable prices, they would be aimed at the large domestic market. The ambiguous objective of "branding for the global market" was largely unintelligible, given that most of the firms were already perplexed by the vulnerabilities of the domestic market itself. Those firms that really had global marketing aspirations and capacities were happy to utilise their own amenities for standardisation, testing, and marketing. Classical drug production has low profit margins and, although it provides an effective means of sustainable subsistence for small and medium-sized companies, offers little incentive for scaling up or branching out due to the rigidities of existing markets and fears related to changing tax rules and departmental raids. The

---

10 Initially, Ayurvedic products were included in a higher Goods and Services Tax category of 12 percent, which was later reduced to a lower bracket following manufacturers' protests.

leading pharmacies compensated for the low profit margins of the classical drug market by relying on the much higher profits available from their reformulated proprietary medicine product lines. The financial liability of the consortium was also aggravated by the attempt to provide infrastructure for the global marketing of proprietary products. The money initially borrowed from government agencies was intended for trading and infrastructural improvements, which the majority of firms had little enthusiasm for.

In practice, then, very few Kerala-based firms produce, or aim to produce, for high-end markets. The market for many of such products may be limited by the locality, culture-specific needs, or unfavourable cost-competitiveness due to high material or transport costs. We suggest that the "success" of a cluster, therefore, need not be measured by whether and to what extent it generates links with the international market. Instead, supportive interventions might better target product diversification and the local technological capabilities of these clusters. Without questioning the importance of exports, the value of global supply chains, or the "entrepreneur-exporters" efforts for enhancing product quality, our intention is to properly acknowledge the strong presence of a large, segmented domestic market for products differentiated by quality and price. This dimension is regularly misrepresented or glossed over in mainstream academic value chain analyses and indeed in many recent governmental strategies and policies.

The role of the government and related public institutions in the initial years of the working of any cluster is crucial. Ideally, the innovation centres located inside an industrial cluster should support SME at a nominal cost, as seen in China (Fratini and Prodi 2013). Links with research activities in universities and public research institutions are also paramount (see Arai et al.; Futaya and Blaikie, this volume). The first major research initiative of CARe Keralam, which was the validation and microbial assessment of the popular formula *nishakatukadi kashayam*, could not gain any leverage because the Ministry of AYUSH showed no interest in its further promotion or extension. Another linkage that did not work effectively was the cluster's engagement with a newly developed industry that supplies customised Ayurvedic medical and massage equipment to the Ayurvedic and health tourism industries. While more than 150 Ayurvedic manufacturers were members of the cluster, it failed to effectively bring tourism firms into the network. Though it was not stated as a distinct aim, the larger intention of integrating Ayurveda into the market by creating a chain of branded Ayurvedic services clearly suggested this forward linkage as a possibility. As far as the development of innovative drugs was concerned, a legal dispute left Kerala's entire Ayurvedic regulatory structure (including new drug approvals) in cessation for three years. Along with the failure to understand the respective structures of the market and institutional governance, rather than contributing to broad-based industrial upgrading and sustainable expansion, this regulatory management disaster left the sector in a state of considerable disarray.

Concluding remarks

This chapter has explored the dynamics, tensions, and struggles of the contemporary Ayurvedic medicines industry through the case of CARe Keralam, which emerged within a policy framework of mainstreaming AYUSH and promoting pharmaceutical development. Building upon earlier industrial analyses (Madhavan 2009; Kudlu 2016), the chapter discussed why such collaborative industrial promotion schemes have not worked effectively within a complicated and fragmented market structure and without the support and follow-up of the central government authorities. In particular, we explained CARe Keralam's underperformance with reference to two main factors, both of them closely linked to the structure of the Ayurveda industry in Kerala. The first is the under-utilisation of the consortium's common facilities, which resulted from a mismatch between the existing structure of the industry and the design of the cluster's main activities. The second factor lies in the inability of the cluster to establish effective links with the medicinal plants and tourism sectors, resulting from the existing institutional structure of raw material supply networks and the lack of any horizontal connections with the requirements of the tourism industry. We also contend that the state government and its concerned officials underestimated these complexities and obstacles while initiating this particular collaborative public-private model, further contributing to its poor outcomes.

From an analytical point of view, it is important to recognise three key dimensions that influence the potential that clustering can hold in a specific context: (1) the nature of the market, both existing and potential *as envisaged by the firms*; (2) the structure and orientation of production regimes; and (3) the macro policy environment. General clustering models help us to understand that the success of horizontal networking with closely linked industries, and vertical stage linking for raw material supply and quality enhancement, depends on the nature of the industry, its structure, and its readiness to embrace change. Progress further depends on how far a cluster-like institutional structure can attract and maintain various services under the same umbrella (in this case, medicinal plant supply networks, pharmaceutical production, and Ayurvedic tourism), in a way that encourages synergy and mutual interdependence. The idea of cluster development in an infant industry like Ayurveda was lauded on the basis of the assumed benefits of collective efficiency for SME (constituting over 95 percent in number and 40 percent in value addition), of constant technical upgradation through networking with larger firms, and common facilitation support through public-private partnership. However, despite initial enthusiasm, the implementation of the cluster did not take proper account of the three dimensions listed above and thus failed to take significant steps towards achieving its stated goals.

A central element of this particular clustering strategy was the provision of common facilities for both large firms and small manufacturing units in Kerala in order to help the latter upgrade their production processes and improve quality standards while encouraging innovation and market expansion across the sector. However, this industry is characterised by a small number of profitable and well-equipped leading companies, a large number of relatively conservative smaller producers, a classical medicine-centred modernisation process, and a strong focus on the domestic market. Because of this deeply entrenched structure, many of the services that CARe Keralam offered – such as support for standardisation, laboratory facilities, or new raw material procurement channels – were either not needed by those involved or did not account for industry realities.

The potential for technological upgradation depends on how firms respond both individually and collectively to the institutional innovations implied by the cluster approach. In this case, the collective approach did not bear fruit for several reasons. All the Kerala-based firms with high turnovers have modern technology such as centrifuges, ovens, incubators, liquid chromatographs, autoclaves, and air sampling machines available in their manufacturing units and in-house R&D laboratories. This enables them to control quality, test existing products and develop new ones without any need for the common facilities provided by the cluster, even though these facilities were of the highest quality. Medium-sized firms that had partly mechanised their production processes and had access only to relatively basic in-house laboratory equipment did not actively participate in the activities of the cluster either, while the smallest production units expressed little need for the advanced technology now available to them, given their limited market aspirations and classical medicine dominated product portfolios. Having said that, some small firms in the central Kerala region were able to scale up classical drug production by making use of the tableting facilities available at the cluster. The initiative of basic research into classical Ayurvedic formulas is also worth mentioning as a successful outcome of the cluster in this field. However, despite considerable investment and laudable aspirations, the cluster's management proved unable to effectively channel these successful strands into any major advances or to have any lasting effect on the industry in terms of its technological development.

Given the existing structure of Kerala's Ayurveda industry, it would appear to have been more important and beneficial for the cluster to have focused on fixing missing linkages and finding new opportunities within the domestic sphere rather than immediately targeting the global market, which is characterised by very different norms, regulatory regimes, and consumption patterns. Local and national markets for both classical and reformulated proprietary Ayurvedic medicines have a very bright growth potential, as evidenced by the steadily increasing demand over recent decades, whereas attempts to break into new overseas markets are expensive, risky, and beset with regulatory challenges that few firms are prepared to undertake. By overlooking this crucial characteristic of the industry and its actual market potential and favouring the aspirational priorities of both central and state governments, costly errors were made, which made it virtually impossible for the CARe Keralam cluster to achieve its core aims. Similarly, CARe Keralam found itself unable to effectively tap the market for medicinal plants because the existing raw material networks in Kerala proved too complicated, horizontally integrated, and resilient.

The relationship between state bodies and industry actors is also crucial to the success of clustering initiatives, as the way these actors understand and respond to each other's actions shapes the long-term impact of any major intervention. Within the broader scope of the governance structure, the CARe Keralam case highlights problems of the Indian state's sectoral understanding and oversight, particularly as it approached Kerala's Ayurveda industry as a singular node of power with a common set of interests and needs. On the contrary, our analysis shows that the hierarchical power structure within the Ayurveda industry created divergent interests and hostility. Ambivalent or weak cooperation from concerned government departments did not help the cluster adapt to industrial and market realities, while the consortium's political structure also played a major role in its failure. The inherent conflict of aims in the cluster's conception – infant industry development vs global market outreach – was exacerbated by complications and disagreements in terms of financial management and allocation. This clearly sounds a note of caution concerning the viability of public-private partnership model at the regional level. Kerala's state government continues to facilitate (through KINFRA) the functioning of the cluster, but how far an increased degree of state ownership works better than a public-private partnership model remains to be seen in the long run. As we have shown, however, the challenges of herbal pharmaceutical industry clustering do not lie solely in any particular ownership or management pattern, but rather in the structure and dynamics of the entire industry, which includes these dimensions but many others besides.

Although CARe Keralam is but one case with very specific features and dynamics, it provides some important resonances and contrasts with the development trajectories of other Asian medical industries. In common with many Asian countries (but not Japan, as shown by Arai et al., this volume), most of the industrial growth and profit potential lies in the reformulated OTC, health products, and cosmetics sectors, which tend to be dominated by larger, well-established firms. Classical formulations remain an important niche market in Kerala and across India, providing the mainstay of a large number of smaller companies, yet offering relatively limited scope for scaling up production volumes or reaching out into new markets. The distinction between classical and non-classical product lines is arguably less clear in many other Asian contexts, where reformulation and regulatory regimes have blurred the boundaries and led to the emergence of numerous hybrid forms (see Chee; Campinas; Futaya and Blaikie, this volume). As Asian medical industries continue to grow, large conglomerates are emerging and dynamic new players are entering the field, while more "traditional" SME continue to remain active. This can lead to tensions between OTC and classical formula production, large corporations and smaller producers, overtly commercial and more traditional approaches, as well as between those producing medicines and those setting policies and regulations. Crucial questions are also increasingly being raised over the sustainability of raw material supplies and the way innovation is harnessed for different industrial, social, and healthcare ends. It is vital that any externally originating policies concerning Asian medical industries appreciate the complexity of the internal structure of the industry itself, as well as its stage of development and capacity to embrace substantive change. Technological facilitation and collaborative linkages can only reach their intended objectives when building upon in-depth understandings of the inherent economic, institutional, political, social, and cultural basis of the industry as a whole, as well as those of raw material supply networks and demand patterns in different sectors and geographical areas.

Acknowledgments

This chapter is based on research funded by the ERC project RATIMED (336932). We are grateful to the officials of CARe Keralam in Thrissur, Kerala and other industry stakeholders for the enriching discussions and sharing valuable information that formed the core of the analysis. Thanks also to Stephan Kloos, Calum Blaikie, and anonymous reviewers for their insightful comments on earlier versions of this paper.

Bibliography

Abraham L (2009) Medicine as Culture: Indigenous Medicine in Cosmopolitan Mumbai. *Economic and Political Weekly* 44(16): 68–75.

Abraham L (2013) From Vaidyam to Ayurveda: Socio-Cultural Transformation of a Regional Medicine. *IIAS Research Newsletter* 65: 32–33, The Netherlands.

Bala P (1992) *Imperialism and Medicine in Bengal: A Socio-historical Perspective.* Newbury Park, CA: Sage Publications.

Bair J and Gereffi G (2001) Local Clusters in Global Chains: The Causes and Consequences of Export Dynamism in Torreon's Blue Jeans Industry. *World Development* 29(11): 1885–1903.

Banerjee M (2008) Ayurveda in Modern India: Standardization and Pharmaceuticalization. In: Wujastik D and Smith F (eds) *Modern and Global Ayurveda. Pluralism and Paradigms.* Albany: State University of New York Press, pp. 201–214.

Banerjee M (2009) *Power, Knowledge, Medicine: Ayurvedic Pharmaceuticals at Home and in the World.* Hyderabad: Orient Blackswan.

Basi M (2012) *Navigating the Medical Market Space: Consuming Ayurveda in Delhi.* PhD Dissertation, Simon Frazer University, Canada.

Belleflamme P, Picard P and Thisse J (2000) An Economic Theory of Regional Clusters. *Journal of Urban Economics* 48(1): 158–184.

Bode M (2008) *Taking Traditional Knowledge to the Market – the Modern Image of the Ayurvedic and Unani Industry 1980–2000.* Hyderabad: Orient Longman.

Confederation of Indian Industry (2018) Ayurveda Industry – Market Size, Strength and Way Forward, Research Report, New Delhi.

Cyransky C (2016) Purifying Purges and Rejuvenating Massages: Ayurvedic Health Tourism in South India, PhD Dissertation, Faculty of Behavioural and Cultural Studies, Heidelberg University.

Dejouhanet L (2014) Supply of Medicinal Raw Materials: The Achilles' Heel of Today's Manufacturing Sector for Ayurvedic Drugs in Kerala. *Asian Medicine* 7(3): 206–235.

Fratini F and Prodi G (2013) Industrial Clusters in China: Policy Tools for Further and More Balanced Development. *European Journal of Industrial Economics and Policy* 9(5). http://revel.unice.fr/eriep/index.html?id=3476

Gereffi G (1999) International Trade and Industrial Upgrading in the Apparel Commodity Chain. *Journal of International Economics* 48: 37–70.

Gereffi G and Kaplinsky R (eds) (2001) The Value of Value Chains. *IDS Bulletin* 32(3), special issue. https://bulletin.ids.ac.uk/index.php/idsbo/issue/view/87

Giuliani E, Pietrobelli C and Rabellotti R (2005) Upgrading in Global Value Chains: Lessons from Latin American Clusters. *World Development* 33(4): 549–573.

GoI (2015) Press Information Bureau on AYUSH Industrial Clusters, Available at: http://pib.nic.in/newsite/PrintRelease.aspx?relid=121432

Government of Kerala (2013) *Ayurveda Health Centres Classified by Kerala Tourism.* Electronic document, https://www.keralatourism.org/ayurvedacentres (accessed 12 February 2016).

Government of Kerala (2015) *Kerala Tourism Statistics 2014.* Electronic document, https://www.keralatourism.org/ pdfs/statistics-2016.pdf (accessed February 9, 2016).

Government of Kerala (2019) Economic Review, State Planning Board, Thiruvananthapuram.

Guerrieri P and Pietrobelli C (2004) Industrial Districts' Evolution and Technological Regimes: Italy and Taiwan. *Technovation* 24(11): 899–914.

Humphrey J (ed) (1995) Industrial Organization and Manufacturing Competitiveness in Developing Countries. *Special Issue of World Development* 23(1): 1–7.

Humphrey J and Schmitz H (2000) Governance and Upgrading: Linking Industrial Cluster and Global Value Chain Research. Working paper n. 120 IDS University of Sussex. http://www.ids.ac.uk

Humphrey J and Schmitz H (2002) How Does Insertion in Global Value Chains Affect Upgrading in Industrial Clusters? *Regional Studies* 36(9): 1017–1027.

Islam N (2008) *Repackaging Ayurveda in Post-Colonial India: Revivalism and Global Commodification*, PhD Thesis, University of Hong Kong.

Kannan S and Frenz M (2017) Seeking Health under Palm Trees: Ayurveda in Kerala. *Global Public Health* 22: 1–11. DOI: 10.1080/17441692.2017.1417458

Kloos S (2017) The Pharmaceutical Assemblage: Rethinking Sowa Rigpa and the Herbal Pharmaceutical Industry in Asia. *Current Anthropology* 58(6): 693–717.

Kudlu C (2016) Keeping the Doctor in the Loop: Ayurvedic Pharmaceuticals in Kerala. *Anthropology and Medicine* 23(3): 275–294.

Kumar A (1998) *Medicine and the Raj: British Medical Policy in India, 1835–1911.* New Delhi: Sage Publications.

Kumar A (2001) The Indian Drug Industry under the Raj, 1860–1920. In Pati B and Harrison M (eds) *Health, Medicine and Empire: Perspectives on Colonial India.* New Delhi: Orient Longman Limited.

Madhavan H (2008) *Home to Market: Responses, Resurgence and Transformation of Ayurveda from 1830s to 1920*, Working Paper no. 408, Centre for Development Studies, Trivandrum.

Madhavan H (2009) Commercializing Traditional Medicine: Ayurvedic Manufacturing in Kerala. *Economic and Political Weekly* 44(16): 44–51.

Madhavan H (2011) *Growth, Transition and Globalization of Traditional medicine: Case of Ayurvedic Pharmaceuticals in Kerala*, PhD Thesis, Centre for Development Studies (Jawaharlal Nehru University), Thiruvananthapuram.

Madhavan H (2014) Innovation Systems and Increasing Reformulation Practices in the Ayurvedic Pharmaceutical Sector. *Asian Medicine* 9(1–2): 236–271.

Menon I and Spudich A (2010) Ashtavaidya Physicians of Kerala: A Tradition in Transition. *Journal of Ayurveda and Integrative Medicine* 2010(1): 245–250.

Naraindas H (2006) Of Spineless Babies and Folic Acid: Evidence and Efficacy in Biomedicine and Ayurvedic Medicine. *Social Science & Medicine* 62(11): 2658–2669.

Panikkar KN (1992) Indigenous Medicine and Cultural Hegemony: A Study of the Revitalization Movement in Keralam. *Studies in History* 8(2): 287–308.

Patwardhan B, Warude D, Pushpangadan P, et al. (2005) Ayurveda and Traditional Chinese Medicine: A Comparative Overview. *Evidence-Based Complementary and Alternative Medicine* 2(4): 465–473. https://doi.org/10.1093/ecam/neh140

Peter M (2000) Location, Competition, and Economic Development: Local Clusters in a Global Economy. *Economic Development Quarterly* 14(1): 15–34.

Planning Commission (2012) Twelfth Plan Document: Social Services, Vol. 3, Government of India. http://planningcommission.gov.in/plans/planrel/12thplan/pdf/12fyp_vol3.pdf

Pordié L (2010) The Politics of Therapeutic Evaluation in Asian Medicine. *Economic & Political Weekly* 45(18): 57–64.

Pordié L and Gaudillière J-P (2014) The Reformulation Regime in Drug Discovery. Revisiting Polyherbals and Property Rights in the Ayurvedic Industry. *East Asian Science, Technology and Society* 8(1): 57–79.

Porter M (2000) Location, Competition, and Economic Development: Local Clusters in a Global Economy. *Economic Development Quarterly* 14(1): 15–34.

Ramesh U and Joseph K (2012) The Holistic Approach of Ayurveda Based Wellness Tourism in Kerala. *International Journal of Advanced Research in Management* 3(2): 29–39.

Reddy S (2002) Asian Medicine in America: The Ayurvedic Case. *The ANNALS of the American Academy of Political and Social Science* 583(1): 97–121.

Sasidharan N and Muraleedharan PK (2009) *The Raw Drugs Requirement of Ayurvedic Medicine Manufacturing Industry of Kerala*. Peechi: Kerala Forest Research Institute, Research Report No. 322.

Schmitz H (1997) Collective Efficiency and Increasing Returns. *Cambridge Journal of Economics* 23(4): 465–483.

Schmitz H (1999) Global Competition and Local Cooperation: Success and Failure in the Sinos Valley, Brazil. *World Development* 27(9): 1627–1650.

Schmitz H and Nadvi K (1999) Clustering and Industrialization: Introduction. *World Development* 27(9): 1503–1514.

Srinivasan K and Frenz M (2017) Seeking Health under Palm Trees: Ayurveda in Kerala. *Global Public Health* (online 2017). DOI: 10.1080/17441692.2017.1417458

Sujatha V and Abraham L (2012) Introduction. In: Sujatha V and Abraham L(eds) *Medical Pluralism in Contemporary India*. Hyderabad: Orient Black Swan.

Wood A (2001) Value Chains: An Economist's Perspective. *IDS Bulletin*, special issue: The Value of Value Chains 32(3): 41–45.

7 Untangling the web of raw material supply for Ayurvedic industry

The complex geography of plant circulations

Lucie Dejouhanet and Sreelakshmy M.

Introduction

Approaching complexity

The 30-year growth of the Ayurvedic sector in the South Indian state of Kerala has been well documented (Madhavan 2006, 2017; Bode 2008; Dejouhanet 2009). The current volume enables this growth to be re-contextualised within the larger transformation processes encountered by medical industries across Asia. As the chapters by Kudlu and Madhavan and Soman illustrate, the Ayurvedic sector has emerged strongly due to both influential private entrepreneurs and Indian government incentives to develop "traditional medicines" in line with the broader emergence of Asian medical industries as competitive pharmaceutical sectors (Craig 2012; Saxer 2013; Pordié and Gaudillière 2014a; Pordié and Hardon 2015; Kloos 2017). To achieve their production objectives, these industries require increasing quantities of raw material while facing rising prices and the diminishing availability of certain important plant species. The sustainability of raw material supply rapidly became a serious concern, shared by industries, traditional practitioners, and institutions.[1] Several research works have collected testimonies reflecting concerns about medicinal resource depletion and rising prices, from Sowa Rigpa practitioners in Tibet (Hofer 2008) and Nepal (Craig 2012) to Ayurvedic industry managers in South India (Dejouhanet 2007) and Chinese herbal markets (Zhen 2011, in Booker 2014). While raw material supply has become a major issue for the sustainability and development of Asian pharmaceutical industries, it has attracted only fragmented scientific attention (Pauls and Franz 2013), focusing either on resource ecosystems, collection practices and cultivation projects, or trade and governance issues[2] (Craig and Glover 2009). Very few studies have tried to gain a precise and detailed understanding of how practitioners or industries actually source their plants, often addressing this issue

---

1 On the urgency of considering the "foundational crisis of raw materials," see Craig's comment on Kloos (2017).
2 For example, see Lele et al. (2010).

DOI: 10.4324/9781003218074-10

through network analyses (Olsen 1998; Belt et al. 2003; Olsen and Bhattarai 2005; Pauls and Franz 2013; Blaikie 2014). The relatively small number of publications investigating Asian medical industries' raw material supply is at odds with the growing importance of this issue. It deserves much closer attention, especially because traceability of raw material and sustainability of its supply are nowadays crucial conditions for the proper development of these rapidly expanding industries (Craig and Glover 2009).

In their attempt to draw out the main issues and arguments relating to the marketing of medicinal plants, Helle Overgaard Larsen and Carsten Smith Olsen (2007) reviewed 119 papers about wild plant collection and marketing in Nepal published between 1976 and 2004 and cross-referenced this with interviews of different stakeholders. They showed that scientists tend to rely on four main assumptions, which are widely diffused and used to legitimise development and conservation projects yet are insufficiently proven. These assumptions, which are also widespread in India,[3] are that:

- *Medicinal plant collection has damaging impacts on natural resources*, because of unsustainable harvesting practices motivated by increasing plant demand, as well as poverty among collectors (GoI Planning Commission 2000; Chominot 2003; Davidar et al. 2008; Madhavan 2009)
- *Medicinal plants are an open-access resource*, since traditional management of common resources collapsed due to nationalisation of forests and market growth (Leaman 1998; Rai 2003)
- *Cultivation of required species can contribute to their protection*, because of the reduction of collection pressure, the guarantee of a stable supply for industry, and the profit obtained by local populations (GoI Planning Commission 2000; Chominot 2002, 2003; Tripathy et al. 2003; Adam and Belt 2009)
- *Collectors are exploited by middlemen*: monetary advances given to collectors drive plant prices down, middlemen are too few and collectors lack information about the real prices of their products (Datta 2001; Ganguly and Chaudhary 2003; van de Kop et al. 2006).

Larsen and Olsen regretted that, because of these four widely disseminated assumptions, political decisions have been driven by ideas of over-exploitation of medicinal plant resources and a lack of local responsibility towards plant conservation. The consequences of this include the implementation of strict rules for the collection and marketing of plants and a condescending perspective towards collectors, who are portrayed as unable to organise themselves for collective resource management.[4]

---

3 We added between brackets some references about India where these assumptions can be found.
4 See van der Valk, this volume for insightful reflections on neoliberal conservation discourse.

The focus on medicinal plant cultivation as a sustainable solution for resource depletion drew attention away from clear reflections on the protection of the resources *in situ*. Although they emerge from the Nepal context, these conclusions emphasise common perspectives on the medicinal plant sector, which are applicable to India and Kerala, as well as to other contexts across Asia (Shahidullah and Haque 2010) and further afield (Hishe et al. 2016).

Research works on the marketing of plants in Nepal share methodological problems with studies conducted in the Indian context. They are based mainly on official statistics – whose precision is difficult to evaluate – and tend to overlook the parallel, informal channels that coexist and interact with formal trade flows (Holley and Cherla 1998; Narendran et al. 2001). Market chain analyses often adopt a vertical perspective, considering the itineraries of plants from collectors to pharmaceutical production units as linear ones (Thomas 1996; Muraleedharan et al. 1997; Shankar 1999; Madhavan 2008). These value chains are characterised by successions of intermediaries contributing to an increase of the plants' value along the channel and therefore to higher prices for pharmaceutical industries (Booker et al. 2012) and "unfair" prices for collectors (Selwyn et al. 2017). This statement could be extended to other types of value chains, but the specificity of the medicinal plant channel here is its complexity and opacity. Considering it only as a commodity chain and through a linear perspective is a reductionist approach for addressing the multi-dimensional sector of raw material supply for traditional medicine industries (Belt et al. 2003; Pauls and Franz 2013). This sector, we argue, is better approached as a complex, multi-layered and dynamic network, which is distinct from but interdependent with the wider "pharmaceutical assemblage" (Kloos 2017). Far from a simple business sector, it operates through a complex and ever-changing combination of factors as diverse as local history, caste and class hierarchy, geographical and social proximity, industrial dynamics, market demands, national and state policies on conservation or socioeconomic development, and interstate relations. This multi-dimensional approach pursues the definition of medicinal plants as "biocultural objects" (Pordié 2002) circulating in complex systems of exchange (Craig and Glover 2009; Saxer 2009). As we will show, these systems are founded in the strong connections, interdependencies, and social and network embeddedness of core stakeholders (Pauls and Franz 2013; Blaikie 2014). Just as Asian traditional medicines have to be considered as holistic systems, the analysis of their raw material supply should not be taken out of context or approached as anything other than a dynamic intersection of many dimensions. This chapter focuses on the geographical and social dimensions of raw material supply to the Ayurvedic industry of Kerala, which opens productive avenues for exploring the dynamic complexity of raw material trajectories that feed medical industries across contemporary Asia.

A watershed moment

In the early stages of Ayurvedic industry expansion, several Indian states tried to structure the raw material supply of this growing production sector.[5] Among them, the Kerala State government, known for its socialist mode of development, created an official channel for the collection and marketing of non-timber forest products (NTFPs) in 1978. This policy had three main ambitions: social improvement by ensuring fair prices to plant collectors; environmental conservation by increasing state control over the use of forest resources; and improvement of public health and medicine production by favouring the development of public Ayurvedic companies. This channel, relying on a cooperative network, was similar to many other crop and natural resource channels created at that time, especially in Southern countries (Hugon 1994, 2005). These channels suffered from the liberalisation policies of the 1990s, but the Kerala state channel for forest plants kept functioning, despite competition from a strong private sector. Today, after a long period of agony, the state system is finally collapsing, revealing the reality of complex supply networks in the twenty-first century.

This chapter examines this key moment, when the state channel is delivered the final blow and the private sector is both comforted in its activity and shaken by new patterns of plant circulation. The supply channels of Ayurvedic companies in Kerala have been described as "the Achille's heel" of the industry (Dejouhanet 2014a) because of the tortuous, virtually untraceable itineraries of the plants from their wild collection to their procurement by the factories. The Ayurvedic industry is indeed extremely dependent on its suppliers, who are mostly local traders working with diverse groups of harvesters. Due to the decreasing availability of natural resources, socioeconomic development in rural areas, and changes in medicine consumption patterns, the raw material supply sector has been forced to adapt. Nowadays, distances between the places where required plants grow and the herbal medicine units that transform them into drugs have widened. The sector as a whole is at a watershed moment when longstanding channels are being forced to recompose, become more complex, and evolve in relation to changing plant availability, market evolution, ever-growing industrial requirements, and new state policies.

Recent shifts in Ayurvedic companies' sourcing practices cannot be properly understood without a clear view of the internal dynamics and functions of their raw material supply networks. To evaluate these changes, we need to untangle the numerous threads that make up these networks, follow plants' itineraries, describe local social structures and dynamics linked to supply activity, and evaluate the level of connectedness within the networks. We argue that the channel perspective, which has been adopted both by

---

5 For an analysis of the system implemented in Uttarakhand, see van de Kop et al. (2006).

state administrations and by most social scientists, has to be decomposed, unfolded, and transformed into a network perspective, because it has never really been a linear construction – even during the formation of the state cooperative system – but rather a complex, multi-layered composition of intertwined flows.

This chapter first focuses on how the state-structured channel for forest plants was organised and why it recently collapsed. Then it describes the different stakeholders involved in Ayurvedic plant supply and analyses the complex connections between them. Finally, it explores the changes in Ayurvedic companies' supply systems and the spatial enlargement of the networks.

Investigating Ayurvedic plant supply in Central Kerala

Our research focuses primarily on two districts of Central Kerala: Thrissur and Palakkad. Ayurvedic units have been highly concentrated in Thrissur district for many years, while the Palakkad gap[6] was the crucial "land road" for the spice trade (Zimmermann 1989). As explained by Madhavan and Soman (this volume), these historical features, combined with the role of local traditional healing families in the development of Ayurveda in Kerala, make these districts central in the regional geography of Ayurveda (Dejouhanet 2009).

Various types of Ayurvedic industrial production units coexist in Thrissur and Palakkad districts:

- Public or semi-public pharmaceutical companies, which are located on the periphery of Thrissur town. These include Oushadhi – The Pharmaceutical Corporation (I.M.) Kerala Ltd. and the much smaller Ayurdhara Pharmaceuticals.
- Large private companies, located mostly around Thrissur town, each with roughly 100 employees. The main ones are Sitaram Ayurveda Pharmacy, SNA Oushadhasala, and Vaidyaratnam Oushadhasala. The biggest private company of Kerala, Kottakal Arya Vaidya Sala (AVS), owns three factories, one in Malappuram district (North Kerala), one in the neighbouring Karnataka State, and one in Kanjikode, which is in Palakkad district. Its Kanjikode factory lies nearby the production unit of another major private company: AVP Coimbatore.
- Middle-sized private companies, with a smaller offering of drugs but providing them to a large market. They are located around Thrissur, on the slopes of forested mountains, or around traditional Ayurvedic places.
- Small pharmaceutical companies producing a smaller range of drugs in limited quantities.

---

6 The Palakkad gap is a topographic corridor, which cuts through the Western Ghats by a plain 30 km wide along a West-East direction. It links Tamil Nadu to the Kerala coast.

Urban areas and main roads, as well as villages traditionally associated with Ayurveda, are the main locations for all types of production units. Further away from urban areas, the size of units decreases. At the foot of the mountains, close to the forest, middle-sized or small units are more numerous, often struggling to maintain their activities in a highly competitive sector. This relative clustering of companies could be expected to have led to homogenisation of raw material supply channels. However, the extreme variety of company sizes, the competition within the Ayurvedic production sector, and also the strong connections between companies and local supply networks created fertile ground for a multiplicity of suppliers to coexist.

Following the itineraries of herbal raw materials reaching traditional medicine production units is not an easy task. Usually, anthropologists choose to follow only a few people – a collector, a trader, or a healer – to figure out how plants circulate (Saxer 2009; Springer 2015; van der Valk, this volume). We chose to spread our research efforts more widely in order to reach the full array of stakeholders and to interview a wide range of actors involved in collecting and marketing multiple items in different places. Our main fieldwork was conducted from 2004 to 2007, followed by regular updates. We visited around a hundred villages in the two districts, which allowed us to conduct more than 180 semi-structured interviews of collectors, alone or in groups. We made more than twenty visits to official plant collection centres, interviewed 10 government officials and 17 private traders, made about 35 visits to Ayurvedic companies, met more than 10 detail shop owners and traditional healers, and 5 medicinal plant cultivators. These investigations allowed us to have precise, as well as diverse, perspectives on the circulations of Ayurvedic plants in the region and on the complex balance between formal and informal transactions.[7]

State vs. private sector supply: An unequal competition

As explained earlier, the government of Kerala started building a regulated channel for medicinal plant supply in the late 1970s and forced all transactions of NTFPs to take place only within this framed system.[8] Many

---

[7] Informal transactions are seldom considered in studies about the Kerala medicinal plant trade, as the "informal sector" is used to refer only to a supposedly large number of small, unregistered pharmaceutical production units, claimed to absorb a large proportion of available medicinal plants (Sasidharan and Muraleedharan 2009; Jayaraman and Anitha 2010). The importance given to this sector appears excessive, as it is comprised mainly of traditional healers providing drugs to local customers, and their consumption of raw material should not be compared to that of Ayurvedic industries (Dejouhanet 2014b).

[8] According to a study by the Kerala Forest Research Institute (Sasidharan and Muraleedharan, 2000), non-timber forest products from local sources represent about 45% of Ayurvedic raw material in Northern Kerala, to which can be added the 20% of material which grows in both forest and countryside. Only 14% comes from non-forest areas.

stakeholders, who were already involved in Ayurvedic raw material supply, were excluded from this channel, because it gave the monopoly over collection to tribal (*adivasi*) collectors and over marketing to a state federation of cooperatives. These people – non-*adivasi* collectors, local intermediaries, and private suppliers – organised themselves into an influential informal sector and, in a manner that we will describe now, managed to subvert the state system and successfully develop their own activities. Even if this competition contributed to weakening the cooperative system, it was the implementation of national policies in favour of tribal development which finally killed off the official channel, which was originally designed to protect local collectors.

The state-structured channel and public Ayurvedic companies

Since 1978, Kerala's cooperative system for collection and marketing of NTFPs has relied on a network of public cooperative societies, named SC/ST (Scheduled Castes and Scheduled Tribes) Service Cooperative Societies, gathered under a State Federation (Figure 7.1). The *adivasi* members of these Societies were granted exclusive rights over collecting and marketing NTFPs, with the obligation to sell them only to their Society. Since 1981, the Federation and its branches have been in charge of marketing the forest products. The public companies, which are Oushadhi – The Pharmaceutical Corporation (I.M.) Kerala Ltd. and Ayurdhara Pharmaceuticals, have prior access to the collected forest goods. The remaining items are sold through monthly auctions,

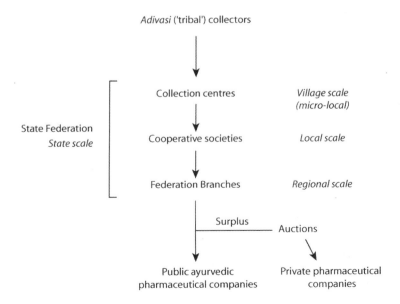

Figure 7.1 The state channel for NTFPs used in Ayurveda (Dejouhanet 2014b).

which are open to private companies, traders, and wholesalers. Successful bidders get a bill from the Federation, which allows them to get a pass from the Kerala Forest Department in order to take items out of the forest areas.

Ensuring a dependable supply of good quality raw materials to government companies was among the main objectives of such a regulated system. Oushadhi was created in 1975, based on the former Thrissur Ayurveda Company of the Raja of Cochin. It grew to become a large company, providing Ayurvedic medicines to Kerala's public hospitals. Thus, securing raw material supplies for this company was a public health issue. This situation led us to hypothesise that Oushadhi, characterised by huge raw material needs, would buy large quantities of forest plants through the Federation, leaving only limited quantities for the auctions. However, when we actually examined the raw material supply of Oushadhi for 2004–2005, the list of items procured from the Federation was quite restricted compared to the potentially available goods. Some of the items supposedly collected by the Societies were even bought from private wholesalers, instead of through the regulated channel. The main reason was that many items needed by the company were not available in appropriate quantities in the Federation branches. However, even some items in high demand by Oushadhi which were available, like the fresh herbs orila (*Desmodium gangeticum*) and moovila (*Pseudarthia viscida*), were not bought through Federation. This incoherence was linked to the difficulties this constraining regulatory system faces in managing fresh items, as well as to the efficiency of the private sector in supplying this type of raw material.

Ayurdhara Pharmaceuticals was created in 2000 by the Federation.[9] It was seen as an opportunity to reinforce the link between NTFP collectors and medicine production, by using the supply potential of the Federation and by hiring *adivasi* workers in the factory. It thus combined the objectives of economic improvement of *adivasis* and development of Ayurveda. Medicines, produced in much smaller quantities than at Oushadhi, were sold in local dispensaries and clinics. Yet despite the strong connection between the Federation and Ayurdhara, this company only obtained 10% of its raw material from the Societies in 2005. Here again, the quantities available through the regulated channel were too small to satisfy the company's needs, forcing Ayurdhara to rely on the private sector. Interestingly, at the same time, Kottakal AVS was getting plants from three SC/ST Societies, two in Palakkad district, and one in Idukki district. It did not participate in the auctions but was negotiating directly with the Societies' management staff.

These observations emphasise deficiencies in the system and the incapacity of the channel both to attract NTFPs and to answer the demand of the

---

9 In Thrissur, the Federation branch office and Ayurdhara Pharmaceuticals office are located in the same building. In Thiruvananthapuram, the Ayurdhara clinic is inside the compounds of the State Federation.

public companies. They show also a diversion of raw materials from the official channel for the benefit of few private stakeholders, which we highlight in the next section.

A captured official channel: Hybrid networks

Serious management problems in the regulated channel were first brought to light during the 1990s (Thomas 1996). Firstly, a large proportion of the NTFPs collected in Kerala was being diverted into the private sector, causing financial losses for the Federation because the quantities collected and the sales profits were too low. Secondly, the marketing system was inefficient, as the Federation did not manage to create appropriate connections with Ayurvedic companies, so they rarely participated in the auctions. The Societies were overstocked, even while the Ayurvedic market was demanding raw materials. The main reasons for this were that the auction system was too constraining, supply through the Societies was irregular, sale prices were not regularly adjusted with the market prices, and the quality of the stocked raw material degraded fast. At the same time, the Societies were struggling financially, especially in the collection season, and suffering from political blockages in their management boards, as well as deficient collaboration with the Forest department (Thomas 1996; Muraleedharan et al. 1997).

Our research work both confirmed these observations and allowed for a more precise analysis of the role of the private sector in the functioning of the official channel (Dejouhanet 2014b). Societies coordinate networks of collection centres. In remote areas, where it is too costly for Societies to have employees, they hire private stock-keepers to take care of their go-downs (warehouses). These "semi-private" stock-keepers are chosen because they can identify the plants and have good relationships with collectors. Many were formerly private merchants. They also have the financial capacity to offer advances to collectors, which the Societies pay back with a delay. They operate mostly in the foothills, where they are also in competition with private outlets. Close investigations showed that some speculation occurs in these go-downs. Stock-keepers could use the cover of being Society commission agents to store extra items and then sell them directly to pharmaceutical industries or wholesalers, thus bypassing the official channel. The profit from these activities allowed them to propose higher prices to collectors and thus to obtain more forest products. As long as the planned quantities of the listed items are in the go-down when the Society manager comes to get them, other transactions remain invisible (Dejouhanet 2014b).

Social capital, as developed by Bourdieu (1980), within the private sector is the key factor in the functioning of this informal, but nevertheless highly structured, network. Many private merchants and stock-keepers are from the Muslim community, which has been traditionally involved in the marketing of forest goods in Kerala (Mathur 1977). Belonging to this socioreligious community and sharing close connections over long periods help to secure transactions and maintain business relationships in the context of an "organised proximity" (Torre and Beuret 2012).

In addition to social relationships between private merchants, collusion between various stakeholders in the private sector contributed to the State-structured channel coming under the effective control of a small number of merchants and wholesalers. In 2007, the secretary of one Society explained to us how wholesalers and commission agents coming to auctions in the Thrissur branch have an agreement between themselves to keep the prices of the sold items low. This allows them to sell the goods back to other wholesalers or merchants with a good profit or to answer tenders from Ayurvedic companies by proposing competitive prices.[10] After the auctions, the Federation provides a bill to the bidder, enabling them to get a pass from the Forest department for transporting the goods out of the forest area. Here again, official certification is used as a cover for greater quantities of forest products to be collected, transported, and sold.[11] This illegal transfer of forest goods is enabled by the private merchants' grip on the marketing stage of the official channel and by circumventing the system's rules. Stock-keepers and merchants have therefore created hybrid networks based on the legal system (Figure 7.2). This situation placed the Societies under a great deal of pressure, and only a few of them were able to continue fulfilling their supporting role to *adivasi* collectors. Deeply weakened, they could not offer much resistance when the Forest department began organising collection activities through village committees, as we shall show in the next section.

The liberalisation of the channel: Towards the end of the State regulation

By 2017, most of the Societies had been closed in Thrissur district. In Palakkad district, the Malampuzha Society is still working with stock-keepers, who take care of collection in the Southern part of the district. The legal system's integration into the informal channel there may have contributed to its durability. The Societies which closed were located

---

10 This analysis confirmed the observations of Shankar and Muraleedharan (1996) concerning the collusion of auction participants, especially in the case of perishable items, and of Muraleedharan, Sasidharan, and Seethalakshmi (1997), who described the system as an oligopsony. The same observations were done in the Forest Department auction centres for medicinal plants in Uttarakhand (Pauls and Franz 2013). This leads to the assumption that everywhere private merchants share the same operating mode for partitioning the legal channels of raw medicinal material.
11 See also van der Valk, this volume.

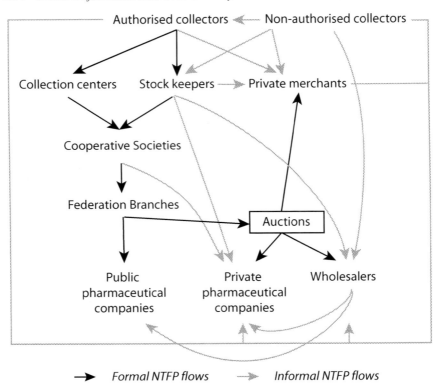

Figure 7.2 Itineraries of NTFPs through hybrid networks.

within forest areas with considerable amounts of collection activity. They were essential providers to the Thrissur Federation branch but suffered from problems of management and, in particular, from competition with the participatory forest institutions created by the Forest department. At the beginning of the 2000s, numerous *Vana Samrakshana Samithi* (VSS) were created in the forest and fringe villages. These are participatory local institutions in charge of protecting the forest area from fire and poachers. Progressively, their agenda incorporated the collection of NTFPs, putting them into direct competition with the collection centres of the Societies. This change at the village level further damaged the already struggling Societies. The coup de grace was delivered by the Kerala Forest Department order dated 7 January 2016, which allowed local tribal institutions (*Oorukoottams*) to market NTFPs to any outlet they wished and therefore to avoid the Societies if their conditions were not considered profitable enough. Coherent with the national Forest Rights Act of 2006, this order gave greater control of the collection and marketing of NTFP resources to *adivasi* populations through their local VSS. The time of state-structured organisation based on a communism-inspired cooperative system is now over, and even though the new rule was aimed to empower local tribal populations, it also officially opened up the marketing of NTFPs to liberalisation.

Nowadays, the Thrissur branch Federation very seldom conducts auctions. None took place in 2016–2017. Collected goods are only supplied to the public company Ayurdhara Pharmaceuticals. Oushadhi and Kottakal AVS are getting forest goods either directly from the collectors, or through VSS when the Forest department makes the arrangements. They still work with the functioning Societies, such as those in Palakkad district. The private Ayurvedic industries did not play a significant role in this liberalisation. Because the vast majority of them never participated in auctions, they seldom interfered directly with Societies and their raw material was mainly procured through the private sector. Even though their supply determined the development of NTFP collection, the shift from a state-structured channel to a local committees' control on marketing was mostly a political choice.

Although *adivasi* collectors have won the right to have their own strategy of marketing, the new system actually reinforces Forest Department control over forest-based activities (Münster and Vishnudas 2012), as the VSS are structurally linked to this Department (the secretary of the VSS is a forest guard). Finally, the liberalisation of the marketing stage offers the greatest benefits to the private sector, which contributed to the collapse of Societies by competing with them harshly and using them for their own profit. In parallel, this change may also redefine power relationships inside the private sector, as the few Federation bidders lost much of their former influence over the marketing of forest goods.

The State channel was designed to improve tribal people's livelihoods, ensure environmental conservation, and help the development of a public Ayurvedic medicine production sector. However, structuring a channel and making it unavoidable by law, without considering the variety of people already involved in supply activity or giving them a place in this channel, made it difficult to maintain in a non-authoritarian State. Nowadays, the idea that middlemen should necessarily be removed from the sector to allow collectors to get better prices is still widespread.

While we have focused so far on the organisation and malfunction of the state channel, we have not yet addressed its true complexity. Non-*adivasi* collectors, who were ignored in the official conception of NTFP collection, work with different outlets, while private merchants not taking part in auctions also continue supplying Ayurvedic companies. Moreover, Ayurvedic production units also need medicinal plants that grow wild outside of forested areas and were thus not included in the State channel. It is thus important to describe the tangible organisation of Ayurvedic raw material supply and the connections between all these stakeholders in a fuller manner, which requires a shift in perspective from channels to networks.

From channels to networks: Understanding multi-layered flows of Ayurvedic plants

> Rather than a simple contrast of being a produce-driven or buyer-driven chains, [value chains in the field of herbal medicines] are likely to be a range of different relationships.
>
> (Booker et al. 2012)

This statement refers both to Chinese and Indian Ayurvedic medicine raw material supply, but is arguably generalisable to other Asian medical industries' supply systems, which rely on a multiplicity of stakeholders and a mixed economy combining state control, private actors, and informal transactions, involving complex plant circulations (Saxer 2009; van der Valk; Blaikie and Craig, this volume). Itineraries of the materials, which are more often tortuous than linear, depend on relationships between stakeholders, on temporary strategies, as well as long-term relations between partners. Looking beyond a channel perspective, raw material supply can be described as a braided network, where nodes play a key role in organising flows. The flow of Ayurvedic raw material can then be described as a dynamic system of (re)negotiated relationships, power confrontations, clientalism, and bypass strategies, as well as a long-lasting system whose stability is built on trust relations, local histories, caste belongings, and social proximities.[12]

The middlemen: A powerful control over collection activity

Many publications portray medicinal plant collectors as exploited by middlemen, unaware of the market situation and the real value of their collected goods, forced to sell their items to these people because of indebtedness, patronage links, and submissive relationships (Shankar 1999; Datta 2001; Ganguly and Chaudhary 2003; Madhavan 2008; Preetha et al. 2015). Many groups of *adivasi* collectors in Kerala are characterised by geographical remoteness, as they live deep in forested areas and only interact with a few outsiders, and social ostracism, based on their lack of education and widely disparaged "tribal" status. While a large number of these groups are indeed suffering from disadvantages and exploitation similar to that described in the literature, the dynamics at play are often more complex than they are portrayed.

Adivasi populations are exposed to frequent social depreciation from other people, be they rural castes, urban families, or government officials (Dejouhanet 2017a). This situation, for certain vulnerable groups, can keep them on the fringe of rural society, as they strive to avoid mockery,

---

12 For a theoretical framework interpreting similar entanglements, see Tsing (2015).

repetitive teasing, or women's harassment. They therefore tend to look for local protection, which can be provided by private merchants. A stock-keeper collecting for a Society explained his incapacity to challenge local private merchants[13] in these terms:

> they drink toddy [palm wine] with the villagers, they sleep and eat in their houses; adivasi always hope good relationships with private merchants, a sense of fellowship, like family members who would take care of them when they are not fine.
>
> (Interview, 2006)

These private merchants are very much involved in the life of these villages: they take care of the "administrative work" – which includes keeping land property documents, managing village rubber plantations, and controlling the bank accounts of villagers (Zacharias 2003). They drive them to town for movie entertainment, or when they want to go to doctor, they are called when any problems happen in the village, and moreover, they take collected items from them regularly, sometimes over many years. They are personally involved in the collection activity, going with the villagers in the forest, setting up forest camps for long stays, and taking items out by jeep. The trust that these collectors give to private merchants is based on this sense of fellowship and on the help and protection they receive in exchange for collaboration and dependence[14] (Dejouhanet 2014b).

Even if cooperative societies were supposed to provide financial assistance and public service proximity to *adivasi* collectors, they could never offer such multi-faceted and trust-based relationships to villagers and were thus not in a position to replace their dependency on private merchants. This system persists in large part because it is maintained by the collectors themselves. Yet when interactions increase with outside communities, when education allows a better understanding of plant prices, and especially when the villagers become politicised, collectors become better informed, get more negotiating capacity, and the influence of private merchants declines accordingly. However, if collectors choose another outlet, they have to pay the bus or jeep rental to get there and spend time to complete the necessary business. They also lose some

---

13 We distinguish here stock-keepers, working for Societies, and private merchants who can be any person buying medicinal plants for their own profit. As we saw, stock-keepers can be former private merchants; their status is attached to a temporary delegation of power by a Society. "Middleman" is used in the broad sense, often as a synonym for "private merchant."

14 This system is reminiscent of the "moral economy of the peasant" described by James C. Scott (1976), where the patronage of landowners is a security for small peasants: the latter obtain protection and financial help for functions, weddings, health expenditures, food, in exchange of their loyalty and constant availability for work.

negotiating power. Having brought their items to a distant place, they may be forced to sell them at a low price because of the expenses already engaged. At the same time, local merchants may admonish them for having chosen another outlet.

The argument we wish to present here is that, even if government, scientists, and experts advise the removal of middlemen from the supply channel of Ayurvedic raw materials, it is nowadays impossible to organise the collection of medicinal plants – or their cultivation (Dejouhanet 2014b) – without some involvement of these local people.[15] Firstly, they have good knowledge of the plants and strong connections with collectors and farmers. Secondly, they have enough influence to systematically capture a part of material flows, either by proposing better prices to collectors or producers or by attracting them through services, cash advances, and other forms of help that no other local structure is able to provide. Thirdly, Ayurvedic companies need such large quantities of items that even organised collectors cannot meet the demand, whereas middlemen work with different groups of collectors and farmers and cooperate together to increase the gathered quantities. They also have the capacity to store and transport raw material so it can be delivered at the appropriate time. The assumption that middlemen are only a barrier to organising sustainable and fair supply channels simplifies and misrepresents their role. These private merchants, categorised as "permanent sub-local traders" by Olsen and Bhattarai (2005), have developed complex, multi-faceted relationships with villagers, they play various roles in local life, have a wide influence, and act as crucial nodes in convoluted supply networks (Pauls and Franz, 2013). Buyback agreements were signed between farmers and Ayurvedic companies, sometimes mediated by NGOs, during Kerala State cultivation projects in the 2000s.[16] However, either the cultivated items were diverted to the private marketing sector because of the better prices they could secure there, or farmers did not manage to supply the correct quality or quantity of items to companies, so their plants were finally rejected (Dejouhanet 2014a). In this situation, the private sector either acted as a fierce competitor or, when it did not get involved in the transaction, could not serve as a safety net to keep production flowing.

---

15 T. Pauls and M. Franz (2013) develop a similar analysis for Uttarakhand. See also Blaikie and Craig, this volume.
16 We chose not to develop the question of cultivation in this chapter: farmers provide agricultural goods to Ayurvedic companies, but medicinal plant cultivation is still at an experimentation stage. Many projects exist, many failed, and if not in factory estates, cultivation of medicinal goods by farmers is seldom profitable (Dejouhanet 2014a). As indicated by Harilal and Soman in this volume, a new project of cultivating twelve plants used in Ayurveda is emerging through a Labour Cooperative Society in Mattathur (Thrissur district); buy-back agreements have been signed with several Ayurvedic companies and government departments are involved in the project. It is yet too early to evaluate its results.

Nevertheless, some collectors did manage to build different relationships with the market, which enabled them to cut out the middlemen. Some of them now sell their items directly at negotiated prices in cities or factories. It is not unusual to see women carrying loads of plants on their heads, supplying the wholesale shops of Thrissur, or waiting at the bus stand close to the Tamil Nadu border. They include *adivasi* and non-tribal rural people, who collect plants on a part-time basis, reflecting the wide diversity of plant itineraries at the collection stage.

Characterising Ayurvedic companies' direct suppliers

Ayurvedic companies, for their part, rely on diverse networks and different types of intermediaries to secure their raw materials. In the previous section, we described the private merchants who are at the first stage of the marketing channel. Their capacity to supply companies, especially large ones, reflects the scale of their business activities. Industries rely on different types of suppliers, who can be described in terms of their contractual relations with companies, the types of items they supply, or the nature of their business.[17] As we will now outline, companies often get their raw material through a combination of local private merchants, "agents," wholesalers, and local collectors.

"Agents": The brokers of the industry

"Agents" are "contractors" who work specifically for certain companies. They can be private merchants, wholesalers, or even farmers, with contract-based ties to industrial producers. Agents do not necessarily work with collectors, and many of them are better described as investors, dealing with networks of private merchants in order to collect together large consignments of raw materials. Local middlemen can also act as agents for companies. To be effective, agents should be able to cultivate long-term relationships and must have a good understanding of the various stakeholders involved in this business and of the connections between them.

Oushadhi's supply relies on a large network of private suppliers, linked by a system of contracts secured through a tender procedure. Tendering is made once or twice a year (especially since the recent implementation of an e-tender system). The agent who offers the lowest price for the full quantity of one material gets the contract for that item. The successful tenderer

---

17 C.S. Olsen and N. Bhattarai (2005) drew a typology of traders for the marketing of medicinal plants in the Himalayan region. Even though their categories are of great relevance, they would require few adjustments for fitting Kerala networks appropriately, especially because Kerala traders combine multi-scale sources of raw material. According to the proposed categories, the "agents" would be "Generalist local traders" or "Specialist central wholesalers."

first pays 5% of the total amount to the company as a guarantee to fulfil their commitment. They must then deliver the proper quantity at the correct time and ensure good quality of the raw material: if not, this amount helps Oushadhi to obtain the material from another source. The activity of Oushadhi agents is therefore quite risky: they must offer low prices to secure the tender, which limits their profit margin, and any problems, like a truck accident or a delay in transportation which leads to the spoiling of the medicinal plants, means they lose both the contract and deposit. If all goes smoothly, taking a tender from Oushadhi is often profitable, as it guarantees an outlet for large quantities of plants. Oushadhi's suppliers are mostly investors who not only have enough financial backing to pay the deposit and organise the supply but also to manage a wide network of local suppliers and to counter any delays or problems arising in the supply process (Dejouhanet 2014a). Similar tender procedures are also used by Ayurdhara Pharmaceuticals and by big companies like Sitaram Ayurveda Pharmacy and SNA Oushadhasala for part of their supply.

Kottakal AVS combines different forms of supply. Most of its dry items come from other Indian states: Gujarat, Maharashtra, Uttar Pradesh, Tamil Nadu, and North-Eastern states. It works with several wholesalers located in Calicut and Thrissur and negotiates plant supply directly with SC/ST Cooperative Societies, as mentioned above, as well as developing medicinal plant cultivation in its own estates. But its main suppliers for fresh items are the ones referred to within the company as "local people." These suppliers, all Muslims, work with their own networks of collectors and local middlemen, providing the company with large quantities of plants at an annually fixed price. Every September, Kottakal AVS establishes its annual need for raw materials and negotiates with its suppliers. The needs are actually so big that it will take any quantity available in order to meet them. It deals directly with 40–50 "agents" spread around Kerala, whose identity is kept secret by the company. They work exclusively for Kottakal AVS, and their relationship with the firm is based on long-term collaboration, which gives both flexibility to the firm (an urgent need can be solved by a phone call) and high dependency on its suppliers whose bargaining power is significant (Dejouhanet 2014a).

Wholesalers: A nodal position in the networks

Wholesalers are also key stakeholders in the supply of Ayurvedic companies. Their specificity is that they are spatially located in one or several shops, which makes them geographically stable and easily accessible both by collectors wishing to sell items and by companies needing material. Wholesalers supply all types of companies. They answer to tenders from Oushadhi, Sitaram Ayurveda Pharmacy, SNA Oushadhasala, and Vaidyaratnam but are also the favourite suppliers for middle-sized, small, or very small companies. The latter know the market prices for medicinal raw materials through the AMMOI's[18] monthly journal *Oushadham*, in which prices are actually checked with a wholesaler in Thrissur. As well as providing raw material to Ayurvedic companies, wholesalers also sell to other wholesalers, detail shops, and Ayurvedic healers. They sell fresh herbs coming from Kerala and Tamil Nadu, as well as dry materials coming from North India or abroad.

The supply capacity of wholesalers relies on them being nodal points in which multi-scale networks converge, from local networks because of their strong connections with collectors, farmers, and private merchants, to national networks through their location at the centre of flows coming from other states. They benefit from interlocked networks not only because of their relationships with local stakeholders at different marketing stages but also from a superimposition of channels at different spatial scales.

Villagers: The "close" suppliers

Finally, there is another type of supplier that is often ignored in value chain analyses but is important for many companies as part of their identity and attachment to their local environment. This involves villagers living in the vicinity of Ayurvedic companies, who collect plants that grow locally and supply them directly to the production units. In many cases, these flows have existed since the production units were first founded and are thus well established. In this way, most companies but Oushadhi and Ayurdhara get raw material directly from their immediate surroundings.[19] Many plants used in Ayurvedic medicines grow in the countryside, at the fringe of forests, in village compounds, or on the roadside. Many collectors of such items are not *adivasi* but villagers, often women, who have garnered some knowledge about specific plants and go, as individuals or in groups, to collect them. Companies ask them for plants on a regular basis and therefore give valuable employment opportunities to the surrounding population, especially during monsoon, which is the low season for agricultural work. The strong link between villagers and Ayurvedic companies through this form of raw material supply illustrates the important role these companies play in the social life, economy, culture, and environment of many villages located in central Kerala.

Complexity of the networks: Mapping the supply organisation

As we have shown, the supply of Ayurvedic plants in Kerala is characterised by a multiplicity of connected, superimposed, and intertwined networks, involving a large variety of stakeholders linked through complex

---

18 Ayurvedic Medicine Manufacturers Organisation of India.
19 Collectors bringing plants directly in Oushadhi or Ayurdhara are sent by an agent.

212 *Lucie Dejouhanet and Sreelakshmy M.*

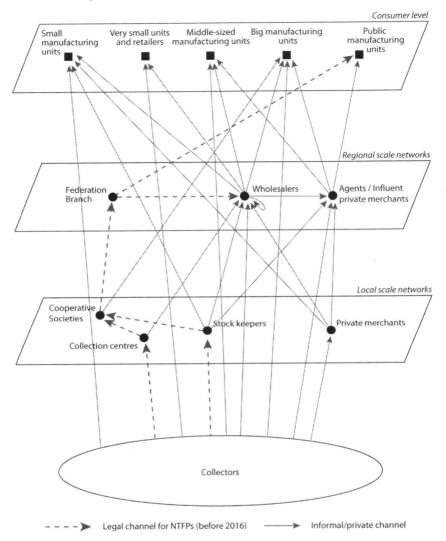

Figure 7.3 The complex organisation of Ayurvedic raw material supply in central Kerala.

relationships. Figure 7.3 graphically summarises the functioning of this sector, both through itineraries of plants and connections between stakeholders. It is built on three levels. The first level shows marketing at the local scale, gathering cooperative societies and their collection centres as well as private merchants. The second tier includes Branch Federations, wholesalers, agents, and important private merchants, who are influential at the regional scale. The third level is that of buyers: small, medium, and large Ayurvedic companies and detail shops that operate at the state scale and beyond. Private merchants are difficult to position, as they work with localised collectors but can also have influence at regional scales, especially those who also work as agents. Even though wholesalers can also be agents, and both appear as central nodes for plant flows, it is more coherent to separate them in this graphic. Clearly, the official channel is but one among many others, and flows of raw material are vertical as well as horizontal.

The organisation of Ayurvedic plant supply shows a complex architecture. It is clearly necessary to go beyond the concept of a single, clearly defined channel and adopt instead a network perspective, including all the complexity of horizontal connections.[20] Some intermediaries act as nodal points connecting multiple marketing networks, organised at different levels, as they function with local, regional, national, and even transnational networks. This is especially true given that networks are geographically expanding and plants are coming from further and further away.

Recent evolution in Ayurvedic supply: Enlarging spatial connections

The Ayurvedic industry is currently facing both a diminution of raw material availability and increasing prices, forcing it to progressively adjust its sourcing and production patterns. Overexploitation of the resources is often considered as the main reason for decreasing availability (GoI Planning Commission 2000; Chominot 2003; Davidar et al. 2008; Preetha et al. 2015), but other reasons must also be considered. Some endangered plant species have been banned from the market by the government (ashoka, *Saraca asoka*, for example), while others have become regularly scarce because of climate change, such as kanjunni (*Eclipta prostrata*) and chittamruthu (*Tinospora cordifolia*). Although destructive collection practices certainly play a role, the lack of availability of plants on the market must also be linked with: the decreasing number of collectors due to new job opportunities and the education of youngsters; biodiversity protection rules forbidding collection in some areas; extension of roads and urban areas into formerly vegetated zones (see van der Valk, this volume); and the National Rural Employment Guarantee Act of 2005, which diverts rural people from collection activity while encouraging the systematic clearing of natural-growth ecosystems of medicinal plants near roads and village grounds (Dejouhanet 2014a). However, it is the suppliers who are facing the greatest difficulties in gathering sufficient quantities and qualities of raw material. Ayurvedic factories procure material from whoever is able to find it at the lowest price. The supply sector is therefore gradually reshaping itself, with some intermediaries rising up and others in decline, contributing to a progressive change in plant circulations.

20 Lazzarini et al. (2001) developed the concept of "netchains" for evaluating interdependence relationships in supply chains and networks.

Mapping the changes in Oushadhi's supply

To explore changing sourcing strategies in the Ayurvedic pharmaceutical sector, we focus on the evolution of Oushadhi's supply. Because it is a public company with a stable market share and no need to continuously increase profits, it may not be the most representative company to analyse the developmental trends in the sector. Nevertheless, it suffers like other companies from decreasing raw material availability and increasing prices, and thus its way of adapting to this context is reasonably illustrative of the choices made by other companies.

Over recent years, large pharmaceutical companies like Oushadhi have shifted to using fewer fresh items and more dried materials in their formulations (Dejouhanet 2014a). It was confirmed in 2017 that commonly used plants such as palmuthuku (*Ipomoea mauritania*), chittamruthu (*Tinospora cordifolia*), and sathavari (*Asparagus racemosus*) are nowadays largely provided in dried form. This may be linked to the increasing production of capsules and tablets in relation to the new consumption modes of Ayurveda (Banerjee 2009; Pordié and Gaudillière 2014a, 2014b). It also signifies a change in the supply of some raw materials, which are less available in fresh form in the surrounding areas and are thus sourced from further away in dried form.

We collected Oushadhi suppliers' list and tender books for the years 2004–2005, 2012–2013 and 2016–2017. Studying the location of suppliers and the evolution of bought quantities and plant prices provides an overview of the evolution of the supply geography of this company. Between 2005 and 2017, the total number of suppliers increased from 32 people or companies to 42, but the number of suppliers located in Thrissur and Palakkad districts remained stable.[21] In 2005, Oushadhi relied mostly on local Thrissur suppliers but also worked with a few agents in Kerala and wholesalers in the neighbouring states of Karnataka and Tamil Nadu. The number of Tamil Nadu agents utilised is irregular throughout the period. While in 2013 these suppliers were numerous, in 2017 Kerala agents seemingly regained attractiveness and the village of Kozhinjampara (Palakkad district), located on the border with Tamil Nadu, emerged as an important place for plant supply. By 2013, in addition to local agents, Chennai and Delhi had become important sources of raw material and by 2017 the market of Kochi-Ernakulam, usually an export port, had also established itself. This illustrates better connections with national marketplaces, confirmed by the recent adoption of an "e-tender" system. This system concerns local plants as well as items from North India and particularly targets expensive plants and those required in large quantities. More and more items are likely to

---

21 Only a few suppliers managed to keep working with Oushadhi over the whole period. A regular supplier may have failed in the auctions for the considered years but may still be active in supplying other companies.

be ordered by e-tender over the coming years, as it simplifies the procedure and considerably shortens the payment delay for suppliers. It allows a larger number of suppliers to respond to the call for tenders and the company to step outside the influence of local suppliers. However, it may also create segregation between people based on their differential access to technology. This gradual digital shift concerns several Ayurvedic companies and represents a major change in the supply organisation.

The quantities of raw material required by Oushadhi have increased steadily in order to meet its growing production output. The highest rise happened for quantities coming from the wholesalers of Thrissur, Tamil Nadu, and North India. The items supplied from these places were also more diverse in 2017 than in 2005. Prices for Ayurvedic raw materials have also increased considerably since 2005. The items brought from North India are mainly high-value ones, like saffron coming from Kashmir through North Indian markets. Many are also dried items, which tend to be more expensive than fresh ones. Thus, even though large quantities of raw material are now coming from Tamil Nadu, the plants collected there are mostly fresh and therefore have lower values. Similarly, although the border village of Kozhimjampara has confirmed its position as a major centre for raw material supply, in diversity as well as quantity, the value of the items supplied there is low. Actually, people from Kozhinjampara collect mainly in Tamil Nadu, where plants are still abundant and manpower is cheap. Collection from Tamil Nadu (Kozhinjampara included) represented 34% of the total raw material quantity used by Oushadhi in 2017, but only 26.4% of the value.

The combination of expanding raw material needs, increasing prices, and the localised depletion of certain plant species has led to the emergence of new procurement sites for the industry. Tamil Nadu in particular has appeared as a reservoir for Ayurvedic plants, which were until recently not being collected in large quantities. Large-scale and systematic collection of plants from Tamil Nadu was organised first through local agents and then through the development of Kozhinjampara as a marketing centre for fresh herbs and local plants: a connector between Kerala-based companies' needs and abundant sources of raw material across the state border.

New spatial connections: Collection in motion

Due to rising prices and demanded quantities of medicinal plants, the business of Ayurvedic raw material supply has become increasingly attractive. The spatial gaps between the collection zones of the influential private merchants, and the forfeiture of the cooperative system, opened up opportunities for middlemen to settle and expand their business. Once again, the role played by private merchants in the development of medicinal plant collection in certain areas has to be emphasised, while their flexibility allows them to enlarge collection zones to new places and to develop efficient transregional flows.

Kozhinjampara is illustrative of these changes in collection patterns and the organisation of supply activities. There was no cooperative society located there, leaving spaces for private merchants to organise collection activity unopposed. They recruited collectors in the villages by showing samples of the required plants, explaining the collection methods, and sending people by vehicle to places they located themselves. Over time, collectors acquired efficiency and autonomy in their activity and private agents became more numerous in Kozhinjampara. Nowadays, more than 80 collectors work there for almost fifteen middlemen. The merchants order plants directly from the collectors, plan their transportation to suitable places, give them cash advances for their expenditures, and do the primary processing of collected items (drying, chopping, bagging, etc.).

Such rural collectors – mainly villagers, often dalit ("untouchable") and Christian – are now emerging as major providers of raw materials to the Ayurvedic industry. In contrast to the downward trend in tribal, forest-based collection, their number has increased over the last ten years. From Kozhinjampara, private merchants send them to Tamil Nadu or even Karnataka, for one or several days, when plants are not available for collection locally. Some items also come from local merchants and collectors actually located in Tamil Nadu. Plants are gathered from many places across the state, some as far as the eastern coastal area, while cultivation is also being developed, especially in Dindigul, 150 km south-east from Kozhinjampara. Appropriate agricultural land is available in Tamil Nadu, as well as cheap manpower. Few agents also now cultivate plants in Kozhinjampara, enabling them to counter the decreasing availability and the seasonality of plants. Their geographical situation also allows them to gather fresh herbs during the rainy season in Kerala and then to cross the border to dry them in Tamil Nadu, where the south-west monsoon rains are blocked by the Ghats.

The activity created in Kozhinjampara village for collecting, cultivating, transporting, and transforming the items is huge. At one merchant's place we visited, 10–20 people were regularly hired for chopping plants, making bundles and maintaining the go-down. In another place, ten people were active in the cultivation fields, helped by two drivers. Go-downs full of plants are spread along tortuous small pathways that crisscross the area, bundles of long stems are stored at the entrance of houses, medicinal plants grow between coconut fields, and people carrying loads of plants on their heads can be seen in the evening time. Village activity is now marked by the rhythm of Ayurvedic plant gathering. The few merchants who have been working there for many years still manage to be competitive because of their long-term relationships with Ayurvedic companies, but some others experience difficulties due to the increasing competition. They now have to deal with young merchants, travelling to distant places in Tamil Nadu, making connections directly with local collectors there, hooked on their cell phones, and trying to anticipate demand patterns. There are a few success stories of youngsters benefitting from a stable financial background and an entrepreneur's mind, becoming highly successful actors in these emerging supply networks. One of them managed to become the sole supplier for more than 40 items needed by Oushadhi within four years.

The enlargement of collection areas is not without ecological consequences, however, as resource harvesting happens at a fast pace in Tamil Nadu. When plants have been gathered from one place, collectors are sent further afield, following the rains and the availability of plants. No strategy for conservation of plants is adopted, collectors from Kerala have no incentives to ensure regeneration of the resources, and people in Tamil Nadu ignored the market value of these plants until very recently. This confirms a widening disconnection between the Ayurvedic sector, on its mission of expansion, and its natural environment.[22] While the Kerala government is involved in the development of medicinal plant cultivation and protection of its forest areas, there does not seem to be any collaboration with the Tamil Nadu state government to regulate the growing flow of vegetal materials between the two states. The Indian National Guidelines on Access to Biological Resources and Associated Knowledge and Benefits Sharing Regulations, promulgated in November 2014, did not give much consideration to inter-state regulations, and Kerala Ayurvedic companies seem to show little interest either in resource conservation in Tamil Nadu or in benefit sharing with material providers there (Dejouhanet 2017b). New circulations of plants emerge, new connections between territories are made and cross-border flows grow, but until now, the traceability issue is still to be addressed, as well as an effective integration of raw material supply to the development strategy of pharmaceutical companies.

Conclusion

Beyond the Himalayan region and India, there is very little literature available on contemporary medicinal raw material supply in Asia.[23] However, Suh's (2008) description of medicinal plant flows between Korea and China in the eighteenth and nineteenth centuries and Bian's (2017) analysis of river

---

22 It is notable that Vaidyaratnam Oushadalayam Pvt. Ltd. chose to remain close to its natural resources by opening a new modern factory in 2009, close to Pollachi town in Tamil Nadu and just a few kilometres from the Kerala border. The relative abundance of raw materials allowed it to specialise there in the manufacturing of export-oriented Ayurvedic medicines and therefore to diversify its activities and enter new markets. Although this strategy was already operating in 1987, when the company opened a factory close to the Peechi forests, it has shifted its focus, as the delocalisation to Tamil Nadu represents more a production expansion than a production sustaining strategy.
23 For example, the book *Medicinal Plants Research in Asia (vol. 1)* inventories research works and projects on medicinal plants in Asian countries, but the sections on collection and trade are extremely limited and weak (Battugal et al. 2004).

transportation of medicinal raw materials in late nineteenth century China show how difficult it was for states to control the trade in medicinal plants, how intricate were the networks structured by governments and private merchants, and how important multi-scaled and systemic analysis is for understanding the issues and challenges of such complex webs. Given what has been presented above, we argue that approaching the raw material supply of the Ayurvedic industry – and of other Asian medical industries – from a linear, channel-based perspective makes it impossible to clearly understand such a complex sector. Such an approach assumes that all plant flows follow a vertical trajectory, bringing them from collectors or farmers to industries through the hands of numerous intermediaries. Although this conception is ultimately correct, it hides the extreme diversity of horizontal flows and the importance of the "range of relationships" (Booker et al. 2012), which connect many different kinds of actors involved in supply activities. Tracing the itineraries of plants is like pulling the threads of an intricately woven social system that is rotating around the supply of medicinal plants to pharmaceutical industries. Untangling this web highlights this realm as a multi-dimensional and multi-scale combination of factors including caste identity, local history, social capital, cultural heritage, industrial strategies, market demands, state policies, and many other elements besides. The dynamic combination of these factors explains and determines both the structure and function of the networks that feed the emergent "pharmaceutical assemblage" (Kloos 2017).

The Kerala State government's attempt to structure its Ayurvedic supply sector is a good illustration of the common assumption that a linear channel is the ideal construction for a fair and sustainable supply. Such a system supposedly allows for a clear understanding of the identities of, and relationships between, resource providers, intermediaries, and industrial producers. The state channel was created as an unavoidable monopolistic system, but the exclusion of large numbers of important stakeholders contributed to its unsustainability and to mounting encroachment by the private sector. In the end, the longstanding competition between state departments, as well as national laws on *adivasi* rights to forest lands and resources, provided the catalyst for the diminution of State Federation control over NTFP collection and marketing. A few SC/ST Cooperative Societies are still functioning today, but *adivasi* collectors are now entitled to market forest goods themselves through their participatory institutions. Finally, the liberalisation of NTFP marketing was the result of several government decisions and marked a dramatic change in the conception of the state's role in framing key sectors, of which the Ayurvedic raw material supply sector serves as an exemplar.

Even if the private sector prospered despite the state channel monopoly, this evolution confirms its dominance in supplying pharmaceutical companies. It remains uncertain whether the empowerment of local institutions to market medicinal items will counterbalance the influence of private merchants. If public companies like Oushadhi work to support direct marketing from *adivasi* populations, helped by the Kerala Forest Department, it may not turn out much different than when cooperative societies existed and flows of forest goods were diverted to the private sector anyway. This situation feeds the common assumption that middlemen should be removed from at least the first level of marketing, if not the whole channel, ignoring the evidence that supply networks of medicinal plants function only because of the private sector. This assumption leads to a misunderstanding of the role of private merchants in the supply networks and also of the role of Ayurvedic industries in the lack of sustainability of their supply. Indeed, suppliers wishing to secure contracts with pharmaceutical companies have to propose the lowest prices, and their transportation and storage costs, as well as the financial risks of the operation, contribute to making intermediaries underpay for the collected items. The system of e-tender now being developed by a few firms will likely reinforce this tendency by increasing competition in the field. Even if the prices paid by the factories for their raw material are increasing, the segmentation of channels by several levels of intermediaries and the intertwining of networks serve to prevent a knock-on effect of this rise on collectors' profits. Instead of the obsession with removing middlemen from the channel, we suggest, in line with very few authors like T. Pauls and M. Franz (2013), that politicians, experts, and scientists should first recognise the complex roles these intermediaries play and their central importance in the functioning of the supply system. Only then would it be possible to set up a realistic framework for formalising[24] their activities, minimising risk factors, smoothing their profits, and securing higher revenues for collectors. Adopting a long-term strategy for sustaining raw material supply is therefore crucial for Asian medical industries, whose expansion is undoubtedly dependent on their capacity to address raw material scarcity as well as to shoulder their social and ecological responsibilities.

The fact that Kozhinjampara middlemen are the most dynamic agents in the area today is because they managed to enlarge their supply networks to Tamil Nadu, where collection is less developed and items are still available in good quantities at low prices. Opacity of plant itineraries and increasing distances between the factories and the places where plants grow tends to weaken even more the sense of responsibility of companies towards the sustainability of medicinal plant resources. While some companies have kept good connections with their immediate social environment, sourcing items from villagers living nearby, there appears to be a general trend towards progressive disconnection from the natural environment, as most of their raw material now comes from far away. This "alienation," described by

---

24 Considering the critical approach to formalisation developed by van der Valk in this volume, we rather use this term to refer to a process of legitimisation, as defined by Blaikie and Craig in their chapter.

Stephan Kloos (2017) for Sowa Rigpa, is questioning the capacity of Asian traditional medicines to fit with the norms of integrated production, epitomised in Good Manufacturing Practices, where the traceability of raw material is a key standard.

Acknowledgements

We are thankful to the Kerala Ayurvedic companies' managers and employees who spent time answering our questions, especially Oushadhi – The Pharmaceutical Corporation (I.M.) Kerala Ltd. for their long-term trust. We thank also all the respondents, collectors, traders, and government officers, who made this research possible. Part of the fieldwork for this chapter was carried out within a doctoral work, undertaken within the French Institute of Pondicherry. Then updates were made possible by post-doctoral funding from the French National Research Agency. We wish to thank the GLOBHEALTH project (ERC Grant) for its recent research funding, and our acknowledgements go to Dr J.P. Gaudillière, director of the Cermes3 (INSERM/CNRS), for his lasting trust. We also thank Calum Blaikie a lot for his insightful comments on the first versions of this paper. We finally wish to thank Sudheesh K. Menon for his precious help in the fields.

Bibliography

Adam G and Belt J (2009) *Developing a Medicinal Plant Value Chain: Lessons from an Initiative to Cultivate Kutki (Picrorhiza kurrooa) in Northern India*, KIT Working Papers Series C5, Amsterdam: Royal Tropical Institute.

Banerjee M (2009) *Power, Knowledge, Medicine. Ayurvedic Pharmaceuticals at Home and in the World*. Hyderabad: Orient Blackswan.

Battugal P, Kanniah J, Lee SY, et al. (eds) (2004) *Medicinal Plants Research in Asia. Volume 1: The Framework and Project Workplans*. Serdang, Malaysia: IPGRI-APO.

Belt J, Lengkeek A, and van der Zant J (2003) *Cultivating a Healthy Enterprise – Developing a Sustainable Medicinal Plant Chain in Uttaranchal – India*. Amsterdam: Bulletin of the Royal Tropical Institute (KIT), No. 350.

Bian H (2017) Between Market and Port: Reconfiguring Traditional Medicine Trade in Late Nineteenth-Century China, *Talk given during the 9th International Congress on Traditional Asian Medicines*, 6–12 August 2017, Kiel, Germany.

Blaikie C (2014) *Making Medicine: Pharmacy, Exchange and the Production of Sowa Rigpa in Ladakh*. PhD Thesis, University of Kent.

Bode M (2008) *Taking Traditional Knowledge to the Market. The Modern Image of the Ayurvedic and Unani Industry 1980–2000*. Hyderabad: Orient Longman.

Booker A (2014) *The Transformation of Traditional Asian Medical Knowledge into International Commodities, the Link between Traditional Medicines and the International Market*. PhD Thesis, University of London.

Booker A, Johnston D, and Heinrich M (2012) Value Chains of Herbal Medicines – Research Needs and Key Challenges in the Context of Ethnopharmacology, *Journal of Ethnopharmacology* 140: 624–633.

Bourdieu P (1980) Le Capital Social. *Actes de la recherche en sciences sociales* 31: 2–3.

Chominot A (2002) L'économie des plantes médicinales en Inde. *Ethnopharmacologia* 29: 54–67.

Chominot A (2003) The herbal drugs economy in India. *Down to Earth*, 31 January, pp. 52.

Craig S (2012) *Healing Elements: Efficacy and the Social Ecologies of Tibetan Medicine*. Berkeley, CA: University of California Press.

Craig S and Glover D (2009) Conservation, Cultivation and Commodification of Medicinal Plants in the Greater Himalayan-Tibetan Plateau. *Asian Medicine* 5(2): 219–242.

Datta SK (2001) Marketing of Wild Medicinal Plants. Tribal Economy in India. *Economic and Political Weekly* 36(38): 3598–3602.

Davidar P, Arjunan M and Puyravaud J-P (2008) Why do Local Households Harvest Forest Products? A Case Study from the Southern Western Ghats, India. *Biological Conservation* 141: 1876–1884.

Dejouhanet L (2007) Les produits forestiers non ligneux et la gestion de la forêt kéralaise: droit d'usage et droit de contrôle. In: Christoph E (ed) *Law, Land Use and the Environment. Afro-Indian Dialogues. Enjeux fonciers et environnementaux: Dialogues afro-indiens*. Pondicherry: IFP, pp. 407–438.

Dejouhanet L (2009) L'Ayurveda. Mondialisation d'une médecine traditionnelle indienne. *Echogéo* 10.

Dejouhanet L (2014a) Supply of Medicinal Raw Materials. The Achilles Heel of Today's Manufacturing Sector for Ayurvedic Drugs in Kerala. *Asian Medicine* 9(1–2): 206–235.

Dejouhanet L (2014b) Secteur informel et réseaux de commercialisation des plantes médicinales au Kérala (Inde). *Économie rurale* 343: 53–70.

Dejouhanet L (2017a) Tourism in the Mountains of Central Kerala (South India): At the Crossroads of Attitudes towards Forest Populations. *Journal of Alpine Research* 105(3).

Dejouhanet L (2017b) Benefit Sharing of Biological Resources in Kerala: The Inextricable Issue of Ayurvedic Raw Material Supply. In: Pradeep Kumar S, Amruth M, Raghu AV, Mohammed Kunhi KV and Raveendran VP (eds) *Medicinal Plants: Benefit Sharing, Development, Conservation*. Peechi: Kerala State Council for Science, Technology and Environment – Kerala Forest Research Institute, pp. 111–117.

Ganguly BK and Chaudhary K (2003) Forest Products of Bastar. A Story of Tribal Exploitation. *Economic and Political Weekly* 38(28): 2985–2989.

Hishe M, Asfaw Z and Gidey M (2016) Review on Value Chain Analysis of Medicinal Plants and the Associated Challenges. *Journal of Medicinal Plant Studies* 4(3): 45–55.

GoI (Government of India) Planning Commission (2000). *Report of the Task Force on Conservation & Sustainable Use of Medicinal Plants*, Delhi.

Hofer T (2008) Socio-economic Dimensions of Tibetan Medicine in the Tibet Autonomous Region, China. Part Two. *Asian Medicine* 4: 492–514.

Holley J and Cherla K (1998) *The Medicinal Plants Sector in India: A Review*. Delhi: MAPPA, IDRC/SARO.

Hugon P (1994) Instabilité et organisation des filières coton en Afrique. *Économie rurale* 224: 39–44.

Hugon P (2005) Les réformes de la filière coton au Mali et les négociations internationales. *Afrique contemporaine* 2005/4(216): 203–225.

Jayaraman K and Anitha V (2010) *Forestry Sector Analysis for the State of Kerala*. Peechi: Kerala Forest Research Institute, Research Report 345.

Kloos S (2017) The Pharmaceutical Assemblage: Rethinking Sowa Rigpa and the Herbal Pharmaceutical Industry in Asia, *Current Anthropology* 58(6).

Larsen HO and Olsen CS (2007) Unsustainable Collection and Unfair Trade? Uncovering and Assessing Assumptions Regarding Central Himalayan Medicinal Plant Conservation. *Biodiversity Conservation* 16: 1679–1697.

Lazzarini S, Chaddad F and Cook M (2001) Integrating Supply Chain and Network Analyses: The Study of Netchains. *Journal on Chain and Network Science* 1(1): 7–22.

Leaman D (1998) Conservation Priorities for Medicinal Plants, in IDRC/CRDI, *Medicinal Plants: A Global Heritage, Proceedings of the International Conference on Medicinal Plants for Survival*, February 16–19, Bangalore: 2–13.

Lele S, Pattanaik M and Rai N (2010) NTFPs in India: Rhetoric and Reality. In: Laird S, McLain R and Wynberg R (eds) *Wild Product Governance: Finding Policies that Work for Non-Timber Forest Products*. London: Earthscan.

Madhavan H (2006) From Home to Market: Responses, Resurgences and Transformation of Ayurveda from 1830s to 1920s, communication paper. In: *The Institutionalisation of Therapeutic Practices in India: Social and Legal Perspectives*. Pondicherry: French Institute of Pondicherry, December 7–8.

Madhavan H (2008) *Linking Tribal Medicinal Plant Co-operatives and Ayurvedic Manufacturing Firms for Better Rural Livelihood and Sustainable Use of Resources*. Munich: MPRA, Paper no. 6954.

Madhavan H (2009) Commercialising Traditional Medicine: Ayurvedic Manufacturing in Kerala. *Economic and Political Weekly* 44(16): 44–51.

Madhavan H (2017) Ayurvedic Pharmaceuticals and the Global Regulatory Context: Complexities and Alternatives. In: Pradeep Kumar S, Amruth M, Raghu AV, Mohammed Kunhi KV and Raveendran VP (eds), *Medicinal Plants: Benefit Sharing, Development, Conservation*. Peechi: KSCSTE-Kerala Forest Research Institute, 93–104.

Mark AS, Deepa GB and Rao JR (2017). Sustainable Harvesting, Value Addition and Marketing Wild Medicinal Plants: Designing Participatory Methods and the Process of Field Implementation – Case Study from Silent Valley and Peechi Wildlife Divisions in Kerala. In: Pradeep Kumar S, Amruth M, Raghu AV, Mohammed Kunhi KV and Raveendran VP (eds) *Medicinal Plants: Benefit Sharing, Development, Conservation*. Peechi: KSCSTE-Kerala Forest Research Institute: 125–135.

Mathur PRG (1977) *Tribal Situation in Kerala*. Trivandrum: Kerala Historical Society.

Münster U and Vishnudas S (2012) In the Jungle of Law. Adivasi Rights and Implementation of Forest Rights Act in Kerala. *Economic & Political Weekly* 47(19): 38–45.

Muraleedharan PK, Sasidharan N and Seethalakshmi KK (1997) *Biodiversity in Tropical Moist Forests: A Study of Sustainable Use of Non-Wood Forest Products in the Western Ghats*. Peechi, Kerala: KFRI, Research Report 133.

Narendran K, Murthy IK, Suresh HS, et al. (2001) Non-timber Forest Product Extraction, Utilization and Valuation: A Case Study from the Nilgiri Biosphere Reserve, Southern India. *Economic Botany* 55(4): 528–538.

Olsen CS (1998) The Trade in Medicinal and Aromatic Plants from Central Nepal to Northern India. *Economic Botany* 52(3): 279–292.

Olsen CS and Bhattarai N (2005) A Typology of Economic Agents in the Himalayan Plant Trade. *Mountain Research and Development* 25(1): 37–43.

Pauls T and Franz M (2013) Trading in the Dark. The Medicinal Plants Production Network in Uttarakhand. *Singapore Journal of Tropical Geography* 34: 229–243.

Pordié L (2002) La pharmacopée comme expression de société: Une étude himalayenne. In: Fleurentin J, Pelt J-M, and Mazars G (eds). *Des sources du savoir aux médicaments du futur*. Paris: Editions IRD–SFE, 183–194.

Pordié L and Gaudillière J-P (eds) (2014a) The Herbal Pharmaceutical Industry in India. *Asian Medicine* 9(1–2).

Pordié L and Gaudillière J-P (2014b) Introduction: Industrial Ayurveda. Drug Discovery, Reformulation and the Market. *Asian Medicine* 9(1–2): 1–11.

Pordié L and Hardon A (2015) Drug's Stories and Itineraries. On the Making of Asian Industrial Medicines. *Anthropology & Medicine* 22(1): 1–6.

Preetha N, Laladhas KP, Oommen OV (2015) Stratagem for Sustainable Utilization of Medicinal Plant Resources, *Proceedings of TIM-Research Conference on Sustainability and Management Strategy*, Bonfring.

Rai ND (2003) *Human Use, Reproductive Ecology, and Life History of Garcinia gummi-gutta, a Non Timber Forest Product in the Western Ghats, India*. PhD Thesis in Biology, University of Pennsylvania.

Sasidharan N and Muraleedharan PK (2000) *Survey on the Commercial Exploitation and Consumption of Medicinal Plants by the Drug Industry in Northern Kerala*. Peechi: KFRI, Research Report 193.

Sasidharan N and Muraleedharan PK (2009) *The Raw Drugs Requirement of Ayurvedic Medicine Manufacturing Industry of Kerala*. Peechi: Kerala Forest Research Institute, Research Report 322.

Saxer M (2009) Herbs and Traders in Transit: Border Regimes and the Contemporary Trans-Himalayan Trade in Tibetan Medicinal Plants. *Asian Medicine* 5: 317–339.

Saxer M (2013) *Manufacturing Tibetan Medicine. The Creation of an Industry and the Moral Economy of Tibetanness*. New York, NY & Oxford: Berghahn.

Scott J (1976) *The Moral Economy of the Peasant. Rebellion and Subsistence in Southeast Asia*. New Haven, CT & London: Yale University Press.

Scott J (1985) *Weapons of the Weak: Everyday Forms of Resistance*. New Haven, CT & London: Yale University Press.

Scott J (1989) Everyday Forms of Resistance. *Copenhagen Journal of Asian Studies* 4: 33–62.

Shahidullah AKM and Haque CE (2010) Linking Medicinal Plant Production with Livelihood Enhancement in Bangladesh: Implications of a Vertically Integrated Value Chain. *The Journal of Transdisciplinary Environmental Studies* 9(2): 1–18.

Shankar A (1999) *A Study on the Economics of Collection, Marketing and Utilisation of Non-Timber Forest Products in Kerala*. PhD Thesis, Peechi: KFRI.

Shankar A and Muraleedharan PK (1996) Marketing of Non-timber Forest Products in Kerala. An Overview. In: Shiva MP and Mathur RP (eds) *Management of Minor Forest Produce for Sustainability*. New Delhi: Oxford & IBH Publishing Co. Pvt. Ltd. 307–314.

Springer L (2015) Collectors, Producers, and Circulators of Tibetan and Chinese Medicines in Sichuan Province. *Asian Medicine* 10(1–2): 177–220.

Suh S (2008) Herbs of Our Own Kingdom: Layers of the "Local" in the *Materia Medica* of Early Chosŏn Korea. *Asian Medicine* 4: 395–422.

Thomas P (1996) *Dynamics of Co-Operative Marketing in Tribal Economies. A Study of Non-Timber Forest Produce Marketing in Kerala*. PhD Thesis, Cochin University of Science and Technology.

Torre A and Beuret J-E (2012) *Proximités territoriales*. Paris: Economica.

Tripathy U, Kaur D and Maheswari R (2003) Sustainable Cultivation of Medicinal Plants. Community Participation in Uttaranchal. *Economic and Political Weekly* 38(10).

Tsing A (2015) *The Mushrooms at the End of the World: On the Possibility of Life in Capitalist Ruins*. Princeton, NJ: Princeton University Press.

Van de Kop P, Alam G and De Steenhuijsen Piters B (2006) Developing a Sustainable Medicinal Plant Chain in India: Linking People, Markets and Values. In: Ruben R, Slingerland M and Njhoff H (eds) *Agrochains and Networks for Development*. Amsterdam: Springer, pp. 191–202.

Zacharias, Sibi (2003) *The Micro-Level Impact of Tribal Development Programmes among the Kadar Tribe of Kerala*. Thiruvananthapuram: Centre for Development Studies (Kerala Research Programme on Local Level Development).

Zimmermann F (1989) *Le discours des remèdes au pays des épices. Enquête sur la médecine hindoue*. Paris: Ed. Payot, Médecine et sociétés.

Part III
Sowa Rigpa industries

8 "Sourcery"
Losing track of Tibetan medicinal plants between commerce and conservation in Northern India

Jan M. A. van der Valk

Asian medical industries fundamentally rely on natural resources, especially plants. This is no different for Sowa Rigpa (Tibetan for "the science of healing," see Craig and Gerke 2016) or, for instance, Ayurveda. In the case of Sowa Rigpa and in agreement with his interlocutors, Kloos (2017: 697) avows that "the greatest challenge today consists in producing sufficient amounts of medicine" in these times of rising popularity and surging demand in India and elsewhere. This "foundational crisis of raw materials" (cf. Craig's comment to Kloos 2017: 707) arises in the context of late capitalism, which feeds on the transformation of traditional knowledge into international, mass-produced cultural commodities (Alexiades 2009). The industrialisation of Ayurveda has been interpreted as *An Indian Path to Biocapital* (Gaudillière 2014a: 412–414) in this context, while economic and cultural property rights systems affecting Sowa Rigpa are also rapidly emerging in both India and China (Madhavan 2017). The notion of Asian medical industries – and the related "pharmaceutical assemblage" (Kloos 2017) – explicitly acknowledges the centrality of capitalism to an extent that was unanticipated by Leslie's (1976) *Asian Medical Systems*, making it visible and available for critique. Looking at Tibetan medicinal plant trade in Northern India through this lens and acknowledging that it is at times impossible to differentiate the material basis of the Tibetan and Indian medical traditions, I argue that the core problem of these industries is neither an inherent shortage of raw materials nor "corruption" and informality/illegality per se. I propose, rather, that the crux lies in the paradoxical situation that ensues as these industries become fundamentally capitalist, profit-oriented endeavours while simultaneously being reframed by the Indian state and regional academic and non-governmental actors as an ideal opportunity for sustainable development through regulation. Recognising that distinctions between the informal and formal economies are blurred, I highlight the labyrinthine nature of Indian medicinal plant trade and the troubling day-to-day interactions between traders and the state's regulatory and bureaucratic apparatus, focusing on the insidious role of neoliberal discourses in the catch-22 between commerce and conservation.

DOI: 10.4324/9781003218074-12

While conservation and capitalism have long been entangled, over the last few decades the global conservation movement has been reinventing itself through the incorporation of a neoliberal ideology, increasingly relying on market mechanisms such as ecotourism, the valuation of ecosystem services, and trade in carbon emissions and biodiversity financial derivatives. Fletcher et al. (2014) aptly describe this new frontier of neoliberal conservation[1] as "Nature™ Inc." An analogous process is taking place in India's medicinal plant policies through the conception of a unified national market and the implementation of measures based on trade surveys. This "green" marketisation was instigated by a newly formed assemblage of state institutions, corporate R&D, NGOs, and academic actors[2] and is driven by the industrialisation of Ayurveda and the emergence of an autonomous social and epistemological sphere of "pharmacy" (Pordié and Gaudillière 2014, but see Kudlu 2016 on the continued prevalence of physician-manufacturers in Kerala). As part of this process fuelled by pharmaceutical globalisation and WHO policies since the mid-1980s (Pordié and Gaudillière 2014: 60–62), Gaudillière (2014b: 176) notices a shift in the actors involved in Indian medicinal plant trade:

> Today, the most visible actors of pharmaceuticalisation are ayurvedic drug companies, at least the bigger ones, which integrate research, formulation, fabrication, and distribution. The emergence of an autonomous world of ayurvedic *materia medica* as component of the reformulation regime, however, mobilises other actors and public institutions. Previously, these were barely associated with Ayurveda but participated in botanical research, bioprospection, agricultural innovation, or forestry and are now increasingly committed to medicinal-plant management.

Corresponding to this shift, a new technoscientific discourse on plant supply and conservation emerged based on the following principles: an assumed link between overexploitation (an economic issue) and gene erosion (environmental damage); mass cultivation as the ideal solution for ingredient quality and scarcity; a focus on commercially – not necessarily clinically – valuable species due to a reliance on trade surveys; and a narrative of exploited rural people, ignorant and greedy harvesters, and secretive, adulterating traders, all caught

---

1 For the purpose of my argument, I define neoliberal conservation, following Büscher et al. (2012: 4), as "an amalgamation of *ideology and techniques* informed by the premise that natures can only be 'saved' through their submission to capital and its subsequent revaluation in capitalist terms". Neoliberalism here refers specifically to "a *political ideology* that aims to subject political, social, and ecological affairs to capitalist market dynamics" through governmentalities, embodied practices, and biopower (ibid.: 5).
2 The references in footnotes 4 and 5 represent the numerous characteristic studies produced by this assemblage in Nepal as well as in India.

up in inefficient informality.³ As Gaudillière (2014b) shows, the National Medicinal Plants Board (NMPB, set up in 2000 in New Delhi) played a major yet contested role in this as a coordinating bureaucratic structure promoting industrial and agricultural management policies, thus forging a "National Plant Market."⁴ My focus on relatively small traders and exporters rather than market-leading firms, however, allows for a much less integrated and managerial vision of raw material supply. This bottom-up ethnographic approach reveals some of the hidden assumptions and contradictions of the abovementioned ideologies and discourses on the ground, questioning authoritarian policy interventions in the trade and conservation of medicinal plants.

The manipulation of markets for the benefit of both people and (endangered) plants – or more cynically to increase state control and revenues – has gained centre stage since the end of the 1980s both in India⁵ and internationally⁶ (Laird et al. 2010: 2–3). Relying on slogans such as "use it or lose it," the underlying assumption was that forests would be left intact despite and because of sustained non-timber forest product (NTFP) collection.⁷ Yet, even though a whole suite of interlinked non-governmental

---

3   Larsen and Olsen (2007) have similarly identified four commonly held assumptions concerning Himalayan medicinal plant trade and conservation based on a survey of 175 collectors, traders, and government staff (Larsen and Smith 2004) and on a literature review of 119 publications by researchers, (international) NGOs, and policy-makers from Nepal: (1) overall degradation of the resource base due to rising demand, (2) the prevalence of open-access harvesting, (3) cultivation as the optimal solution, and (4) that harvesters are cheated by middlemen. None of these preconceptions turned out to be well-supported by empirical evidence. Refer to Dejouhanet and Sreelakshmy in this volume for publications on India reporting these assumptions.
4   In the last two decades, four national reports on India's medicinal plant trade were published, which largely align with the neoliberal conservation discourse outlined here, albeit with several reservations (Holley and Cherla 1998; Subrat et al. 2002; Nagpal and Karki 2004; Ved and Goraya 2008).
5   See Lele et al. (2010) for a national overview of historical shifts in Indian state policies on "non-timber forest products" (NTFPs), or "minor forest products" (MFPs) as they are commonly referred to across South Asia, observing a large and problematic gap between rhetoric and reality. Sustainability, under the form of "ecological balance", only entered the agenda in 1988. In the past two decades, several pieces of legislation pronounced the devolution of ownership and control towards forest, rural, and tribal communities, but actual shifts in power have not been implemented in practice or even acknowledged; most interpretations of existing forestry law still take the state to be the owner of all NTFPs.
6   Based on an extensive review of the NTFP literature, Pierce (2010) shows that NTFP commercialisation as a conservation-development tool is currently still the number one topic of interest. The number of NTFP studies has grown steadily during the last two decades, with the majority being published during the last few years (Shackleton et al. 2015). "Developing countries" and rural areas are the most prevalent study sites, whereas Asia and India in particular have the most papers (Shackleton et al. 2011).
7   This assumption ignores the high complexity of NTFPs (e.g. Neumann and Hirsch 2000), the many challenges of their commercialisation (Belcher and Schreckenberg 2007), as well as the multiple and often confusing and inconsistent nature of NTFP-relevant laws and policies (Laird et al. 2010).

organisations and state institutions aims to understand and streamline the herbal industry, it often remains unfathomable. Studies alternatively emphasise its elaborate organisational structure (usually in the form of supply chains, cf. Booker et al. 2012) or the rampant secrecy, informality, and illegality (e.g. Pauls and Franz 2013). Dejouhanet (2014), for example, concludes that the refusal of state (and industrial) actors to really understand the functioning of ayurvedic raw material supply networks is the Achilles heel of the sector in Kerala. She underscores the "desperate need" for cultivation and supply chain integration while at the same time witnessing the "enormous obstacles" posed by informality and complexity as well as the widening gap between collectors and manufacturers. These contradictions between state- and corporate-led modernisation and standardisation on the one hand and commodity chain heterogeneity on the other, however, are a basic characteristic of supply chain capitalism; where subcontracting, outsourcing, and "scandalous economies and ecologies" have become the norm (Tsing and Matsutake Worlds Research Group 2009: 349). Supply chain capitalists actively "search for niches of diversity within the cracks and ruins of state and corporate management" (ibid.: 363), which also implies that supply chain integration may not be desirable for everyone. Moreover, alarmist conservation language framed in economic terms masks the inconvenient truth that "environmental (and other) crises increasingly are themselves opportunities for capitalist expansion" (Büscher et al. 2012: 7). As such, neoliberal "win-win" conservation-development interventions have the tendency to serve the dominant ideology and the interest of elites by paradoxically promoting marketisation and economic growth as solutions, alienating us from systemic causes and "the materiality of plants themselves and the (social) ecologies from which they come" (Craig in Kloos 2017: 708).

In this context, the neoliberalisation of environmental knowledge production – and of universities in general – is worrisome on multiple levels, relying on the epistemological foundation of the market as supreme information processor (Lave 2012: 21–24). Adams' (2002) tour de force on the application of "Randomised Controlled Crime" to Sowa Rigpa, based on Comaroff and Comaroff's (1999, 2000) millennial capitalism, can thus be extended to (Tibetan) medicinal plant trade and conservation in India, as I will show: in both cases market interests fuse with scientific knowledge practices in the production of globalised truths (i.e. the neoliberal conservation discourse), shifting ownership and profit while criminalising local actors (collectors and traders). In her monograph chapter titled *Cultivating the Wilds*, Craig (2012) explores intersections between political ecology and medical anthropology as Sowa Rigpa practitioners interact and at times clash with conservation-development organisations and the commodification of Himalayan natures and cultures. *Amchi* (*am chi*) offer local critiques of conservation[8] by pointing out the complicity of the government and big-business Tibetan medical factories in stimulating mass for-profit collection, while they feel that governments seem to care more about the plants than the practitioners who rely on them for healing (see also Blaikie 2009). The larger issue at hand is aptly summarised in the introduction to the Special Issue titled *Conservation, Cultivation, and Commodification of Medicinal Plants in the Greater Himalayan-Tibetan Plateau* (Craig and Glover 2009: 227):

> [E]conomic growth and improved livelihoods are also supposed to facilitate the conservation of natural resources and Earth's biodiversity. Yet [...], it is quite difficult to square concepts of "sustainability" with efforts to scale up the Tibetan medical industry, either from the perspective of commodification and sheer resource use or from the perspective of a moral economy of *gso ba rig pa* practice and the standards of medicinal potency and benefit that practitioners of this tradition espouse.

This chapter is based on fieldwork with the suppliers of two seemingly unrelated manufacturers of Tibetan "alternative pharmaceuticals:" PADMA – a Swiss pharmaceutical company – and Men-Tsee-Khang, the largest exile institution for Tibetan medicine in India.[9] Situated in a "core" and a "periphery" of modern Western technoscience, respectively, these producers nevertheless face similar issues when it comes to matters of manufacture (van der Valk 2017). One important bundle of connections, flows, and frictions they share is the sourcing of raw materials: both get a significant amount of dried bulk herbs from Indian suppliers. My initial aim was to trace a handful of herbs from PADMA and Men-Tsee-Khang all the way back to their places of origin. To their roots. This turned out

---

8   Tibetan conceptions of "conservation" (often translated as *srung skyob*) rely on a markedly different construction of "nature", premised on spirit-mediated relationality and Buddhist ethics (Craig 2012: 188). This does not imply that Tibetan sacred sites cannot be refugia of biodiversity (Anderson et al. 2005; Salick et al. 2007; Shen et al. 2012), for instance, but it does hint at a fundamental issue when recruiting *amchi* for joint conservation-development projects (cf. Aumeeruddy-Thomas and Lama 2008; Law & Salick 2007).
9   Men-Tsee-Khang refers to the Tibetan Medical and Astrological Institute (originally in Lhasa), which was re-established in exile in India in the 1960s (Kloos 2008: 16–24), while PADMA AG is the only company in Europe producing medicines and food supplements based on Tibetan formulas (inherited from a Buryat-Russian Sowa Rigpa family lineage, cf. Saxer 2004). The former positions itself as a guardian of tradition and the Tibetan culture and nation (Kloos 2013), whereas the latter is a pioneer caught up in-between the mainstream pharmaceutical industry and contentious European Complementary and Alternative Medicine (Schwabl and Vennos 2015; van der Valk 2017: 277–286).

to be a daunting task.[10] Tracing Tibetan *materia medica* through Indian supply chains, one can easily lose touch with Sowa Rigpa altogether as it dissolves into the much larger Ayurveda-dominated trade.[11] Both producers put me in touch with some of their major suppliers in India, who I subsequently visited in Delhi (October 2013, March 2014, and August 2015), Gurgaon (March 2014, August 2015), Amritsar (July 2015), and Manali (July–August 2015). Because and sometimes in spite of this personal introduction from one of their important customers, these traders were surprisingly supportive of my research and open to enquiries. I also explored the large wholesale markets of Delhi and Amritsar independently, buying herb samples and questioning a number of sellers on trade names, quality, (incredibly inflated) prices, and (vague descriptions of) sourcing. The jump from wholesale markets to harvesting areas is a quantum leap that can only occur within a rare configuration of trust between harvesters, traders, manufacturers, and the researcher.

I succeeded in physically following the trail of only one plant back to where it grows and is harvested: *ruta* (*ru rta*, here equated with *Saussurea costus*, or "costus"), one of the few high-altitude Tibetan medicinal plants to be cultivated successfully in fields (Blaikie 2009). Cultivation obviously makes the plants easier to locate, but it still took us nearly two days of driving from Manali to reach the farms deep in Lahaul Valley. The trader who drove us there was also a cultivator, and incidentally he was selling to both PADMA and Men-Tsee-Khang. Following these tracks, I came across alleged instances of "bribery" and "corruption." These proved to be fertile for critiquing the moral high ground taken in the neoliberal conservation discourse promulgated by Indian regulators and the majority of medicinal plant trade analysts, which is based on a reified division between formal and informal economies and the concomitant assumption that strictly regulated, legal markets are always more beneficial for people and plants. In an increasingly formalised but highly dysfunctional state governance regime, however, practices branded as illegal or corrupt may be the only viable option to stay in business. To drive this point home,

---

10 Methodologically, I adopt a multi-sited – or more precisely translocal (Hannerz 2003) – ethnographic approach of "following the thing" (Marcus 1995), being aware that the "following" metaphor appears to imply a pre-existing field and submission to a laid-out track rather than active co-production. However, I not only question the singular identity of the things I am following but equally the existence of neatly organised supply chains, thus frequently losing track(s) altogether. See also Harris (2013: 24–26) on the practical impossibility of tracing the complex and far-flung origins of commodities such as Tibetan wool carpets.

11 A minority of Tibetan medicinal plants fall outside the remit of the mainstream Indian herbal trade, which means that Tibetan medicine producers must rely on alternative sources. This was for instance the case for *Meconopsis* spp. (*tsher sngon*, *utpal*, etc.), which are sourced by Men-Tsee-Khang from Tibet via Nepal or wild-harvested by staff and students in Himachal Pradesh.

I apply "sourcery"[12] as an analytical descriptor for the risky practice of sourcing medicinal raw materials from Indian markets by crossing convoluted legal and moral grey zones, and through ambivalent economies of favours. This term invokes the occult nature of the trade by alluding to witchcraft, which anthropologists have argued shares some essential characteristics with corruption, as I elaborate under the next heading. "Sourcery," the idea of a risky and occult practice of sourcing raw materials, is the manifestation of a failed formalisation; it is the *alter ego* of the state-sanctioned neoliberal "herbal sector."

"Corruption" and "sourcery:" Neoliberal capitalism and its occult economies

In India, corruption has received ample consideration, particularly since the ground-breaking work by Gupta (1995, 2005). His analyses of popular narratives and media and fictional discourses of corruption in North Indian villages and beyond unravel their contributions to reified, fetishised representations of "the state" and "civil society" as stable, unitary entities. Popular knowledge of the state is inextricably linked to notions of corruption as poor and illiterate villagers aim to cope with the structural violence inherent in bureaucratic encounters. Based on fieldwork in the East Indian industrial belt city of Jamshedpur, Sanchez (2012, 2016) furthermore collapses distinctions between corruption and organised crime, showing how criminal entrepreneurs act as valves between "licit" and "illicit" economies. In an insightful blogpost (South Asia @ LSE, 12 May 2016) titled *"Corruption is both a symptom of the basic structures of capitalism, and a technology that supports them,"* he summarises the argument of his book (2016) as follows:

> Far from operating at the fringes of the state and economy, corrupt actors are usually enmeshed within long-term negotiations with an array of specialists in organised crime, industrial capitalism, financial services, labour contracting, development and the judiciary. [...] [R]ather than sporadically diverting capital to the informal peripheries of capitalism and the state, corruption is a systematic series of negotiations between institutional authority, corporations and violence. These criminal practices are instrumental acts of elite class struggle, whose object is accumulation by dispossession.

There is thus a need to move away from provincialising public discourses on petty bribery – as in Gupta (1995), where villagers "imagine" a core of state accountability at higher levels – to practices that are integral to India's

---

12 I borrow this term from Terry Pratchett's fantasy novel titled *Sourcery*, which was first published in 1988.

political economy and national politics. Both Jamshedpur's industrial steel workers and the peri-urban North Indian herbal traders I worked with offered what Sanchez (2016) terms "systemic corruption discourses." I was struck by the prevalence of allegations of corruption towards state institutions and bureaucrats by traders on the one hand and accusations of illegal/informal and unethical practices towards harvesters, cultivators, and traders from within Indian policy and research circles on the other. However, I am cautious not to assume that "informal," "illegal," and "corrupt" activities are necessarily hidden or occult. As noted by Ledeneva (2014) for late and post-communist Russia, networks of mutual help are a tacitly accepted "open secret." Economies of favours outwit the constraints of centralised distribution systems while also evidencing that it is infeasible for the state to fully enforce its own far-reaching regulations. They thus simultaneously support and undermine the workings of establishment, fading the boundaries between corruption and informality.

Several anthropologists have compared corruption to witchcraft, arguing how both can re-establish a moral order in times of profound institutional instability and how occult practices provide an alternative access to knowledge and power (Bähre 2005; Bubandt 2006; Blundo 2007; Turner 2007; Rudnyckyj 2009). Bubandt (2006) for instance contends that magic is an extension of politics on another level, as he witnessed how both sorcery – which I retain as a fuzzy notion and use synonymously with witchcraft – and corruption are part of the same occult politics of the ongoing democratisation of Indonesia. Both are politically efficacious yet morally ambivalent, often go together, and share the common dilemma of the unknowability of the other. Anthropological research on sorcery evidences its circularity (witchcraft can best be dealt with by witchcraft), ambivalent figures and their moral ambiguity (precarious distinctions between positive and negative forms), a troubled relationship with nation-states and capitalist economy, and paradoxical interactions with modernity (Geschiere 1997). Without delving deeper into this body of literature,[13] I use these generalised common traits of sorcery and corruption to paint an alternative picture of how the Indian trade in medicinals operates. By considering these occult practices as both artefacts of and an attempted escape from

---

13 In India, women are common targets of witchcraft accusations and witch hunts in tribal communities (Chaudhuri 2012, Mullick 2000). These have been analysed as the result of profound socioeconomic changes and gender inequalities that manifest as these indigenous societies integrate more into the Hindu-dominated patriarchy (Mullick 2000), whereas police and other state actors attempt to stamp out these activities, which they regard as "backward" (Desai 2009). Gender discrepancies also play into the Indian herbal industry: a large portion of the collectors are female (who are blamed for indiscriminate wild-harvesting, which is low-prestige and arduous work), while middlemen and wholesalers are nearly exclusively male (who are blamed for exploiting the harvesters; cf. Olsen and Larsen 2003; Larsen and Olsen 2007).

millennial capitalism and its neoliberal reforms, my argument parallels Comaroff and Comaroff's (1999, 2000) striking analyses of "the enchantments of modernity." I build on their definition of "occult economies:" "the deployment of magical means for material ends or, more expansively, the conjuring of wealth by resort to inherently mysterious techniques, techniques whose principles of operation are neither transparent nor explicable in conventional terms" (Comaroff and Comaroff 1999: 297, footnote 31). However, the economies I describe are more mundane. The two traders I track in the following sections are not considered witches, but their role as "profiteering middlemen" has been cursed repeatedly in surveys aiming to make herbal trade legible to conservation/development-justified state control. In what follows, I aim to map the murky waters of their sourcing strategies, showing how these are caught up in a contradictory field of finger-pointing and tensions within shifting bureaucratic interests, emerging neoliberal conservation agendas, and the idealised structures of industrial "upgrading" (as laid out and critiqued by Madhavan and Soman for South India, this volume).

An exporter in Gurgaon

I first met Dr Saini (pseudonym) in March 2014 at his parental home in Gurgaon. Belonging to the gardener sub-caste by birth, he studied botany in Germany and obtained a doctoral degree in plant pathology. After his studies he started working as a consultant for the Swiss multinational Sandoz (which later became Novartis), writing a report on the precarious state of the agricultural sector in India. Along the way he became interested in medicinal plant cultivation as a potentially pesticide-free income alternative for farmers. Pursuing this interest with a critical mind, but as a newcomer, Dr Saini learned a lot about the herbal industry the hard way. A friend suggested that he should make use of his expertise by going into medicinal plant exports. He first contacted PADMA in 2003 and was consecutively employed as a consultant between 2004 and 2006, gathering information and herbarium specimens of PADMA 28 ingredients (cf. Schwabl and Vennos 2015: 110) growing in India. Because of his friendly nature, scientific background, and familiarity with both Europe and India, he became an essential transcultural middleman and supplier.

Gurgaon city can be reached with the Delhi metro in less than an hour. Also called "Millennium City," its sprawling urbanisation and numerous skyscrapers testify its role as one of the leading financial and industrial centres of India over the last decade. Dr Saini and I had a leisurely lunch in a fancy restaurant with table linen and an extensive buffet, where we discussed his work with PADMA. He regularly exports dried myrobalan fruits (*Terminalia chebula*, Tib. *a ru ra*), pomegranate seeds (*Punica granatum, se 'bru*), bael fruits (*Aegle marmelos, bil ba*), cotton tree flowers (*Bombax ceiba*, nā ga ge sar), and country mallow (*Sida cordifolia*).[14] He sources chebulic myrobalan from the forests of Madhya Pradesh in central India, where "tribals" (*adivasi*)[15] collect and dry the fruits. He found that he could not trust the Delhi wholesalers, especially since "he is not a local" (even though Gurgaon is right next to Delhi), and since he needs to supply PADMA with batches of consistent high quality.[16]

> I never buy from them. I went to these markets; you cannot rely on them. I thought, better to go to the place where it is produced, find a local man, give him a bit more money, tell them what material we need, and go from there. It is easier to travel there, see the material, take what you want, and take money in cash and then transport. This is what I do. We need a middleman, but not the big wholesaler.

A similar setup has worked for him for pomegranate, which grows abundantly on private farmer land on the hills of Himachal Pradesh, and for bael fruits. When the materials arrive at his place, however, several days labour are often still required to manually clean, sort, and dry them further to reach PADMA's standards. After lunch, we drove over to his parental house in the much quieter and older Gurgaon village. There, he had a small herb processing unit: a shaded drying area with two fans, two storage rooms, and more space to dry herbs on top of the roof. An older man and his son who had a room on the premises were employed as caretakers, and their work was overseen by Dr Saini's wife. For some plants, however, he was not able to find any reliable source.

I went on a *Sida cordifolia* (Sanskrit name *bala*, Unani name *khireti*) collection trip with his most senior worker during a second visit to Gurgaon more than a year later (August 2015). The monsoon was hitting hard, and

---

14 *Sida cordifolia* is not commonly identified in contemporary Tibetan *materia medica* works; it is part of the innovative reformulation of Gabur 25 ("Camphor 25") in Switzerland in the 1960s, which is based on a Buryat family lineage. It is part of PADMA 28, PADMA's flagship product (see van der Valk 2017: 258).

15 *Adivasi* is a Hindi umbrella term for often rural ethnic minorities. In the Indian Constitution these are categorised as "Scheduled Tribes" and granted certain exclusive land rights such as the harvest of "Minor Forest Products" (at least on paper, cf. Lele et al. 2010).

16 Visiting Old Delhi's spice market (Khari Baoli) several times, I experienced first-hand what the trade is like for the uninitiated. A buyer needs to be aware of the current names, prices, and what exactly s/he wants in advance in order not to get the wrong item (perhaps an inferior substitute or a counterfeit) at an incredibly inflated rate. There will likely be several types of the same raw material, with each type subdivided further into quality grades. The quality, timing (year, season), and volume will all influence the price. There is not one standard name, no standard price, nor quality. This further implies that trade surveys are only rough approximations and puts "market ethnobotany" in a different light (as herbal markets are often assumed to be a rather straightforward context for research, but see for instance Albuquerque et al. 2014: 370–375).

many streets were flooded for days. While driving outside the city centre for about 40 kilometres, Dr Saini tried to assure me that there was no pollution in Haryana, saying that there was no heavy industry with smoking chimneys in the area (although the air quality is record-breakingly bad in nearby Delhi). He admitted there was some waste disposal here and there but held that at least it is not spoiling the air. It had initially taken him a lot of effort to locate the area to which we were headed and to pinpoint the good patches that lay scattered across abandoned fields. Initially, he had attempted to organise a small group of local youngsters to do the harvesting, but this experiment failed. They found the work too hard, harvested indiscriminately, and soon lost interest. When Dr Saini came with his own men to collect, the locals resisted, so they looked for another spot a bit further along the road. It was "vacant land," and here no questions were asked. The first time they harvested was in 2005, and the last *Sida* order from PADMA that came through in 2012 was 500 kg. On a normal harvesting day during the second half of August, a group of three to five men would reach the area around 11 a.m. and finish about five hours later. Using scissors – not sickles as these are less selective – the group can gather roughly 30–35 kg of dried material a day (80% of the weight is lost during drying and sorting), so the whole operation would usually take about a month.

We arrived in the harvesting area. We drove by one of the better patches, but the recent construction of a bus stand had obliterated it. New hotels, warehouses, a school, a hospital, and a *mandir* had all been constructed over the past few years along the main road, and more were underway. We stopped at a small shack on the roadside. Over some tea, Dr Saini noted how congress grass (*Parthenium hysterophorus*) – a well-known invasive species that arrived in the country with imported wheat – was increasingly dominating the landscape. The shopkeeper, dressed in a bright pink sari, agreed: she had suffered from severe allergic skin reactions after handling these plants. I joined the senior worker on a walk to assess the amount of *Sida* remaining. It emits a particular smell, which helps in locating patches. The looming presence of transmission towers and cables marks the area, which lies near an electrical power distribution hub. The outcome was not very encouraging. Dr Saini concluded that they probably would not be able to collect the necessary amount of one thousand kilos of dried material this year, even though we located some more promising patches later on. This failed harvesting excursion is but one example that helped me to re-evaluate the ubiquitous commercial overharvesting discourse as a small piece of a much larger puzzle: rapid urbanisation and concomitant land grabbing, commercial agriculture, invasive species, and complex socioenvironmental interrelations between harvesting, disturbance, and regeneration cycles. These aspects could easily be more damaging to NTFP populations and forests than "overharvesting." The collection area itself also diffuses romantic distinctions between urban and "pollution-free" rural spaces and between wild and cultivated plants while showing that "forests" are but one amongst many sourcing habitats and that *adivasi* are not the only harvesters.[17]

After the *Sida* plants have been fully dried, they would usually be stored in large polyethylene bags that go into sealed drums for export. Dr Saini has to prepare the invoice and the packing list. After customs, the materials travel Delhi-Mumbai by train, where it is then shipped to Hamburg. This process, however, is fraught with difficulties. For export, Dr Saini must prove by means of receipts and purchase orders at which prices he bought and will sell his materials to satisfy the Gurgaon Excise (inland tax) and Income office. Before the last national elections (it was cancelled by ruling politicians to win votes), it was obliged to fill in "Form 38" each time raw materials were purchased from another state at a cost of more than 20,000 rupees (300 USD). Dr Saini would usually employ an accountant to take care of this, but one day he wanted to find out why his accountant asked for thousands of rupees to take care of this, even though the official rate for the five forms requested was negligible. As he arrived at the office to get the blank forms, his contact and a lawyer were already waiting. He was served tea and waited for two hours. Finally, the officer arrived and was ready to receive them. First, he disputed that the address given was not Dr Saini's home address. But after some convincing, he backtracked. The officer invited him for some more tea. After another hour of waiting, a second officer came in. A series of more non-sense arguments followed. In the end Dr Saini agreed to pay the officer 700 rupees (10 USD). His lawyer also wanted 200 (3 USD) for his presence, and the clerk who had to process the file another 100 (1.5 USD).

> It is organised. There are rates fixed for everything [...] You waste your day and still have to pay money. Or if you don't pay, you don't get the form even after three or four days [...] You cannot complain to anyone, where will you go? The highest official sitting in that building is involved in that.

"Harassment," "unnecessary botheration," "long queues," and "corruption" are how Dr Saini describes this structural violence, which is also part of exporting herbs abroad. Even though he pays someone a "documentation fee" to arrange the permits and certificates in his place, the transit permit may already cause trouble before the consignment even reaches the customs office. Normally, there are no problems at this stage, as he hires a specialised private company that transports the materials in sealed trucks

---

17 Ved and Goraya (2008), the most recent herbal trade survey with a national focus, identified wild harvest from wastelands as a critical supply issue since it is unmonitored and unregulated as opposed to forest areas (see Gaudillière 2014b: 192–193).

across state borders. But about four years ago there was "a conspiracy" between the transport manager, the driver, and an officer at the border checkpoint of Haryana. The consignment was blocked; he was summoned and asked to pay 55,000 rupees (820 USD) or alternatively 25,000 rupees (373 USD) if no receipt would be involved. Dr Saini requested a receipt to win time. He had made a phone call to the father-in-law of his daughter, a big boss in the administration, to settle the matter. Alas, this intervention came 15 minutes late. He had already paid the fee. One officer came running after him, apologising and blaming the driver. Officially, the reason why the materials were confiscated was that he could not provide a receipt documenting the purchase. This was the case because the middleman who organised the harvest of the pomegranate seeds in two or three Himachali villages was not an authorised salesperson. Getting a license and paying taxes would be difficult for this man belonging to a deprived family, who only went through basic education. The actual situation, however, is that the large majority of all transactions in this business are cash payments without receipts. The law is only strictly applied arbitrarily when local bureaucrats want a piece of the cake: "It is a big trouble in India, to be a taxpayer: the system is corrupt!"

A third example narrated by Dr Saini of failed state involvement in the medicinal plant sector revolved around cultivation subsidies for farmers. As a botanist and agricultural scientist, he was initially genuinely interested in promoting organic cultivation of herbs as an alternative income strategy for farmers. He soon abandoned this idea entirely. One trader even told him directly, "please don't advise any farmer to cultivate [medicinal plants]:" as big wholesalers "are supporting two hundred families, they owe them." "If I start buying from farmers, what will happen to the families which have been working with them for hundreds of years. It is the local people still who collect. It works better I think." Nonetheless, Dr Saini discovered that "cunning, dishonest money-minded private consultants" were promoting the cultivation of expensive herbs to farmers and doing a good business out of selling seedlings. But after two to three years of growing nobody was interested in buying the crop, especially since it was often available cheaper wild-sourced on the market. On top of that, government subsidies to support farmers who cultivate medicinal plants were abused by corrupt entrepreneurs. At the mortgage bank that finances cultivation projects, Dr Saini learned about how a loan could be obtained and what the charges and profit levels would be. But the banker did not want to give him details on who was cultivating what, how much, and where. Even if on paper ten hectares would be in cultivation, in reality there would only be a few plants there, as Dr Saini saw later with his own eyes. The local department of horticulture inspector who has to supply a certificate was also involved in this lucrative business, as I was told, sharing the subsidy money with the bankers, consultants, nurserymen, and so on. As a result, "only fake people that submit fake papers" would be granted funds, not benefitting farmers (let alone biodiversity) at all.[18] Nevertheless, Dr Saini maintains that the government is at least making some progress, hoping that the then-current Prime Minister Narendra Modi would keep some of his promises.[19]

A cultivator and trader from Lahaul

Costus (Tib. *ruta*) has been cultivated as a cash crop for almost a hundred years. It was first described botanically, as a new species with a binomial name, by Dr Hugh Falconer (1808–1865, Falconer 1841: 456–457), who was the superintendent of the East India Company's botanical garden at Saharunpur (Uttar Pradesh) at the time. As was also noted by Falconer, costus is endemic to a geographically restricted part of the Western Himalayas, growing wild in small patches on 2600–4000 m high moist slopes in Kashmir and Himachal Pradesh, Uttarakhand and Northwest Pakistan. NMPB scientists prioritised *Saussurea costus* as 1 of the 32 "important medicinal plants in short supply" (Kala et al. 2006).[20] It is currently cultivated in small fields by families from Lahaul Valley and Uttarakhand who obtained export permits, as well as in Ladakhi herbal plots (cf. Blaikie 2009). Described by Kuniyal et al. (2005) as "the oldest cash crop in the cold desert environment," *kuth* – the most common Hindi name for costus – cultivation was found to be in a bottleneck due to factors such as the lengthy reproductive cycle (up to three years), small land holdings, and fluctuating and low market prices that led to farmers shifting to the more profitable cultivation of peas, potatoes, and hops. Based on their *Review of the Status of Saussurea Costus*, TRAFFIC India (2011: 15) concluded the following (see Kuniyal et al. 2015 for a similar conclusion):

> [t]here is little evidence to suggest that the uplisting of the species into Appendix I [of CITES, the Convention on International Trade in

---

18 See Dejouhanet (2014: 225–232) for examples of medicinal plant cultivation project failures and success stories, which she relates to market integration. See also Alam and Belt (2009).
19 In the five years since 2014, Modi's National Democratic Alliance government "introduced a series of changes in the country's environmental and forest laws which civil society groups termed as a dilution of the rules, attack on tribal rights and opening up of forest sector for private players," which continues along the same populist neoliberal lines since his party's victory in the 2019 general election (Aggarwal 2019).
20 Kumar et al. (2011) researched the distribution of medicinal and aromatic plants in Ladakh, discussing and listing endemic and endangered species and their use in common Tibetan medical formulations. Besides coming up with a technocratic model for the conservation and sustainable development of "the trans-Himalayan medicinal plant sector," Kumar et al. also ranked *ruta* as the single most important trans-Himalayan medicinal plant used in Tibetan medicine, based on the number of times it was mentioned as an ingredient in available English-language formularies.

Endangered Species of Wild Fauna and Flora] 25 years ago has done much to conserve the species in the wild in India. [...] On the contrary, the high and often complex level of regulations has only deterred potential cultivators with the result that commercial cultivation has also not picked up. [...] In the case of cultivation, there is great uncertainty whether permits will be granted or not. There is also some confusion regarding the government agency responsible for issuing the permits. This is compounded by a lack of transparency regarding the rules and regulations and an unclear process of decision-making. This has led to a situation where Indian cultivators, those who venture into *S. costus* cultivation, do not find buyers while the market is flooded with Chinese imports from cultivated sources.

It was *amchi* Dolkar, the younger daughter of Ama Lobsang (see Josayma and Dhondup 1990), who introduced both Men-Tsee-Khang and PADMA to the costus grower, trader, and exporter I got acquainted with in July 2015. Both described Mr Mishra (pseudonym) to me as an honest man. Mishra was born into a Brahmin family of four brothers and four sisters in a small hamlet along the Lahaul valley more than fifty years ago. His father owned farmlands and also cultivated some costus and *Inula racemosa* (*ma nu* in Tibetan), just like his grandfather. He remembers taking these roots on horseback over the pass to Manali to sell them there. In seventh class, during the two-month summer holiday, they also went into the mountains, on steep ridges, to harvest *kutki* (Tibetan: *hong len*, mostly identified as *Neopicrorhiza scrophulariiflora*). They did not have a clue on prices and would just sell it to a man from Amritsar passing by, and then buy some candy. In 1993, a researcher from Lucknow came to their village looking for hawthorn berries. Young Mishra helped him find some shrubs in the vicinity, which was the beginning of a fruitful business relationship. The researcher quit university and founded his own company, and soon both men were prospering. In 1998, they started officially by securing legal documentation, which Mishra learned how to obtain from the academic. He then started exporting costus for the French perfume industry in 2005, at first via a commission agent in Delhi. As he was new in the trade ("at that time we were not skilled") he was taken advantage of by the agent, whose profit margin was up to five times higher than his. When he found out this collaboration ended, but luckily the buyer sent him a direct purchase order later, cutting out the middleman. From then onward, he was exporting directly to companies in France, Germany, Switzerland, Yemen, and Dubai. Over time he also started supplying big domestic manufacturers such as Himalaya and Organic India, as well as more Tibetan doctors in Dharamsala and Delhi. He now rents several plots of land in two hamlets deep in Lahaul valley, where a manager oversees the maintenance and harvest of the crop in the growing season (May to October). Costus is the main crop, followed by *Inula*, and a small number of far less abundant fields containing *Aconitum heterophyllum*, *Podophyllum hexandrum*, and *kutki*. He has attempted to grow *jatamansi* (*Nardostachys grandiflora*, Tib. *spang spos*) for several years but has failed so far. To supplement the cultivated stock, Mishra maintains contact with a network of (mostly part-time) gatherers in Ladakh and the Kulu and Chamba valleys in Himachal from whom he buys directly or via an agent. When we met, he was only selling crude, dried herbs, even though he had a small distillation unit and was very keen to go into costus oil. On average, Mishra can harvest between 20 and 40 metric tonnes of costus a year.

Mr Mishra related experiences similar to Dr Saini's in his dealings with the NMPB, AYUSH, forest department offices, and the wildlife crime control bureau in Delhi. He had tried to contact AYUSH for a long time. I saw a pamphlet in his office advertising a "Centrally Assisted Scheme" that provides financial assistance for the cultivation of medicinal plants. Even though he is formally cultivating, trading, and exporting a critically endangered plant, he was unsuccessful in getting any support, or even a written response, to his queries. Mishra's explanation is that:

> Only if you know a good politician, then you will find benefits. These people are so dirty, the people who are running the Indian country: politicians and bureaucrats. Both are corrupted. [...] Every Indian says "we are independent". The people are not, only two [groups of people are]. Who? One is the bureaucrat, one is the politician. They are doing everything, and have lots of money. Laws are nothing [to them], they make the law! The law is for poor people.

He made clear that AYUSH has no influence on his work; all their schemes and guidelines remain in the realm of paper. The forest department on the other hand does enforce rules and regulations, and sales taxes have to be paid even though export itself is free. Harvesting permits specify the what, when, where, how much, and by whom of wild collection. These should be obtained from the local forest officer, who confirms which areas are open for harvest. The problem here is that many high-value plants such as *Nardostachys*, Neo*picrorhiza*, and *Dactylorhiza hatagirea* (Tib. *dbang lag*) are rare and only grow in specific, restricted habitats. It is therefore likely that one obtains a permit for an area that is "open to harvest" but where the species you are after don't even grow. The forest officer may be aware that there is nothing in that area but can be swayed with a bribe. As there is no effective policing of the often difficult-to-reach harvesting areas themselves, the collection party is free to harvest in a neighbouring "closed area." Mishra ensured me that this is a common strategy, only a tiny portion of wild-collection is legal, and most harvesters do not get any form of approval.

After we had returned from our road trip to Lahaul, I was staying at the Mishra family residence near Manali for a while. On the third day, we drove past Mandi to Gohar, where forest items confiscated by the Nachan Forest

Division (FD) of Himachal Pradesh were being sold by auction. Mr Mishra had received an official notification letter from the forest department, which listed what was on offer: a dozen quintals (1.2 tonnes) of *Taxus baccata* leaves and *Berberis aristata* roots. He had predicted that the quality of these goods would be poor and added that most buyers would only be interested anyway in the "very good documents" that came with the purchase. They could then burn the original goods or get rid of them cheaply on the domestic market and replace it with high-quality material sourced illegally from elsewhere for which they now had official export documents.[21] Indeed, the *Berberis* roots were lying piled up outside in the open air on the soil of a courtyard in Mandi. This would negatively affect its berberine content, the yellow-coloured alkaloid that is commercially extracted from the roots. The FD in Gohar was situated in a manicured garden of trees and flower patches and consisted of offices, a residence, a parking space, and a store. The staff consisted of a few forest officers (FOs) in uniform, clerks, assistants, workers, and several armed guards. I was not allowed to accompany Mishra into the office, where he had to negotiate with the FO. In the end, it turned out he was the only potential buyer. The other people around were only there for timber. He sighed:

> There is no system at all here in India. The FD captures goods and just dumps them somewhere. It is like taking an apple out of someone's hand and then throwing it [away]. The FO is also not knowledgeable on herbal trade. He only wanted to provide a transport permit to Delhi or Amritsar, but I need a legal procurement certificate as well since this is required by my buyer [a commercial extractor]. He had never issued that before and had to make enquiries first.

While Dr Saini deputes someone to take care of export documents, Mr Mishra takes care of that himself in Delhi. There, he has to interact with five separate offices before the materials can go through customs. Certificates of Origin, Non-Objection Certificates (NOCs), phytosanitary documentation, CITES, and tax exemptions all have to be arranged. The more people are involved, the worse it becomes:

> We have everything. We have the net, mobile, laptop, but it's useless! You have to go personally. Sometimes [there is a] corrupted officer, they want something. "Where is your invoice?" "This is your invoice! Ooooh, a lot of money. What is [in there] for me?" [...] Everyone sees the invoice. This man is exporting for 40,000 euro. They don't know how we

---

21 Dejouhanet and Sreelakshmy, this volume, also report how official certificates are used as a "cover" that allows merchants and stock-keepers to circumvent the rules in Kerala, creating a hybrid supply network.

obtained this. He thinks, "he purchased this at some little cost, wants to send and get a big profit." [...] This is a big problem.

The sentiment that there is no functioning system was a recurring theme in my interviews. The formal trade channels are practically impossible to navigate as a private trader (and particularly exporter) without resorting to informal exchanges and economies of favours to get through the highly dysfunctional bureaucracy. Dr Saini and Mr Mishra blame corruption for this sorry state of affairs while official policies and surveys lament the informal, secretive, and unsustainable nature of the trade, labelling harvesters and cultivators as ignorant, middlemen as parasitic, and wholesalers as greedy. The ethnographic vignettes above, however, indicate how these distinctions between state and different economic actors are blurred. Mr Mishra, for instance, started out as a small collector and cultivator. He now oversees several cultivation plots and maintains large stocks of these and other crops for the domestic market as well as for export. He also purchases directly from local collectors, organises harvesting parties for specific orders (with the help of local agents), buys from auctions, and intends to directly tap into the essential oil market by means of his recently installed distillation unit. He is highly mobile, travelling between the fields in his ancestral Lahaul, his company and storage in Manali, going to Delhi to do the paperwork, and visiting important customers regionally and abroad. Even on the basic level of categorising these savvy entrepreneurs as "economic actors" with clearly delimited operations and scales, trade surveys largely fail to grasp the dynamic complexity at hand. This is reflected in the ambiguous application of the term "middlemen" and their vilification. From the perspective of the small-scale traders I followed, officials repeatedly turned out to be the "parasites," with arbitrarily implemented regulations and documents serving both as facilitators and as cover-ups of occult yet ubiquitous sourcing practices. In these legal grey zones, several technocratic medicinal plant protection and cultivation measures appeared to be scams, becoming tools of accumulation by dispossession in which institutional authorities collude with elite criminal entrepreneurs to extract wealth through an interdependent web of taxes, fees, bribes, subsidies, and loans.

Failed formalisation: The dark art of sourcing, the blinding light of governance

The Executive Summary of *The Medicinal Plants Sector in India* (Holley and Cherla 1998: xi–xii), funded by the International Development Research Centre and the World Bank, claims that:

> Current practices are unsustainable and many studies have emphasized rapid depletion of the natural resource base. This problem is further compounded by the inequitable nature of the harvesting and marketing of the plants, thereby perpetuating impoverishment for those charged

with stewarding and gathering the resource. Evidence points to a limited number of people profiting in dramatic disproportion to their inputs. Nonetheless, India, known to be a storehouse of biological diversity, has to focus on sustaining the resource base of medicinal plants. Efforts to relieve pressure on wild plants through cultivation have made a good start but have a long way to go. [...] Although the overall sector is largely informal, it works in practice. However the constraints are likely to have an increasing impact, resulting perhaps in a crisis situation. [...] It is clear that a set of interventions at various levels could lead to the promotion of the sustainable and equitable development of the sector and help to avert a crisis. These could pave the way for sharply focused strategic planning for the future. The report outlines a number of these interventions.

Government interventions in the lives of NTFPs, including medicinal plants, have generally made things worse for both people and plants (Laird et al. 2010). Formalisation – defined as "the replacement of informal ownership, access, and economic activity through the recognition and inscription by the State of rights and conditions of access" (Putzel et al. 2015: 457) – is a defining characteristic of NTFPs globally as well as in India. The neoliberal conservation discourse identified in the introduction has fostered a set of unfounded assumptions on the nature of India's medicinal plant "sector," leading to a problematic marriage between state and market that obviates the multi-layered "braided networks" of raw material supply (see also Dejouhanet and Sreelakshmy, this volume). In line with Wynberg et al.'s (2015) findings in Southern Africa, many actors seek alternative economic opportunities and a lighter regulatory load in the face of strict measures, becoming creative *bricoleurs* of the multi-layered regulatory landscape by necessity. Ingram et al. (2015: 50) therefore count "institutionalised corruption" and the resulting (mal)governance as a distinct but parallel NTFP governance chain or layer "shadowing and nested around statutory and customary structures" and ranging "from additional payments 'to get things done' in business, to elites engaging in state and power capture, and as a deliberate strategy of clientelism by state officials and traditional authorities". My findings further align with Saxer's (2009: 327) conception of "border regimes" as a liminal space of unruly and malleable state power, and his observation that "the survival of a border regime rests, ironically, on both officials and traders breaking its rules in order to make it work." Many regulations are confusing, only partly enforced, and come with unintended side effects which eventually undermine their intended goals. This is "the secret of law:" "Corruption is thus at the very core of order, inscribed into the law of the nation-state. [...] The possibility of its transgression or perversion is always already inscribed into the law as hidden possibility" (Nuijten and Anders 2007: 12). A situation of ambivalence ensues in which reliance on the principles of an economy of favours may be the only feasible option, as is reflected in the first-hand struggles of Dr Saini and Mr Mishra. Both of these men are sourcerers: crafting their own chains, filling in voids in the pluralist patchwork of regulations in unpredictable ways. Interactions with state institutions and their officers cannot be avoided altogether as companies need to be registered and pay taxes, obtain legal documents and permits, and as goods pass by various checkpoints before reaching their destinations. These points of contact could be considered as nodes of formalisation, intersections where the usual informality is transformed – at least partially and temporarily – by forced official interventions that shine some light on the otherwise occult paths followed by herbs in India. The flash that produces this formal snapshot, however, often creates unrealistic artefacts that can only be dealt with by going back into the darkroom of informality. The herbal sector is at the most a quasi-formal economy: sourcing is sourcery. This "magical" reality seems far removed from the disenchanted, formal vision promulgated by bureaucratic governmental institutions and medicinal plant trade studies invested in paradoxical neoliberal control.[22] The reformulation occurring on the market is the transition from living organism to commodity, but governing the wilds is only possible if one concedes the true nature of the beast. The examples above illuminate a significant aspect of how Asian medical industries operate at the intersection of capitalism and state regulation, showcasing how the heterogeneity of global "supply chains" reinforces yet at the same time eludes the logic of neoliberal conservation discourses. To discover how these industries really (mal)function and to understand the situatedness of capitalism(s), critical anthropological approaches are vital.

National trade surveys – an early, rather ironic example is quoted above – have profoundly shaped the regulatory landscape of medicinal plants in India. Newly empowered institutions such as the National Medicinal Plants Board are now supposed to simultaneously boost the economy, fight inequity, and save nature from an impending overexploitation crisis. Building on the technocratic conception of a unified industrial sector, however, these schemes and guidelines take the market as an ideological starting point, key instrument, and ultimate goal. This neoliberal strategy effectively reduces complex socioecological issues to managerialism while ignoring the contradictory realities of India's occult herbal economies. This is clearly not a straightforward example of increasing "free trade," to the contrary: the traders I tracked faced numerous bureaucratic obstacles in their struggles to harvest, cultivate, buy, transport, sell, and export plant raw materials.

---

22 Neoliberalism as an ideology is not restricted only to trade liberalisation. As defined by Comaroff and Comaroff (2000: 292), it features "the odd coupling, the binary complementarity, of the legalistic with the libertarian; constitutionality with deregulation; hyperrationalization with the exuberant spread of innovative occult practices." Neoliberalism, and neoliberal conservation, in particular, are inherently contradictory (cf. Büscher et al. 2012: 13–16).

At the same time, their earnest attempts to receive any kind of state support for the cultivation of endangered plants such as costus – which is the ideal policy solution, according to mainstream scientists and regulators – failed miserably. The formalisation of Indian herbal trade has largely failed, and so has neoliberal conservation; at least, that is, if saving nature is really its intention. The herbal entrepreneurs I followed were especially frustrated by this "accumulation by conservation" (Büscher and Fletcher 2015) and explained this phenomenon to be part and parcel of India's systemically corrupt state bureaucracy and its unholy alliance with powerful criminal capitalists (as confirmed by the work of Sanchez).

Can Asian medical industries be "sustainable," and if so, on whose terms? Formulating an answer to this conundrum requires much more than the quantification of demand–supply gaps. Protectionist "fortress conservation" measures (including restricted areas and blacklists of endangered species) may look good on paper but tend to protect state interests and the premises of the industrial model while alienating other people-plant relationships and covering up deeper inequalities. As Blaikie and Craig note in this volume, alienated modes of making Tibetan medicines, relying on mechanised mass production and legalistic conceptions of quality and efficacy, tend to ignore the precarity of the multi-species entanglements in which pharmaceutical assemblages are enmeshed. Tibetan medical and Buddhist sensibilities and moral economies, on the other hand, could serve as an inspiration for alternative ways of relating to our life-worlds, mending the destructive dissociation from conviviality. While a lack of government recognition and support for Sowa Rigpa creates its own forms of precariousness, as is the case for Nepal's physician-pharmacists, this chapter showcases how trade policies that are supposed to create "win-win" scenarios become tools of state-facilitated alienation, and the convoluted ways in which Indian suppliers of Tibetan *materia medica* navigate the murky waters of the resulting occult economies. Given the fundamental limitations of the current regulatory apparatus, Tibetan medicine producers sourcing from India – such as Men-Tsee-Khang and PADMA – clearly cannot rely on the "invisible hand" of the market for ensuring sustainability, nor can their suppliers. If the supply of raw materials is the fragile Achilles heel of the Ayurvedic industry (Dejouhanet 2014), then the catch-22 I described between commerce and conservation is like covering up the whole foot in an overly tight, contaminated plaster, leading to malformation. As my journeys with two North Indian entrepreneurs have pointed out, the "realist" economic logic of trade surveys, policies, and documented transactions proved to be all but realistic – let alone "sustainable" – in practice. In this vein, my attempt at a counter-hegemonic argument in this chapter sought to highlight the ruptures, incommensurabilities, and messiness hidden underneath the stabilising structures and discourses of predatory capitalism.

Acknowledgements

I kindly acknowledge Men-Tsee-Khang and PADMA for facilitating my doctoral fieldwork. My heartfelt thanks also go to my PhD supervisor Miguel N. Alexiades and to Laura Rohs, Viola Schreer, Barbara Gerke, and Lucie Dejouhanet for their insightful comments on earlier versions of this piece. Lastly, I am grateful to Stephan Kloos and the entire RATIMED team for their hospitality and the many fruitful exchanges. The publication of this chapter was supported by the Austrian Science Fund (FWF), grant 30804.

Bibliography

Adams V (2002) Randomized Controlled Crime. *Social Studies of Science* 32(5–6): 659–690.

Aggarwal M (2019) *NDA 2.0: What it means for India's environment?* Environment and Elections, Hewing the Regulatory Tree Series, Mongabay India. Published online on 24 May 2019, https://india.mongabay.com/2019/05/nda-2-0-what-it-means-for-indias-environment/

Alam G and Belt J (2009) *Developing a Medicinal Plant Value Chain: Lessons from an Initiative to Cultivate Kutki (Picrorhiza kurrooa) in Northern India*. KIT Working Papers Series C5, Amsterdam: Royal Tropical Institute.

Albuquerque UP, Vital Fernandes Cruz da Cunha L, Farias Paiva de Lucena R et al. (eds) (2014). *Methods and Techniques in Ethnobiology and Ethnoecology*. New York, NY: Humana Press, Springer.

Alexiades M (2009) The Cultural and Economic Globalisation of Traditional Environmental Knowledge Systems. In: Heckler S (ed) *Landscape, Process and Power: Re-Evaluating Traditional Environmental Knowledge*. New York, NY: Berghahn Books, pp. 68–98.

Anderson D, Salick J, Moseley R, et al. (2005) Conserving the Sacred Medicine Mountains: A Vegetation Analysis of Tibetan Sacred Sites in Northwest Yunnan. *Biodiversity and Conservation* 14(13): 3065–3091.

Aumeeruddy-Thomas Y and Lama YC (2008) Tibetan Medicine and Biodiversity Management in Dolpo, Nepal: Negotiating Local and Global Worldviews, Knowledge and Practices. In Pordié L (ed) *Tibetan Medicine in the Contemporary World: Global Politics of Medical Knowledge and Practice*. London: Routledge, pp. 160–185.

Bähre E (2005) How to Ignore Corruption: Reporting the Shortcomings of Development in South Africa. *Current Anthropology* 46(1): 107–120.

Belcher B and Schreckenberg K (2007) Commercialisation of Non-Timber Forest Products: A Reality Check. *Development Policy Review* 25(3): 355–377.

Blaikie C (2009) Critically Endangered? Medicinal Plant Cultivation and the Reconfiguration of Sowa Rigpa in Ladakh. *Asian Medicine* 5(2): 243–272.

Blundo G (2007) Hidden Acts, Open Talks: How Anthropology Can "Observe" and Describe Corruption. In: Nuijten M and Anders G (eds) *Corruption and the Secret of Law: A Legal Anthropological Perspective*. Aldershot: Ashgate, pp. 27–52.

Booker A, Johnston D and Heinrich M (2012) Value Chains of Herbal Medicines – Research Needs and Key Challenges in the Context of Ethnopharmacology. *Journal of Ethnopharmacology* 140(3): 624–633.

Bubandt N (2006) Sorcery, Corruption, and the Dangers of Democracy in Indonesia. *Journal of the Royal Anthropological Institute* 12(2): 413–431.
Büscher B and Fletcher R (2015) Accumulation by Conservation. *New Political Economy* 20(2): 273–298.
Büscher B, Sullivan S, Neves K, et al. (2012) Towards a Synthesized Critique of Neoliberal Biodiversity Conservation. *Capitalism Nature Socialism* 23(2): 4–30.
Chaudhuri S (2012) Women as Easy Scapegoats: Witchcraft Accusations and Women as Targets in Tea Plantations of India. *Violence Against Women* 18(10): 1213–1234.
Comaroff J and Comaroff J (1999) Occult Economies and the Violence of Abstraction: Notes from the South African Postcolony. *American Ethnologist* 26(2): 279–303.
Comaroff J and Comaroff J (2000) Millennial Capitalism: First Thoughts on a Second Coming. *Public Culture* 12(2): 291–343.
Craig S (2012) *Healing Elements: Efficacy and the Social Ecologies of Tibetan Medicine*. Berkeley, CA: University of California Press.
Craig S and Gerke B (2016) Naming and Forgetting: Sowa Rigpa and the Territory of Asian Medical Systems. *Medicine Anthropology Theory* 3(2): 87–122.
Craig S and Glover D (2009) Conservation, Cultivation, and Commodification of Medicinal Plants in the Greater Himalayan-Tibetan Plateau. *Asian Medicine* 5(2): 219–242.
Cross J (2010) Neoliberalism as Unexceptional: Economic Zones and the Everyday Precariousness of Working Life in South India. *Critique of Anthropology* 30(4): 355–373.
Dejouhanet L (2014) Supply of Medicinal Raw Materials. The Achilles Heel of Today's Manufacturing Sector for Ayurvedic Drugs in Kerala *Asian Medicine* 9(1–2): 206–235.
Desai A (2009) Anti-"anti-witchcraft" and the Maoist Insurgency in Rural Maharashtra, India. *Dialectical Anthropology*, 33(3): 423–439.
Falconer H (1841) Aucklandia. *Annals and Magazine of Natural History, Including Zoology, Botany, and Geology*. 6: 456–457.
Fletcher R, Dressler W and Büscher B (2014) Nature™ Inc.: The New Frontiers of Environmental Conservation. In Büscher B, Dressler W and Fletcher R (eds) *Nature™ Inc.: Environmental Conservation in the Neoliberal Age*. Tucson, AZ: University of Arizona Press, pp. 3–21.
Gaudillière J-P (2014a) An Indian Path to Biocapital? The Traditional Knowledge Digital Library, Drug Patents, and the Reformulation Regime of Contemporary Ayurveda. *East Asian Science, Technology and Society* 8(4): 391–415.
Gaudillière J-P (2014b) Herbalised Ayurveda? *Asian Medicine* 9(1–2): 171–205.
Geschiere P (1997) *The Modernity of Witchcraft, Politics and the Occult in Postcolonial Africa*. Charlottesville: University Press of Virginia.
Gupta A (1995) Blurred Boundaries: The Discourse of Corruption, the Culture of Politics, and the Imagined State. *American Ethnologist* 22(2): 375–402.
Gupta A (2005) Narratives of Corruption: Anthropological and Fictional Accounts of the Indian State. *Ethnography* 6(1): 5–34.
Hannerz U (2003) Being There … and There … and There!: Reflections on Multi-Site Ethnography. *Ethnography* 4(2): 201–216.
Harris T (2013) *Geographical Diversions: Tibetan Trade, Global Transactions*. Athens: The University of Georgia Press.

Holley J and Cherla K (1998) *The Medicinal Plants Sector in India*. New Delhi: International Development Research Centre.

Ingram V, Ros-Tonen M and Dietz T (2015) A Fine Mess: Bricolaged Forest Governance in Cameroon. *International Journal of the Commons* 9(1): 41–64.

Josayma TT and Dhondup K (1990) *Dolma & Dolkar: Mother and Daughter of Tibetan Medicine*. New Delhi: Yarlung Publications.

Kala CP, Dhyani PP and Sajwan BS (2006) Developing the Medicinal Plant Sector in Northern India: Challenges and Opportunities. *Journal of Ethnobiology and Ethnomedicine* 2: 32.

Kloos S (2008) The History and Development of Tibetan Medicine in Exile. *Tibet Journal* 33(3): 15–49.

Kloos S (2013) How Tibetan Medicine in Exile Became a "Medical System". *East Asian Science, Technology and Society* 7(3): 381–395.

Kloos S (2017) The Pharmaceutical Assemblage: Rethinking Sowa Rigpa and the Herbal Pharmaceutical Industry in Asia. *Current Anthropology* 58(5): 693–717.

Kudlu C (2016) Keeping the Doctor in the Loop: Ayurvedic Pharmaceuticals in Kerala. *Anthropology & Medicine* 23(3): 275–294.

Kumar GP, Kumar R, Chaurasia OP, et al. (2011) Current Status and Potential Prospects of Medicinal Plant Sector in Trans-Himalayan Ladakh. *Journal of Medicinal Plants Research* 5(14): 2929–2940.

Kuniyal CP, Rawat YS, Oinam SS, et al. (2005) Kuth (*Saussurea lappa*) Cultivation in the Cold Desert Environment of the Lahaul Valley, Northwestern Himalaya, India: Arising Threats and Need to Revive Socio-Economic Values. *Biodiversity & Conservation* 14(5): 1035–1045.

Kuniyal CP, Rawat DS and Sundriyal RC (2015) Cultivation of *Saussurea costus* cannot be Treated as "Artificially Propagated". *Current Science* 108(9): 1587–1589.

Laird S, McLain R and Wynberg Rachel (eds) (2010) *Wild Product Governance: Finding Policies that Work for Non-Timber Forest Products*. London: Earthscan.

Larsen HO and Olsen CS (2007) Unsustainable Collection and Unfair Trade? Uncovering and Assessing Assumptions Regarding Central Himalayan Medicinal Plant Conservation. *Biodiversity and Conservation* 16(6): 1679–1697.

Larsen HO and Smith PD (2004) Stakeholder Perspectives on Commercial Medicinal Plant Collection in Nepal. *Mountain Research and Development* 24(2): 141–148.

Lave R (2012) Neoliberalism and the Production of Environmental Knowledge. *Environment and Society: Advances in Research* 3: 19–38.

Law W and Salick J (2007) Comparing Conservation Priorities for Useful Plants among Botanists and Tibetan Doctors. *Biodiversity and Conservation* 16(6): 1747–1759.

Ledeneva A (2014) Economies of Favours or Corrupt Societies: Exploring the Boundaries between Informality and Corruption. *The Baltic Worlds* 2014(1): 13–21.

Lele S, Pattanaik M and Rai ND (2010) NTFPs in India: Rhetoric and Reality. In Laird S, McLain R and Wynberg R (eds) *Wild Product Governance: Finding Policies that Work for Non-Timber Forest Products*. London: Earthscan, pp. 85–112.

Leslie C (ed) (1976) *Asian Medical Systems: A Comparative Study*. Berkeley, CA: University of California Press.

Madhavan H (2017) Below the Radar Innovations and Emerging Property Right Approaches in Tibetan Medicine. *The Journal of World Intellectual Property* 20(5–6): 239–257.

Marcus GE (1995) Ethnography in/of the World System: The Emergence of Multi-Sited Ethnography. *Annual Review of Anthropology* 24(1): 95–117.

Mullick SB (2000) Gender Relations and Witches among the Indigenous Communities of Jharkhand, India. *Gender, Technology and Development* 4(3): 333–358.

Nagpal A and Karki M (2004) *A Study on Marketing Opportunities for Medicinal, Aromatic, and Dye Plants in South Asia.* New Delhi: International Development Research Centre.

Neumann R and Hirsch E (2000) *Commercialisation of Non-Timber Forest Products: Review and Analysis of Research.* Bogor: Center for International Forestry Research.

Nuijten M and Anders G (eds) (2007) *Corruption and the Secret of Law: A Legal Anthropological Perspective.* Aldershot: Ashgate.

Olsen CS and Larsen HO (2003) Alpine Medicinal Plant Trade and Himalayan Mountain Livelihood Strategies. *Geographical Journal* 169(3): 243–254.

Pauls T and Franz M (2013) Trading in the Dark – the Medicinal Plants Production Network in Uttarakhand. *Singapore Journal of Tropical Geography* 34(2): 229–243.

Pierce A (2010) NTFP Law and Policy Literature: Lie of the Land and Areas for Further Research. In Laird S, McLain R and Wynberg R (eds) *Wild Product Governance: Finding Policies that Work for Non-Timber Forest Products.* London: Earthscan, pp. 375–384.

Pordié L and Gaudillière J-P (2014) The Reformulation Regime in Drug Discovery: Revisiting Polyherbals and Property Rights in the Ayurvedic Industry. *East Asian Science, Technology and Society* 8(1): 57–79.

Putzel L, Kelly A, Cerutti PO, et al. (2015) Formalization as Development in Land and Natural Resource Policy. *Society & Natural Resources* 28(5): 453–472.

Rudnyckyj D (2009) Spiritual Economies: Islam and Neoliberalism in Contemporary Indonesia. *Cultural Anthropology* 24(1): 104–141.

Salick J, Amend A, Anderson D, et al. (2007) Tibetan Sacred Sites Conserve Old Growth Trees and Cover in the Eastern Himalayas. *Biodiversity and Conservation* 16(3): 693–706.

Sanchez A (2012) Questioning Success: Dispossession and the Criminal Entrepreneur in Urban India. *Critique of Anthropology* 32(4): 435–457.

Sanchez A (2016) *Criminal Capital: Violence, Corruption and Class in Industrial India.* Abingdon: Routledge.

Saxer M (2004) *Journeys with Tibetan Medicine. How Tibetan Medicine Came to the West: The Story of the Badmayev Family.* MSc Dissertation, University of Zürich, Zürich.

Saxer M (2009) Herbs and Traders in Transit: Border Regimes and the Contemporary Trans-Himalayan Trade in Tibetan Medicinal Plants. *Asian Medicine* 5(2): 317–339.

Schwabl H and Vennos C (2015) From Medical Tradition to Traditional Medicine: A Tibetan Formula in the European Framework. *Journal of Ethnopharmacology* 167: 108–114.

Shackleton C, Pandey A and Ticktin T (eds) (2015) *Ecological Sustainability for Non-Timber Forest Products: Dynamics and Case Studies of Harvesting.* Abingdon: Routledge.

Shackleton S, Shackleton C and Shanley P (eds). (2011) *Non-Timber Forest Products in the Global Context.* Dordrecht: Springer.

Shen X, Lu Z, Li S et al. (2012) Tibetan Sacred Sites: Understanding the Traditional Management System and Its Role in Modern Conservation. *Ecology and Society* 17(2): 13.

Subrat N, Iyer M and Prasad R (2002) *The Ayurvedic Medicine Industry: Current Status and Sustainability*. New Delhi: Ecotech Services and International Institute for Environment and Development.

TRAFFIC India (2011) A Review of the Status of Saussurea costus, Nineteenth Meeting of the Plant Committee (CITES), Geneva.

Tsing A and Matusutake Worlds Research Group (2009) Beyond Economic and Ecological Standardisation. *The Australian Journal of Anthropology* 20(3): 347–368.

Turner S (2007) Corruption Narratives and the Power of Concealment: The Case of Burundi's Civil War. In: Nuijten M and Anders G (eds) *Corruption and the Secret of Law: A legal Anthropological Perspective*. Aldershot: Ashgate, pp. 125–142.

van der Valk JMA (2017) *Alternative Pharmaceuticals: The Technoscientific Becomings of Tibetan Medicines in-between India and Switzerland*. PhD Dissertation, University of Kent, Canterbury.

Ved DK and Goraya GS (2008) *Demand and Supply of Medicinal Plants in India*. New Delhi and Bangalore: National Medicinal Plants Board and Foundation for Revitalisation of Local Health Traditions.

Wynberg R, Laird S, van Niekerk J et al. (2015) Formalization of the Natural Product Trade in Southern Africa: Unintended Consequences and Policy Blurring in Biotrade and Bioprospecting. *Society & Natural Resources* 28(5): 559–574.

9 Making Tibetan medicine in Nepal

Industrial aspirations, cooperative relations, and precarious production

Calum Blaikie and Sienna R. Craig

The production of Tibetan medicines[1] has become increasingly industrialised over recent decades. This trend has been starkest in Tibetan areas of China, where large and medium-sized factories churn out thousands of tons of medicines and herbal products each year for sale in Tibetan-speaking areas across China, regionally, and worldwide (Adams 2001; Janes 2001, 2002; Craig and Adams 2008; Hofer 2008a, 2008b; Schrempf 2015). What was, only two decades ago, a field dominated by small-scale manufacture, carried out by individual practitioners and localised organisations using simple technology and manual labour, has rapidly morphed into a multi-million dollar industry involving high levels of mechanisation and specialisation, advanced product development, modern packaging, clinical trials, and quality control mechanisms such as Good Manufacturing Practices (GMP) (Adams 2002; Craig 2012; Saxer 2013; Kloos 2017a; Kloos et al. 2020). On a smaller scale, factory-based mass production also predominates in Bhutan (McKay and Wangchuk 2005; Wangchuk, Pyne and Keller 2013; Taee 2017) and Mongolia (Kloos, this volume), while output volumes are increasing steadily in Tibetan-speaking enclaves of India (Kloos 2017b; Blaikie 2018; Prost 2009).

The rise of large factories has been driven by the source-forces of state and private investment, directly linked to capitalist development, nationalist ideologies, and regulatory policies that aim to standardise, modernise, and control "traditional medicine production" in technoscientific and profit-yielding ways. However, despite this ascendency, cottage industry production remains vibrant across much of the Tibetan cultural area (Craig 2012; Blaikie 2013, 2015; Blaikie et al. 2015). Small pharmacies contribute significantly to the total output, not only in peripheral or "underdeveloped" areas but also in regions where large factories are flourishing (Kloos et al.

---

1 "Tibetan medicine" is the term best-known worldwide for the medical tradition usually referred to as "Sowa Rigpa" (Tib. *gso ba rig* pa) in the Tibetan language. Various names are used for this tradition in different places and nomenclature is a contested issue (see Craig and Gerke 2016). In this chapter, we use "Sowa Rigpa" to refer to the tradition itself, and "Tibetan medicines" when speaking of the drugs and the industry that produces them.

DOI: 10.4324/9781003218074-13

2020. The coexistence of various modes of Tibetan medicine production challenges standard models of industrialisation, which predict the decline of smaller producers as larger firms take over. The complex dynamics shaping Sowa Rigpa medicine production thus demand further scholarly attention, particularly concerning the various ways industrialisation is understood and engaged with by producers working at different scales and in different socioeconomic and political contexts.

It has been argued that, although firmly rooted in each national context, Tibetan medicine production is cohering into a transnational industry, which constitutes a "pharmaceutical assemblage" (Kloos 2017b). As Kloos describes this phenomenon, "Emerging realities, such as traditional pharmaceutical industries, are special kinds of assemblages because they are contingent upon the particular yet global dynamic of pharmaceuticalisation, and because they revolve around the specific object of the drug" (2017b: 694). Kloos outlines four interdependent domains of material production and scholarly inquiry that he sees as crucial to the Sowa Rigpa pharmaceutical assemblage: *raw materials, manufacturing processes, the market,* and *intellectual property rights*. Ethnography plays a vital role in ensuring that the interconnections between these domains do not fade from view, especially given that definitions of the "assemblage" in social theory emphasise contingency and differentiation as well as totalising or synthetic visions that may, or may not, be reducible to a single logic on the ground (Deleuze and Guattari 1987; Collier and Ong 2005; DeLanda 2006; Sassen 2008).

Our ethnographic research on Tibetan medicine production in Nepal reveals distinct aspects of the pharmaceutical assemblage, but it also encourages us to foreground embodied knowledge and ethics as elements that can easily be overlooked when reaching for an assembled "bigger picture." While contributing to a more representative understanding of the "pharmaceutical nexus" (Petryna et al. 2006; Van der Geest 2006) with respect to Asian medicines, our work reinforces the importance of a "moral economy" of Sowa Rigpa (Saxer 2013; Hofer 2018), but in some new ways. Our focus is on what we call the "clinic+pharmacy" mode of production, in which one *amchi* (Sowa Rigpa practitioner) procures raw materials and produces medicines at a small scale, using simple technology and a few hired labourers working under close supervision. The vast majority of medicines made in this way are prescribed directly to patients in clinics run by the *amchi* physician-pharmacists themselves, with any surplus sold at low cost to other *amchi* through personal networks. The *amchi* who work in this way tend to describe this clinc+pharmacy model in ethically inflected terms that contrast their locally oriented, artisanal activities with what they see as the growth and profit-maximising imperatives of the factory sector. This prompts an analysis that is at once rooted in the pragmatics of political economy and in ethical imagination: How and why do non-capitalist forms of production exist alongside, and in response to, more "alienated" capitalist modes? (Gibson-Graham 2006; Muehlebach 2013; Fassin 2014).

In relation to these themes, this chapter also contributes to anthropological discussions of precarity. *Amchi* engaged in the clinic+pharmacy model recognise the medical and cultural value of their mode of production, even as they acknowledge its precarity in the face of industrialisation. We argue that different forms of precarity – political and economic, cultural and ecological – are shaping cottage industry production in Nepal. This precarity arises from decades of unstable governance and social upheaval, from the government's lack of recognition for Sowa Rigpa as a medical system, and from increasingly tenuous raw material supplies, as well as the larger geopolitical context. Acknowledging the contingency and interdependence inherent to Tibetan medical production in such a setting, we follow Stewart (2012), who writes about the ways precarity "take[s] form as a composition, a recognition, a sensibility, some collection of materialities or laws or movements" (518).

We also take inspiration from the work of Anna Tsing (2015) and others writing multi-species ethnography (Ogden et al. 2013). Although lacking the space to fully engage in this kind of analysis in this chapter, we argue that the Sowa Rigpa industry – and specifically the clinic+pharmacy model – emerges from dynamic interactions between human and non-human actors. This includes the embodied knowledge of practitioner-pharmacists, pharmacy labourers, physicians, and patients, as well as the plants, animals, and minerals that comprise Tibetan medicines, the environments from which they are sourced, and the routes they follow from Tibetan and Himalayan environments into formulas. As Nepali physician-pharmacists consider the future viability of their practice within the larger phenomenon of Tibetan medicine industry scale-up, they often make comments to the effect that "Without the plants, there can be no medicine and thus no Sowa Rigpa" (Ghimire et al. 2021). We are curious about how *materia medica* from within and beyond Nepal circulate and are being transformed from "homemade" pills and powders into "readymade" drugs, which then recirculate through various kinds of socioeconomic networks, with new value judgments about quality and efficacy, cost and benefit attached. Tsing notes that precarity demands flexibility, enables new connections to be made within assemblages, and shapes multi-species entanglements. She also writes that "a precarious world is a world without teleology" (2015: 20). Likewise, rather than viewing Nepal's Sowa Rigpa physician-pharmacists and their medicines as moving inexorably along a preordained trajectory of industrialisation, we see a coherent, adaptive, and valid mode of production in its own right, which also offers a unique perspective on the traditional medicine industry in Asia and beyond.

In what follows, we trace the emergence of Nepal's Tibetan medicine cottage industry and describe how it is organised in Kathmandu, including its relationship to the country's "peripheries" and to the flows of people, raw materials, money, and ideas across its northern and southern borders. This is followed by a more detailed account of a single clinic+pharmacy, the

Kunphen Tibetan Medical Centre, which is in many ways exemplary of this mode of operation while being exceptional in others. We then explore the range of viewpoints surrounding the scaling up of production, highlighting points of tension that are coming to the fore as this nascent industry articulates itself in new ways within the Sowa Rigpa pharmaceutical assemblage.

The lack of stable governmental structures that recognise, support, and account for Sowa Rigpa in Nepal shape both medicine production and clinical practice. Unlike for Ayurveda (Cameron 2008, 2009, 2010; Subedi 2018), no central agencies or specific government regulations exist in today's Nepal to which Sowa Rigpa pharmacies are directly accountable; neither is there a singular body representing practitioners and producers at the national level. The Himalayan Amchi Association (HAA) has lobbied for nearly two decades to secure official state recognition, but with limited success (Craig 2008, 2012). The more recent establishment of the Sowa Rigpa International College (SRIC) has increased the visibility of Sowa Rigpa in the eyes of the state (Craig and Gerke 2016), but the creation of a unified Sowa Rigpa Council within Nepal's Ministry of Health remains as an unrealised aspiration. Even so, private clinic+pharmacies have proliferated, particularly in Kathmandu, playing important roles in health care provision in urban but also rural areas, where *amchi* have been producing their own medicines for centuries.

The growth of a Kathmandu-based cottage industry entails complex relationships between urban and rural *amchi*; younger and older generations; lineage and institutionally trained practitioners; and between Nepali citizens and those hailing from Tibetan areas of China, diasporic Tibet, or Bhutan, but now living in Nepal. Even as the legal status of these pharmacies remains unclear, rural *amchi* are increasingly dependent on them to meet clinical needs. This cottage industry is reaching new patients and markets and envisioning futures that link medicine manufacture to *amchis'* continued abilities to practice. In addition, pharmacy growth and the potential to further scale up production not only reflects changing domestic health policy and practice but also wider regional political-economic dynamics, rehashing the country's (in)famous self-representation as a "yam between two boulders" of India and China.[2] These powerful neighbours are vying for influence and competing for resources in Nepal while offering various models of pharmaceutical development and inputs into this process, including raw materials, expertise, technologies, and potential consumer markets.

We argue that although artisanal and cottage industry-scale Tibetan medicine production remains important in other Asian contexts (Hofer 2008a; Blaikie 2011, 2018; Kloos et al. 2020), historical, geographic, economic,

---

2 See this recent *Washington Post* story for an overview of current politics: https://www.washingtonpost.com/world/asia_pacific/nepal-votes-thursday-will-china-or-india-come-out-the-winner/2017/12/05/41473934-d550-11e7-9ad9-ca0619edfa05_story.html?utm_term=.c69c222305f3

ecological, and cultural particularities make the Nepali model unique. While meriting attention as such, it also serves as an exemplary case study that can further understanding of the persistence of smaller scales of production in other locations within the Sowa Rigpa pharmaceutical assemblage. The rapid growth of commercial Tibetan medicine production is by no means without vexing questions and critical voices elsewhere, but these take on a particular tenor in Nepal. The concept of the pharmaceutical assemblage is helpful in capturing the open-ended, emergent, and contingent nature of these developments. Furthermore, Gibson-Graham's work (2006), as well as scholarship that highlights the "moral economy" of Tibetan medical production (Saxer 2013; Hofer 2018; Gerke et al. 2019; Kloos 2020), help us think about the relationship between expanding markets, the commodification of raw materials to the point of ecological precarity, and increasingly alienated modes of production, on the one hand and claims to artisanal production and dynamics of exchange that challenge or contravene capitalism, on the other.

Some *amchi* see pharmaceutical "development" as a way to promote Sowa Rigpa in Nepal, making it more acceptable to the state, increasing chances of official recognition, and, importantly, providing financial resources to support education and clinical practice. Indeed, many *amchi* observe the booming Tibetan pharmaceutical, cosmetic, and supplement industries in neighbouring countries and see the smaller-scale emulation of such efforts as essential to their own definitions of success – if not survival – in this precarious socioeconomic landscape. They reckon Nepal's inability to create such industries as a reflection of governmental weakness and collective short-sightedness, noting with irony how medicinal plants are cultivated or wildcrafted in Nepal, exported to factories in India and China where they are made into medicines, and then sold back to Nepalis as readymade commodities at higher prices. At the same time, many *amchi* are critical of the industrialisation taking place elsewhere, portraying it as the triumph of profit and scale over quality and integrity, which debases their medical ethics and, crucially, the ecologies on which medicine production depends. They see excessive mechanisation and regulatory regimes imported from biomedicine as reducing the potency and efficacy of formulas, unskilled labour on production lines replacing the skilful mastery of physician-pharmacists and their apprentices, and the debasement of valued connections between plants, medicine making, doctors, and patients. The majority of Nepal's practitioners stand somewhere between these two positions, in a state of ambivalence and uncertainty. As Stewart notes, precarity's forms are both "compositional and decompositional" (2012: 524). These debates are at the centre of our ethnographic analysis.

Terrains of production

The phrase "terrains of production" describes the numerous components involved in making and circulating medicines. It points to both physical and ideological domains; to geographies, fields of knowledge, and social dynamics across various scales. Terrains of production exist within larger "social ecologies," a term that helps to capture the interrelationships among the environmental, socioeconomic, biological, political, and cosmological dimensions in which illness and healing occur (Craig 2012: 5). The clinic+pharmacy mode prevalent in Nepal is linked in many ways to more industrialised, commercialised modes that dominate in other Asian contexts, yet it resists teleologies of modernisation.

Over recent decades, terrains of production have shifted significantly in Nepal. Localised, lineage-based models of education, practice, and medicine production – in which most practitioners were both physician *and* pharmacist – have given way to hybrid institutions and new ideas about what it means to be an *amchi*. It is now more common than it was even ten years ago for rural *amchi* to purchase medicines rather than make their own. These practitioners increasingly struggle to secure resources, time, and labour to make their own formulas. Some feel pressure to stock a wider range of medicines than in former times, reflecting shifting disease patterns and patient expectations. Most *amchi* now make some essential drugs themselves and buy others from urban pharmacies. For example, in the early 2000s, *amchi* from Lo Kunphen school and clinic in Mustang District routinely made between 60 and 70 individual formulas each year, limiting the purchase of readymade medicines to those which demanded pharmacological mastery and expensive ingredients. Today, this same institution produces fewer than half as many formulas and purchases the rest from Kathmandu-based clinic+pharmacies.

The conditions behind this transformation point to key concerns in political ecology, or what West has called "a sophisticated contemporary theory of accumulation by dispossession and the vast effects of this ongoing process" (2012: 30; see also van der Valk, this volume). The depletion of high-altitude medicinal plants, driven both by market demands and climate change, the increased regulation of non-timber forest products (NTFP) in Nepal, and the rising cost of raw materials and transportation have all contributed to the decline of home production in rural areas. Nepal's political instability and related rural-to-urban and international outmigration have also had an impact. Concomitantly, the clinic+pharmacy model has risen to prominence in urban areas. These institutions take advantage of better access to new technology (especially grinding and pill making machines), financial capital, and transportation networks than those in rural areas. Such material transformations are affecting understandings of what it means to be a "professional" *amchi*. Urban practitioners are moving towards a full-time physician model, with the expectations of a steady salary and a predictable schedule. They are also serving diverse patients – not only culturally Tibetan people familiar with Sowa Rigpa but also other Nepalis as well as foreign tourists and expatriates – and are operating with the shifted cultural expectation that patients should pay for medicines, along with nominal medical examination fees. This is a departure from historical expectations and therapeutic economics founded in principles of reciprocity (Craig 2012; Blaikie 2013; Hofer 2018; Pordié and Kloos 2022). At the same time, the clinic+pharmacy model allows both rural and urban *amchi* to sustain more personalised, artisanal claims about the efficacy, potency, and safety of the medicines they prescribe to patients since they recognise that production processes are different than those of large factories in China. In Nepal, claims over the efficacy of medicines are still linked to claims of physician-pharmacist expertise and, in turn, to an ethics of production that relies on embodied skill and experience rather than national regulatory standards. This holds important implications for the scaling-up of production.

Most of Nepal's cottage industry pharmacies are overseen by a single *amchi* who determines which medicines to make and when, sources raw materials, makes compounding decisions, supervises each stage of the process, and manages sales. In the smallest pharmacies, some *amchi* still contribute manual labour as well. However, it is more common for senior *amchi* to employ non-*amchi* staff to perform the physical work: operating grinding machines, preparing pills, packaging, etc. For example, Shechen Clinic employs two full-time pharmacy workers, while Kunphen Medical Center employs ten individuals who work in shifts. The Phentok clinic+pharmacy, run by a senior physician-pharmacist who has trained many of Nepal's most successful *amchi*, formerly employed novice *amchi* but today has just one full-time worker. Shelkar Monastery's clinic+pharmacy employs three non-*amchi* workers, while the head *amchi* of Phende Himalayan Sorig Center, which now has three branch clinics across Nepal, oversees seasonal production with the help of two non-*amchi* assistants.

Paid non-*amchi* staff have become central to cottage industry production. Employing such labourers instead of relying on the donated or bartered labour of *amchi* students or local villagers represents a significant shift in the terrain of production, one that mitigates against certain forms of precarity while introducing others. Although this change marks a transition toward a more "alienated" mode of production, it does not necessarily imply a pre-ordained industrialisation process. As is the case in larger factories in other Asian countries, technical specialties (such as making incense, cosmetics, and medicinal teas as well as medicines), vocational training, and standardised manufacturing systems are becoming established in Nepal, albeit on a small scale. Maintaining a reliable, trustworthy non-specialist labour force is increasingly difficult across many sectors.[3] Finding non-*amchi* workers

---

3 Explanations for this include much greater uptake of higher education, growing distaste for manual labour, and wage labour opportunities that pull millions of working-age Nepalis to India, the Gulf States, Southeast Asia, and beyond. More than 30 percent of Nepal's GDP comes from remittances.

for cottage industry medicine production is challenging, requiring proactive recruitment and competitive salaries. While production schedules become more predictable as a result of these new labour relations, the social commitments to making good medicines may be reduced.

Although many of Kathmandu's senior cottage industry *amchi*-pharmacists were born and trained in Nepal, others hail from India, Tibet, or Bhutan, and some do not have Nepali citizenship documents. This introduces yet another form of precarity and can make a difference in their ability to help officially shape efforts to recognise and support Sowa Rigpa at the national level, if not to practice and produce medicine. While several such individuals were trained in a lineage-apprenticeship model in Nepal, others were educated at Tibetan exile institutions in India (Men-Tsee-Khang; Central Institute for Higher Tibetan Studies; Chagpori). Although several elder *amchi* studied with individual teachers or within institutions in Tibetan areas of the People's Republic of China (PRC), it is rarer for the up-and-coming generation to have trained in Tibet. These facts illustrate the truly transnational nature of Sowa Rigpa and its pharmaceutical industry: at once rooted within and existing beyond the nation-state. Terrains of production, per force, cross borders. *Amchi* born or trained elsewhere enrich Sowa Rigpa and its pharmaceutical production in Nepal while connecting it to other locations in Asia and beyond.

Ngawang Namgyal's journey illustrates these dynamics well. A Tibetan refugee born in Nepal, he learned to make medicines from a private physician in whose clinic he worked as a novice. After two years, the HAA hired Ngawang Namgyal to serve as their association *amchi*. He worked for four years in their Boudha clinic, which itself did not produce medicine. During this time, he established a private pharmacy in collaboration with one of the pharmacists working at the Shechen Clinic: "In the daytime, I went to HAA and he went to Shechen Clinic. Then after [in the evenings and on weekends] we made medicine together." The medicines they produced served several rural clinics, particularly in Solukhumbu and Humla districts, as well as other private clinics in Kathmandu and Delhi. They also sold raw materials to the Men-Tsee-Khang and private *amchi* in India. Then, after several years of working together, Ngawang Namgyal's pharmacist partner migrated to Europe and he no longer had time to maintain both a clinical practice and pharmacy. He chose the pharmacy and now sells medicine to seven clinics in urban and rural Nepal.

Let us now consider the Shechen Clinic, an integrative medical institution and charitable hospital founded in 2000. Offering biomedical, homeopathic, and Sowa Rigpa services, Shechen is run by a non-*amchi* management team. This contributes to, but does not fully explain, its somewhat distinctive mode of pharmaceutical production. Sonam Pelmo, the current *amchi* in charge, is a Bhutanese woman who studied medicine and pharmacy at the Central Institute for Higher Tibetan Studies in India, then completed a one-year clinical internship before being hired at Shechen. This cosmopolitan

Making Tibetan medicine in Nepal 261

practitioner-pharmacist demonstrates many of the characteristics of the new generation of institutionally trained, outward-looking *amchi*, described by Pordié (2008) as "neo-traditional."

When Sonam took this job, Shechen hospital management had recently reduced the Sowa Rigpa staff from one physician, one pharmacist, and one raw materials manager down to just one *amchi*, with responsibility for all areas, supported by two full-time, non-*amchi* pharmacy workers. As Sonam described these individuals, "They do not know how the pharmacology really works, or how to actually compound the medicines." Put another way, they can follow technical directions, but Sonam is solely responsible for overseeing production, and she is always present when raw materials are weighed and mixed. Workers manage the processing, grinding, drying and finishing, under her close supervision. Sonam receives a printed stock list every week and uses it to manage medicine production: "If there are less than 1000 pills of any of the popular medicines, then we must start the process of making more. We can go below this for the less popular medicines, which we do not use so much. For the really popular ones, even if we have 2000 pills, I need to think about the next batch." She explained that if they are running low on a particular medicine, "first I look at the herbs that we have – there is also a printout of this. I calculate all that I will need to make the medicine, then see what else I need to get. Once I have all the raw materials, we can make more." This computerised stock control system for raw materials and medicines resembles those found in pharmaceutical factories in India and China, but there is nothing comparable among other Kathmandu producers.

Shechen produces a total of 130 herbal products, including medicines, incense and massage oils. Sonam explained that they make 10–20-kilogram batches of the more popular medicines several times each year and 1–3 kilograms of the less popular formulas once. "It is not beneficial to make medicine in huge quantities. That way it does not stay fresh. I make smaller amounts and that means the medicine never sits for too long in the packaging." Soon after arriving, Sonam altered the production manifests, adding several medicines with which she was familiar but were not made at Shechen and removing several with which she was unfamiliar and was not using. In keeping with an artisanal ethos and a patient-centred practice, Sonam explained that she sometimes adjusts formulas according to her own experience and feedback from patients: "If I see that my patients are not responding well to a particular medicine, then I change the formula a little, or add some *khatsar* [additional ingredients], then wait to see if the effect improves." Sonam's curious, experimental approach to pharmacy stands in contrast with the more conservative methods of many physician-pharmacists, who tend to stick as closely as possible to the classical formulations. She also noted that one of the things she finds most challenging about her multi-faceted job is accessing raw materials. "With some of them, it is so hard to get. Like for two years I could not get any *pangyen* [Gentianaceae] at all.

It was not available. This was very difficult. We could not make several medicines for a long time." Here in this not-for-profit clinic+pharmacy, Sonam is engaging in the raw materials market in new ways and introducing a range of innovations while holding fast to an ethics of manufacture that centres on the links between production, prescription, and patient response.

As Sonam Pelmo's comment indicates, the lynchpin in Nepal's terrains of production – and their place within the larger Sowa Rigpa pharmaceutical assemblage – are raw materials. Difficulties accessing *materia medica* and rising herb market prices represent major impediments to scaling-up production. Many Kathmandu-based pharmacies formerly relied on networks of villagers and rural *amchi* to provide them with key ingredients. This, in turn, demands that local people maintain tacit and locally specific knowledge about where and how to collect, within an ethics of care that we might gloss as "sustainability." However, these generations-old patterns of resource exchange have not only shifted as village demographics have transformed and climate change impacts upon mountain ecologies, they have also become dangerous business. Consider this description from Ngawang Namgyal: "Before there was no problem with the Forestry Department. Villagers could bring 10 or 20 kilograms, no problem on the way. But four years ago, the new Forestry Minister came and it became very tight. Now you need documents, but the village people don't have these documents." Ngawang Namgyal mentioned particular problems with procuring two key medicinals: Himalayan orchid (Orchidaceae, T. *wanglak*) and *Picrorhiza kurroa* root (T. *honglen*). "One year it was fine and then suddenly the police start taking people to jail, taking a lot of money and punishing them [for possession and transport of these plants]."

This situation bespeaks multi-species entanglements with economic, ecological, legal, cultural, medical, and infrastructural implications on local, national, and transnational levels. With expanding road networks throughout rural Nepal (many of them funded by Chinese or Indian government aid) and a greater desire on the part of the state to capture income from NTFP, vehicles coming to urban centres from the mountains are subject to frequent searches and check posts, making documentation from the Ministry of Forests and Soil Conservation paramount. Due to barriers of language and culture, geography, and economic disparity, it is virtually impossible for most villagers from Nepal's high mountains to understand these requirements, let alone navigate these regulatory regimes and secure such documents. Increasingly, entrepreneurial *amchi* and traders pay local herb collectors in advance (who may or may not have training in sustainable harvesting techniques), obtain the documents, and then transport the plants to Kathmandu by jeep or truck. Ironically, conservation laws and state enforcement practices are forcing moves away from more sustainable collection through personal networks under the supervision of local *amchi*, towards industrialising commodity chains (cf. Dejouhanet and Sreelakshmy; van der Valk, this volume). In addition, while many *amchi* are aware that medicinal plants are becoming severely depleted in the wild, leading to higher prices and fears of extinction, they often wish to stick with classical formulae and avoid substitution (T. *tshabs*) (Craig 2012: 205–213; Blaikie 2013, 2018; Blaikie et al. 2015). Coupled with a relative dearth of medicinal plant cultivation efforts, such trends render high altitude *materia medica*, and all that relies upon them, increasingly precarious.

Cross-border flows of *materia medica*, and the vast networks that channel them, are crucial elements of Sowa Rigpa's transnationality. Nepal's position in the centuries-old *materia medica* trade between South Asia and the Tibetan Plateau is well established. However, in all directions, ingredient flows between more and less powerful stakeholders are shaping terrains of production in uneven ways. Pharmaceutical firms and industry lobbies are much larger and more influential in China and India, so state and bureaucratic infrastructures work in their favour. Raw material prices are rising steeply, and questions of quality, adulteration, and counterfeit ingredients are coming to the fore (Gerke 2015; van der Valk, this volume). As Saxer (2013) has shown, policies and regulations regarding the Nepal-China plant trade are out of step with on-the-ground realities. There are many reports of large-scale commercial herb collection taking place in Nepal by Indian Ayurveda companies and, to a lesser extent, Tibetan medicine companies based in China, who can pull strings with officials in order to avoid scrutiny or simply bribe their way around enforcement efforts. What we call "Big Pharma with Traditional Characteristics" has particular implications in Nepal, feeding the fears of some *amchi* that the skill of small-scale production is itself becoming endangered (Blaikie 2011), and the understandable desire on the part of other physician-pharmacists to scale up or risk being swept away.

These entanglements between people and plants should not be reduced to economic transactions, although they frequently are (Olsen and Bhattarai 2005; Kala et al. 2006). They depend on social networks and forms of embodied expertise as well as place-based knowledge (Dejouhanet and Sreelakshmy, this volume), all of which are becoming increasingly precarious. For example, Kathmandu-based pharmacies are heavily reliant on high-altitude plants brought from Tibet, mainly by one prominent middleman who has engaged in this trade for four decades. Navigating both the Nepal-China and Nepal-India borders requires particular sociolinguistic and bureaucratic acumen, as well as a host of documents from various state agencies in three nations. However, as this man grows old, a crucial raw material supply channel becomes tenuous. It is worth noting how heavily dependent the production of Tibetan medicines in both Nepal and India have been on *one person* to supply so many vital high-altitude ingredients. This shows what a massive understatement it was when one Kathmandu-based *amchi* commented: "When [this trader] stops doing his work, pharmacies in Nepal and India will have a big problem."

This section has shown how particular historical, socioeconomic, bureaucratic, medical, and ecological dynamics, characterised by various forms of precarity, have shifted terrains of production in Nepal, resulting in the decline of micro-scale production and growth of cottage industry manufacture. We have seen how several features of industrial pharmacy, such as paid labourers, computerised stock control systems, basic mechanisation, and commercial raw material sourcing have been adopted within this cottage industry mode, yet also how resistance to further industrialisation remains strong. We have also glimpsed the deep interconnections that hold the Sowa Rigpa pharmaceutical assemblage together while allowing for various industrial trajectories and scales in different locations.

Kunphen Medical Centre: Borders, state recognition, and quality control

In order to further illustrate the development and current dynamics of cottage industry production, we describe the story of Kunphen Medical Centre (henceforth "Kunphen"), a pioneer of the clinic+pharmacy model for more than 30 years. In many ways, Kunphen exemplifies this mode of operation, yet it also incorporates some unique features that contrast with other similar institutions in Kathmandu. Kunphen's long existence, excellent reputation, diverse clientele, and quasi-legal status vis-à-vis the Nepali state, as well as its close relations with a large Tibetan medicine factory across the border in the Tibet Autonomous Region (TAR) of the PRC, put it in a highly favourable position for pharmacy expansion. However, although output has increased over the years, Kunphen resolutely remains on a cottage industry scale and those involved extol the virtues of artisanal medicine making as an explicit counterpoint to factory mass production.

The story of Kunphen begins with Dr. Kunsang (1924–2006), a Tibetan-born student of the great monk-physician and long-time director of the Lhasa Mentseekhang, Khyenrab Norbu (1883–1992). Building on this master's training, Dr. Kunsang became not only a highly skilled physician in his own right, but also an expert pharmacist adept in complex techniques, including the creation of *tsotel* (mercury sulfide organometallic complex) and the production of *rinchen rilbu*, or precious pills (cf. Gerke 2013, 2017). In the early 1950s, shortly after Dr. Kunsang left Tibet and settled in Kathmandu, he was called to Nepal's Royal Palace to treat the late King Tribhuvan, who was suffering from a liver disorder. Dr. Kunsang's successful treatment of this most important individual was the beginning of a long relationship of patronage between the Palace and what became Kunphen,[4] including unprecedented state support for Sowa Rigpa and the granting of a peculiar quasi-legal status to this institution.

From the late 1950s onwards, Dr. Kunsang made medicines and treated patients from all social strata at his Kunphen clinic, located in the Chettrapati neighbourhood in the heart of old Kathmandu. His clientele

---

4 In Tibetan, *kunphen* means "doctor to the king."

and reputation grew. In 1963, His Majesty's Government of Nepal granted Dr. Kunsang "Traditional Health Trainer" status, supporting the facilitation of training courses for local *amchi* from rural areas across Nepal. In the mid-1980s, Dr. Kunsang established the God Monkey Medicine Industry in Nyalam, TAR, near the region of his birth in Tingri. This institution has grown into a highly successful Tibetan medicine factory, mass-producing medicines for local and national markets (Saxer 2013).

In addition to the practical exchange of raw materials, processed ingredients, and medicines between pharmacies in Nyalam and Kathmandu, as discussed below, Dr Kunsang also facilitated the cross-border exchange of knowledge. Several renowned Tibetan medical experts, including the late Troru Tsenam and Jampa Trinley, visited Kathmandu, allowing Nepal-based practitioners to learn directly from some of Tibet's most revered Sowa Rigpa scholars. Nepal-based *amchi* also travelled to Nyalam, where they were exposed to a very different model of Tibetan medicine production. However, such exposure did not result in Kunphen following Nyalam's lead by scaling up its own production processes. On the contrary, it appears to have galvanised a discourse of artisanal, small-scale pharmacy among those working at Kunphen so that the two entities follow parallel but distinct trajectories rather than a course of convergence.

In 1973, facilitated by close connections with the palace and the state, the Kunphen Medical Center was recognised by the Nepal Health Department (now the Ministry of Health), leading to government registration of the clinic and pharmacy. The pharmacy was formally registered as *Kunphen Aushadi Udhyog* (literally "Kunphen Medicine Factory"), distinguishing it neither as a specifically "Tibetan" concern nor as an institution falling under the "Ayurveda" category within the Ministry of Health, as is the case for several other cottage industry factories in Kathmandu and elsewhere in Nepal. This special categorisation was significant because it meant Kunphen could continue producing medicines outside the auspices of the Ayurvedic authorities or biomedical regulatory regimes, while also sidestepping the problems that often accompany political association with Tibet in Nepal. At the same time, the registration of almost 100 specific formulas and annual official inspections of the pharmacy also began.

Today, as before, Kunphen is a busy clinic treating more than 50 patients each day from a wide array of backgrounds. The majority are Nepali-speakers and Himalayan Nepali citizens, but many foreign tourists and Nepali dignitaries also visit. Several years ago, Kunphen opened a branch clinic at Boudha, which serves a predominantly Tibetan clientele as well as tourists, many of them hailing from the former Soviet Union and Eastern Europe. Arguably, Kunphen's success is the combined result of the strong personal reputation of Dr. Kunsang in Nepal, his and his family's unique positioning vis-à-vis a shifting Nepali state, good management of the clinic and pharmacy, and the cross-border connections with Tibet, sustained through many moments of political transition.

Let us look in more detail at the Kunphen pharmacy. When Dr Kunsang passed away, his nephew, Kunsang Dorjee, became the head pharmacist at Kunphen, where he is responsible for pharmacy administration and the compounding of each formula through to quality control and packaging. Dr Kunsang's daughter, Dr Tashi Pedon, also plays a major role within the pharmacy, while Dr Nyima Tsering, a young Tibetan exile *amchi* trained at the Men-Tsee-Khang in Dharamsala, married into the family and today works as both a physician and assistant pharmacist. They are supported by a team of ten non-*amchi* labourers, most of whom have been working there for many years and are skilled in raw material processing, grinding, mixing, and pill making. Kunphen produces a total of 171 medicines and herbal products, around 120 of which are made regularly in reasonable quantities. Among these, approximately 15 are medicines developed at Kunphen and not available elsewhere. Dr Kunsang took well-known formulas from Tibetan pharmacological texts, adapted the proportions, and added extra components (*khatsar*) to make "new" medicines with highly specific indications. Several of these have become very popular due to their effectiveness, bolstering Kunphen's reputation. Nyima Tsering explained:

> These are new medicines for me also. When I worked in Dharamsala, we did not have these medicines, but through my practice here I have started prescribing them and the results are good. For example, there is one pill called *shang drum men,* which is specifically for hemorrhoids, of which there are many cases in Nepal due to the spicy food. This medicine works very well and is very popular with patients – many come here just asking for that.

Of the total annual medicine production, roughly 80 percent is used in the two Kunphen clinics, while 20 percent is sold in bulk to other *amchi* in Nepal and internationally. Kunphen-made medicines have a good reputation among many diasporic Tibetan physicians and are prescribed to patients from New York City to Mexico City and beyond. Diasporic *amchi* order medicines by email or telephone, often every 3–4 months. All Kunphen medicines are listed on their website and although not offered to patients directly via "online shopping," practitioners and patients can order them by email and they are then delivered "by special request" anywhere in the world. These direct sales involve only a tiny fraction of annual output, but global availability via the internet is a sign both of Kunphen's strong current position and its scope for growth. Together with regular bulk exports to practitioners, it further distinguishes Kunphen from other clinic+pharmacies in Kathmandu, few of which have websites, let alone aspirations towards global distribution.

Kunphen's production, import, and export activities are made substantially easier and less risky through its longstanding connections to the Nepali state. Kunphen exists in a state of quasi-legitimacy: not fully "legal" due to the lack of central recognition of Sowa Rigpa, but without fear of state sanction. As they have done for over 30 years, representatives from the Ministry of Health still conduct annual, unannounced inspections of the pharmacy. Because the inspectors are biomedically trained and "know nothing about Tibetan medicine," according to Kunphen staff, these visits remain largely symbolic but nevertheless offer a degree of legitimacy and protection. Because almost 100 formulas were registered with the Ministry of Health in Kunphen's name during the 1960s, they can easily procure the papers needed for export. Kunphen's patronage by the state and its familiarity to the bureaucrats signing the documents also expedite the import and export of medicines and raw materials between Nepal, the TAR, China and India. Such advantages are not available to other pharmacies in Kathmandu, who must either struggle to get official clearance for each batch to be imported or exported or operate in the shadows (cf. Saxer 2013: 109–113). While not exactly avoiding capitalist accumulation or state regulation, Kunphen is able to maintain a great degree of control over how its medicines are produced and who uses them, adhering to an ethics of practice that can also be seen to challenge more bureaucratised and alienated modes.

The relationship between the Nyalam factory and Kunphen was crucial to the development of Nepal's clinic+pharmacy model but it also represents a unique case of successful cross-border institutional collaboration in the field of Tibetan medicine production. It is at once a straightforward and curious arrangement. While Kunphen produces medicines at a relatively modest scale for a diverse patient population, the God Monkey Medicine Industry has grown into a large, state supported Tibetan pharmaceutical enterprise, mass-producing drugs for sale across the region. What is the nature of the relationship between these two entities, both of which owe their existence to the same individual? Why has Kunphen remained small-scale while the Nyalam factory has expanded dramatically? How can these linked but contrasting trajectories help us to understand the resilience of the clinic+pharmacy model in Nepal and its role in the larger Sowa Rigpa pharmaceutical assemblage?

In earlier decades, the Kunphen and Nyalam pharmacies would supply raw materials to one another in quantities ranging from a few kilograms to a truckload. Kunphen acted as a conduit for lowland Nepali and Indian materials into Tibet, while Nyalam sent consignments of high altitude plants harvested across the PRC to Kunphen. In line with general trends in the cross-border movement of raw materials, these exchanges became more difficult around the turn of the millennium (Saxer 2013), although they continue on a smaller scale today. Such exchange relations reflect differential access to materials in distinct geographical locations and are conducted pragmatically in the mutual interest of both parties.

Since its founding, the God Monkey Medicine Industry has ridden several waves of political tumult and change in the state regulation of Sowa

Rigpa. Today, it clearly engages in industrial mass-production, using the latest technology, quality control methods, and packaging, while marketing its medicines widely both within the TAR and across China. In many ways, the Nyalam factory represents "Big Pharma with Traditional Characteristics," yet certain features set it apart from other large factories in the PRC. Crucially, the business is entirely Tibetan owned, with 60 percent of shares held by its workers, 20 percent by the current director, and 20 percent by Dr. Kunsang's Kathmandu-based family (Saxer 2013: 47). Those at Kunphen consistently stress the absence of Chinese owners as vitally important. In their discursive model of the moral economy of Tibetan pharmacy, Chinese-owned or heavily Chinese-influenced factories are mainly get-rich-quick schemes, sacrificing quality and authenticity for profit. Such an approach is seen to ignore the "correct" way to prepare medicines, leading to lower standards, ineffective medicines, and, ultimately, the debasement of Sowa Rigpa. Viewed from Kunphen, the Nyalam factory mitigates some of the negative side effects of industrial production through the lineage of their mutual founder and the ongoing intentions of the current management, who try their best to maintain high standards despite the scale of their manufacture.

In contrast with Nyalam, the Kunphen pharmacy remains in many ways resolutely "traditional." *Amchi* oversee the entire operation and closely supervise the paid staff who perform the manual labour. Many procedures are still carried out by hand; compounding is done on specific days and at certain times, according to the Tibetan calendar. Medicines are finished in classical forms – pills and powders as opposed to tablets and capsules – and supplied in simple packaging rather than blister packs as at Nyalam. Medicines are made frequently and in small batches to ensure the highest possible potency and efficacy. The institution has resisted moving toward highly mechanised production because, as Nyima Tsering explained:

> If you make huge amounts of medicine, of course there will be problems, like the materials will not be mixed together properly. We use sunlight to dry the pills, not artificial heat like in the big factories, because that also makes a big difference to the potency. Using too many machines is not good: the medicine loses a lot of potency. People say that food made on wood is tastier than with gas – it's like that also with medicines [...] We see directly in our practice that a small quantity has more potency and works better for the patients. Because of this, we make each medicine two or three times each year. This consumes a lot of time, but makes a big difference in terms of potency.

Kunphen does what it can to maintain artisanal production processes that will sustain its good name. Although its clinical reach both within Nepal and internationally is expanding and its medicine output increases each year, it continues to resist moving further towards mechanised mass production.

A particularly complex and compelling aspect of the Kunphen-Nyalam relationship has to do with the production of *tsotel* and *rinchen rilbu*, many of which have *tsotel* as a key ingredient. Following Dr. Kunsang's instruction, the Nyalam factory continues to make *tsotel* in large amounts on an occasional basis and to send some of what they make to Kunphen. Kunphen uses this *tsotel* to produce *rinchen rilbu* and sends several boxes of them back to Nyalam each year. Dr Kunsang did not instruct those at the Nyalam factory in the production of *rinchen rilbu* themselves – only one of their key ingredients. Why? Was this insight into the political economy of production and the desire to invest in the Kathmandu-based operation with a source of reliable and significant income? Was it about moral economies of scale and the need to produce the highest quality *rinchen rilbu* by limiting industrial processes and profit motivations? Could it be about ensuring quality by reducing biomedically derived state regulatory interference? Or was it connected to the complex ritual requirements for consecrating *rinchen rilbu*, which may not have been accessible in Nyalam? We are not yet sure of the answers – and perhaps each of these questions could be answered with a "yes" – but such inquiry remains important. It focuses attention on the specificities involved in producing certain rare and precious components and medicines that require humans, plants, animals, and minerals to intermingle through complex practices of pharmacology and religious ritual, on the hidden complexities of cross-border collaboration, and on the territorialised components of the Sowa Rigpa pharmaceutical assemblage.

Very close connections over three decades, combined with a clear trend towards industrialised pharmaceutical production across the Tibetan-speaking world, make it remarkable that the Nyalam factory has not become a model for the Kathmandu operation. The two exist in very different socioeconomic, political, and medical spaces, which goes a long way towards explaining their parallel trajectories but does not explain them entirely. Nyalam has certainly benefitted from China's policies of liberalisation, state support for the expansion of traditional medicine industries, and a favourable environment for private investment (see Chee; Campinas, this volume). Nepal, on the other hand, has offered a more precarious basis for pharmacy growth due to the lack of official recognition or state support for Sowa Rigpa, negligible private capital investment, and a small, tightly circumscribed marketplace. This recalls Stewart's conceptualisation of precarity's forms, which "magnetize attachments, tempos, materialities, and states of being … [and ask that we] attune to how things are hanging together or falling apart or wearing out in time that compresses or stretches out into an endurance" (2012: 524). Although its context of precarity has significantly shaped the way Kunphen makes medicine, we contend that the continuation of cottage industry production is as much, if not more, to do with their discourse of the quality, efficacy, and integrity of small-scale manufacture as a counterpoint to the perceived negative impacts of industrial mass production. Although the two entities remain distinct in terms of outlook and mode of operation, they contribute in equally important ways to the emergent Sowa Rigpa pharmaceutical assemblage.

Contested discourses of scaling-up and the quest for recognition

For Nepal's urban *amchi*, investment in cottage industry production can work in their favour, given economies of scale. As we have seen, these pharmacies are becoming a crucial point of access to medicines for rural and urban *amchi* alike. Notably, readymade Nepali formulas are less expensive and often considered of higher quality than imported equivalents from India or China. The market for such medicine has begun to grow: demand feeds increased supply, which feeds more demand. Cottage industry production can be lucrative, and yet, due to the moral economy underlying Sowa Rigpa and to other cultural expectations that shape how one speaks of success, profit is rarely discussed as a motivation for pharmacy expansion. The fact that it is downplayed, however, does not mean that it can be ignored. Deemphasising profit and critiquing industrialisation take place within a context in which people are also keenly aware of the social power, recognition, and, indeed, economic benefit that can come from scaling up production. This is coupled with Nepali practitioners' understanding of a rising national demand for Tibetan medicines among diverse patient groups – despite the lack of state recognition – and a keen attunement to the need for their practices to appear "modern" or "developed" (N. *bikasit*) in the eyes of the state in order to pursue formal recognition. These are enduring characteristics of Nepali development discourse (cf. Pigg 1992, 1996) recast through the particular lens of Sowa Rigpa. After hydropower and tourism, the herb trade is often cited as the best source of potential GDP growth for Nepal.[5]

Kathmandu's physician-pharmacists largely earn their living from cash sales of medicines, so they seek to increase output and their share of the national market while remaining attuned to norms established and perpetuated by what has been called elsewhere a "Sowa Rigpa sensibility" (Adams et al. 2011). Essentially, this is a cultural discourse that frames *amchi* as compassionate healers and Sowa Rigpa as fundamentally about the alleviation of suffering rather than material gain. It is a form of ethical imagination. In this framework, the pursuit of profit must not be too obvious and should not be seen to compromise quality. Prices must remain affordable not only to rural *amchi* clientele but also to patients. Herein lie some important tensions, which resonate in Himalayan India (Blaikie 2011, 2013, 2018; Pordié and Kloos 2022) but contrast starkly with industrial production in China

---

5 Subedi (2006); http://www.myrepublica.com/news/21627/

(Saxer 2013). Most importantly, among Indian and Nepali *amchi* alike, there remains a vibrant, critical discourse about the disadvantages of industrialised production. These critiques include a sense that mass production can lead to poor quality medicines due to ingredient substitution, lack of oversight, and damage to the potency of medicines from the use of certain kinds of machines. Adding to this is cultural and ideological commentary about the intrusive importation of biomedical concepts of quality, safety, and efficacy into Tibetan medicine production, epitomised in GMP regulations.

Amchi also recognise that industrialisation regimes are expensive and that, while state recognition of Sowa Rigpa in Nepal remains a goal, it is likely to involve compliance with new governmental manufacturing standards that would make cottage industry production unaffordable. As Wangchuk, a senior Kathmandu-based physician-pharmacist put it:

> Right now, I make medicines in my small pharmacy with papers from the Department of Ayurveda. The government does not see this as 'Sowa Rigpa' but I can still produce. In the future, if we want to make factory medicines under 'Sowa Rigpa' we will need different papers and more money. Without investment from sponsors or the government we cannot make big factory medicine. And if we want to change how we make medicines into this factory type, the government will make more laws. They will pay more attention and then maybe make us change how we mix and compound – like they do in China with GMP. This would not be good for quality and would make medicines more expensive.

While Wangchuk and others operate through the Department of Ayurveda, and Kunphen navigates permission through their longstanding special agreement with the Ministry of Health, others have registered their clinic+pharmacy operations as "natural" or "herbal" product companies. These various modes of registration reflect attempts to minimise legal risks in the absence of state recognition. At times, cottage producers collaborate by mixing and grinding at one location, then making pills and packaging somewhere else. Arguably, the productive nature of precarity that allows for this sort of adaptive flexibility would change with increased industrialisation.

Uncertainties about scaling up and anxieties about the future of small-scale production featured prominently in an event that brought together physician-pharmacists of diverse backgrounds. In 2011, we helped to facilitate a Kathmandu-based workshop that gathered 40 *amchi* from Nepal, India, and Tibetan regions of China to engage in medicine making and discuss issues of safety, efficacy, and quality in light of these regional trends away from small-scale production (Blaikie et al. 2015). We witnessed how some Nepali *amchi* were impressed by the technological sophistication and state investment enjoyed by Tibetans involved in industrial production, yet they remained critical of mass production, citing a preference for cottage industry scales and methods. Furthermore, some of the Tibetans who have borne witness to transformations in production practices in China since the early 2000s were also critical of these trends, even as they were deeply embedded within them.

Through their participation in events such as the 2011 workshop, as well as their own global networks and exposure to Sowa Rigpa institutions and developments, Nepal's *amchi* are increasingly aware that factory production has become the dominant mode, corresponding with a decline in small-scale production, particularly in rural areas. They know very well that market logic is replacing logics of reciprocity, barter, and regional self-sufficiency. Added to this are ideologies of development, including desires to produce medicines that appear "modern" in form and that reach new patient-consumers, and how scaling up commercial production in Nepal may generate funds for other activities such as education and clinical practice, neither of which receives state support. Just as there are competing discourses and deep political-economic divisions among the "major players" in Tibetan medical industries in China (Saxer 2013) and complex socioeconomic and political dynamics between Ladakhi and diasporic Tibetan producers in India (Blaikie 2016; Kloos 2016), Nepali *amchi* are not unified in their conceptions of how the industry should develop and are ambivalent about possible futures. However, many are keenly aware that the "status quo" is changing, reflecting and determined by shifting relationships between capitalist markets and the ethical imaginaries that at once resist and are couched within them. In other words, *amchi* understand that these entanglements are precarious, given the particular conjunctions of economy, ecology, politics, and culture they imply.

Practices of cottage industry packaging and marketing highlight some of these points of tension. For example, Sonam Pelmo remains enthusiastic about the new products Shechen is developing, including medicated pain relief oils, ointments, nasal drops, and herbal teas. She pointed to a bottle of ointment, saying that the product was ready, but the packaging remained a problem:

> Look at this bottle! It is not nice, not attractive. They look cheap and not good quality. Packaging is very important. It must look attractive or people will think it is low quality. There is no use putting this high-quality medicine in bad packaging. Also, labels are very important. It takes a long time to design the label, make it look nice and tell all the right information.

Others among Nepal's physician-pharmacists have also embraced this push towards the development of new forms for medicines, as well as a focus on packaging, labelling, and marketing. Tenzin Dharkye, the *amchi* director of Phende Sorig, noted that he added expiry dates to the packaging he uses, not because of any top-down regulation but due to patient feedback and his own sense of what evokes quality and efficacy. "People that I was treating were happy with my medicines, with their positive effects. But some would

Making Tibetan medicine in Nepal 273

come to me and say 'Doctor, we like your medicines but they don't have *date* on them and we know that medicines are supposed to have *date* so that we know if they are still good or not. So, we request to you to put *date* on medicine.' I also thought this is a good idea." Tenzin Dharkye noted that this is how Tibetan medicines are packaged in China, but that he felt he could be even more specific, adjusting expiry dates depending on the formula's ingredients and the form (pill, powder, or capsule) as well as recommending ideal conditions for storing medicines. He had also followed scientific debates about the damaging health effects of bisphenol-A (BPA) as found in plastics. Without any state mandate but with a concern for the quality and reputation of his burgeoning brand, he sought out BPA-free plastic containers in which to bottle the 20–30 formulas that he produces.

Sometimes the issue of packaging can cause tension, at times heightened by generational divides. For example, while Wangchuk's medicines are revered by other *amchi* and his clinic+pharmacy remains one of the busiest in Kathmandu, he invests virtually nothing in packaging and marketing. His clinic is located down a darkened corridor, past currency exchange kiosks and souvenir shops, off the main circumambulation path at Boudha. It is one room, painted the colour of corn flour. The wall opposite the door is lined with cabinets in which his pills and powders rest in glass and plastic jars, each with a handwritten label. He uses squares of torn up newspaper or white printer paper in which to wrap prescriptions, on which instructions for use are handwritten. Canvas and plastic bundles sit on shelves behind his simple desk, bringing with them the smell of the mountains – dried, unprocessed herbs and minerals – some of which have been offered by patients in lieu of cash. These are indications of a non-market-driven moral economy that exists alongside the markets he must also navigate to make medicine.

After the earthquakes of 2015, Wangchuk's formula for *nagpo guchor* was in particularly high demand. This nine-ingredient formula is a non-consumable pill wrapped in black cloth, worn against the skin to ward off infectious disease and offer protection during times of epidemics. As was the case with certain Tibetan incense during the SARS outbreak in China (Craig and Adams 2008), Wangchuk had trouble keeping up with the demand for *nagpo gujor* since the earthquakes. His unadorned version sold for 30 rupees per pill. Another physician-pharmacist's version of this same formula, for which he had produced an elaborate plastic package with written instructions in English, was selling for 100 rupees per pill.[6] When Gyatso, a village-based physician-pharmacist and current chairman of the HAA, discovered this discrepancy, he was not amused. After noting that the only difference between the two pills was the packaging and indicating that he still thought Wangchuk's were of the highest quality, he said, "In twenty years, we will be lucky if we have even half the medicines like these ones," gesturing to

6 Notably, an online retailer was selling *nagpo guchor* pills for 36 USD each, or the equivalent of 3600 NPR, a 100-fold increase over Wangchuk's prices.

Wangchuk's pharmacy. "It is more likely that our medicine will only be available for rich people in India, China, and the West. People say they like *traditional medicine* these days, but do not think enough about where the plants come from. They want things that they can feel are *natural* but they don't think deeply about what this means .... People don't realize that they cannot buy good health. They are buying an illusion of health." Wangchuk nodded in agreement. "As time goes by, we make fewer medicines. The prices of plants are going up. Mountain plants are becoming rare. The changing environment is part of it," Gyatso continued, recognising the potential impacts of climate change on Sowa Rigpa production, "but so is greed. And Nepali stupidity. We send our medicinal plants out of this country for 10 rupees per kilo and buy them back as *readymade* for 100 rupees. It will keep going like this unless Nepal and other places where the plants grow use some intelligence."

Gyatso trusts in the power of Tibetan medicines and wants Sowa Rigpa in Nepal to thrive, including – but not limited to – its capacity for medicinal production. His comments not only critique capitalist logic, as revealed through the relationship between packaging, marketing, and pricing, but also illustrate the precarity of the Sowa Rigpa pharmaceutical industry as a whole, as well as the ethical, pharmacological, ecological, and economic concerns about scaling up that he shares, at least in part, with many other *amchi* in today's Nepal.

Conclusion

Nepal's Tibetan medicine industry is firmly rooted within its borders but is also profoundly shaped by flows of people, ideas, and materials that extend beyond them. The predominant clinic+pharmacy model forms part of a transnational industry yet illuminates aspects – multi-species entanglements, forms of precarity, notions of quality and integrity – that are not easily visible from the more economically or politically powerful nodes of this assemblage. Nepal's physician-pharmacists are well aware that large, profit-oriented factories and biomedically derived notions of quality and efficacy are increasingly dominant in neighbouring countries. They are influenced by these trends and some want to move in a similar direction. Yet scaling up faces severe material limitations in Nepal, as well as critique from within the *amchi* community. In this sense, our ethnography illustrates the points made by Gibson-Graham (2006) with respect to the ways that many forms of production can persist alongside, or at times resist, capitalist accumulation. It also points to the ways that multi-species entanglements can help to make sense of, if not check, the possibilities for making good medicine within conditions of precarity brought on, at least in part, by these self-same dynamics of capital (Tsing 2015).

Although *amchi* pharmacists in Kathmandu invest in production and make their livelihoods from it, they do not think or operate strictly as capitalists, and in many ways, actively resist (in discourse and practice) the elevation of profit, growth, and market share over embedded, ethical imaginary notions of quality, tradition, lineage, compassion, and service. As such, while Tsing's concept of "salvage accumulation" works for the large factories in the PRC, which draw resources from non-capitalist formations into their capitalist supply chains, such an argument does not work so well in Nepal. Instead, it remains important for Nepali *amchi* that links between source, producer, product, physician, and patient are kept as close as possible. Nepal's *amchi* are aware that these connections have been compromised elsewhere (Kloos 2017b:713), and their discourses and practices emerge in part from this awareness. In fact, we argue that they often leverage such connections as a conscious counterpoint to industrialisation and commodification as part of a strategy for maintaining aspects of medicine making and not only as an excuse for not being "developed" enough.

Conversations with Nepal's *amchi* reveal that many are thinking about these questions and are attuned to the stakes involved. Some are considering models of cooperative pharmacy production, connected with efforts to link conservation, cultivation, production, and supply across Nepal's different ecological zones. This cooperative model could present, if not an "anti-capitalist" framework, then at least an engagement that recognises more overtly both the points of precarity within the Sowa Rigpa pharmaceutical assemblage and the multi-species entanglements through which it is created. The possibility of such a cooperative model – reflecting a particular sociotechnical imaginary – would necessitate new forms of trust – new ethical imaginaries – between Nepal's *amchi* and, most likely, increased engagement with state regulatory agencies. Unlike India or China, Nepal remains a precarious political state, and Sowa Rigpa itself is officially and legally precarious within this context. The resources from which Tibetan medicines are made are also increasingly precarious, largely due to the scaling up of production elsewhere. Kathmandu's *amchi*-pharmacists live within these various forms of precarity and negotiate through them on a daily basis. Their production of medicines reflects these circumstances.

As medicines move and change, they constitute shifting multi-species entanglements that vary widely in their meaning, significance, and perceived attributes, but which are not reducible to "market transactions," "commodity chains," or "industrial processes," although these have been the primary focus of much conventional analysis of the Himalayan medicinal plant trade (Olsen and Bhattarai 2005; Kala et al. 2006) and Asian traditional medicine industries (Bode 2008; Banerjee 2009; Pordié and Gaudillière 2014). Multi-species work is "attuned to life's emergence within a shifting assemblage of agentive beings" (Ogden et al. 2013: 6). Just as the question of what makes for efficacious medicine is dictated not only by the embodied skill of producers but also by the innate potencies of ingredients themselves and the circumstances of their harvest and transit, multiple pathways coexist to give meaning and value to these formulas and the modes of production which underlie them (Blaikie et al. 2015).

Given such conditions, we argue that it is inappropriate to view Nepal's clinic+pharmacy mode of production as a transitory, proto-industrial form that will inevitably morph into industry proper, or to present such a trajectory as inherently desirable for those involved. Indeed, Kunphen's relationship with the Nyalam factory and Shechen's adoption of certain features of industrial production and rejection of others show the inaccuracy of such a view. Instead, Tibetan medicine production in Nepal can be seen as a sophisticated, adaptive response to the absence of state pressure, support, and regulation and the uncertainties this produces; to limited marketing and investment conditions; to Sowa Rigpa's historically marginal but growing presence within Nepal's healthcare milieu; and to Nepal's position at the margins of Asia's booming traditional medicine industry.

The clinic+pharmacy model represents a distinctive "alternative modernity" (Gaonkar 2001) that has allowed for growth, but that still privileges discourses of potency, quality, and efficacy linked to artisanal production, embedded in lineages and localised social ecologies. Despite the seemingly inexorable rise of industrial Tibetan medicine production across much of the tradition's geographical range, cottage industry production continues vibrantly in some Tibetan regions of China, in Himalayan India and in the Tibetan exile communities based around Dharamsala. The situation in Nepal is different from these other regions in many ways, as we have shown, but at the same time serves as an exemplar. It makes crucial aspects of the tensions and debates surrounding the scaling up of medicine production visible and comparable without losing sight of historical, social, and spatial specificities. Through its emergent and contingent nature, its multiplicity, its shifting yet somewhat stable and distinct fields, the Nepal case also makes an important contribution to the assemblage concept. The pharmaceutical assemblage comes into focus in particular ways when we see Nepali *amchi* borrowing from and adapting elements of mass production (stock control systems, paid labourers, grinding and pill-making machines, internet advertising, etc.) but not others (impersonal raw material ordering, novel packaging, microwave drying of *materia medica*, large production batches, etc.). In so doing, Nepal's practitioner-pharmacists emulate some aspects of mass production, but curtail their scale of application, while rejecting outright other techniques for reasons that are at once ethical and economic, rooted in particular social-ecological and geopolitical realities. Neither relic nor halfway house, Tibetan medicine production in Nepal is rather a thoughtful and effective approach that is very much part of the emergent pharmaceutical assemblage of transnational Sowa Rigpa. In fact, the particular forms of hybridity maintained in Nepal – a dynamic bricolage in a situation of great precarity – makes it a crucial site, both for the future of Sowa Rigpa and for the advancement of scholarly understanding of Asian medical industries.

Acknowledgements

Both authors would like to thank all of the *amchi* whose knowledge contributed to this chapter. Blaikie acknowledges the European Research Council funded *Reassembling Tibetan Medicine* project (ERC 336932) based at the

Institute for Social Anthropology, Austrian Academy of Sciences for supporting this research. Craig acknowledges the Claire Garber Goodman Fund for Anthropological Research, Department of Anthropology, Dartmouth College for sustained support of research related to Sowa Rigpa in Nepal and Tibetan regions of China over many years, including in ways that contributed to this chapter.

Bibliography

Adams V (2001) The Sacred in the Scientific: Ambiguous Practices of Science in Tibetan Medicine. *Cultural Anthropology* 16(4): 542–575.

Adams V (2002) Randomized Controlled Crime: Postcolonial Sciences in Alternative Medicine Research. *Social Studies of Science* 32(5–6): 659–690.

Adams V, Schrempf M and Craig S (eds) (2011) *Medicine between Science and Religion: Explorations on Tibetan Grounds*. Oxford: Berghahn Books.

Banerjee M (2009) *Power, Knowledge, Medicine: Ayurvedic Pharmaceuticals at Home and in the World*. Hyderabad: Orient Blackswan.

Blaikie C (2011) Critically endangered? Medicinal plant cultivation and the reconfiguration of Sowa Rigpa in Ladakh. *Asian Medicine* 5: 243–272.

Blaikie C (2013) *Making Medicine: Materia medica, Pharmacy and the Production of Sowa Rigpa in Ladakh*. PhD Dissertation, University of Kent.

Blaikie C (2016) Positioning Sowa Rigpa in India: Coalition and Antagonism in the Quest for Recognition. *Medicine, Anthropology and Theory* 3(2): 50–86.

Blaikie C (2018) Absence, Abundance and Excess: Substances and Sowa Rigpa in Ladakh since the 1960s. In: Deb Roy R and Attewell G (eds) *Locating the Medical: Explorations in South Asian History*. New Delhi: Oxford University Press, pp. 169–199.

Blaikie C, Craig S, Gerke B and Hofer T (2015) Co-producing Efficacious Medicines: Collaborative Ethnography with Tibetan Medicine Practitioners in Kathmandu, Nepal. *Current Anthropology* 56(2): 178–204.

Bode M (2008) *Taking Traditional Knowledge to the Market: The Modern Image of the Ayurvedic and Unani Industry*. Hyderabad: Orient Blackswan.

Cameron M (2008) Modern Desires, Knowledge Control, and Physician Resistance: Regulating Ayurveda Medicine in Nepal. *Asian Medicine* 4: 86–112.

Cameron M (2009) Untouchable Healing: A Dalit Ayurvedic Doctor from Nepal Suffers his Country's Ills. *Medical Anthropology* 28(3): 235–267.

Cameron M (2010) Feminization and Marginalization? Women Ayurvedic Doctors and Modernizing Health Care in Nepal. *Medical Anthropology Quarterly* 24(1): 42–63.

Collier S and Ong A (eds) (2005) *Global Assemblages: Technology, Politics and Ethics as Anthropological Problems*. Malden, MA: Blackwell.

Craig SR (2008) Place and Professionalization: Navigating *amchi* Identity in Nepal. In: Pordié L (ed) *Tibetan Medicine in the Contemporary World: Global Politics of Medical Knowledge and Practice*. Abingdon: Routledge, pp. 62–90.

Craig SR (2012) *Healing Elements: Efficacy and the Social Ecologies of Tibetan Medicine*. Berkeley, CA: University of California Press.

Craig SR and Adams V (2008) Global Pharma in the Land of Snows: Tibetan Medicines, SARS, and Identity Politics across Nations. *Asian Medicine* 4: 1–28.

Craig SR and Gerke B (2016) Naming and Forgetting: Sowa Rigpa and the Territory of Asian Medical Systems. *Medicine, Anthropology, Theory* 3(2): 87–122.

DeLanda, M (2006) *A New Philosophy of Society: Assemblage Theory and Social Complexity*. New York, NY: Continuum Books.

Deleuze G and Guattari F (1987) *A Thousand Plateaus*. Minneapolis, MN: University of Minnesota Press.

Fassin D (2014) The Ethical Turn in Anthropology: Promises and Uncertainties. *Journal of Ethnographic Theory* 4(1): 429–435.

Gaonkar D (ed) (2001) *Alternative Modernities*. Durham: Duke University Press.

Gerke B (2013) The Social Life of Tsotel. *Asian Medicine* 8(1): 120–152.

Gerke B (2015) Moving from Efficacy to Safety: A Changing Focus in the Study of Asian Medical System. *Journal of the Anthropological Society of Oxford* 7(3): 370–384.

Gerke B (2017) Tibetan Precious Pills as Therapeutics and Rejuvenating Longevity Tonics. *History of Science in South Asia* 5(2): 204–233.

Gerke B, Craig SR and Sheldon V (2019) Sowa Rigpa Humanitarianism: Local Logics of Care within a Global Politics of Compassion. *Medical Anthropology Quarterly* 34(2): 174–191.

Ghimire S, Bista G, Lama NS et al. (eds) (2021) *"Without Plants, We Have No Medicine": Sowa Rigpa, Ethnobotany, and Conservation of Threatened Species in Nepal*. Kathmandu: World Wildlife Fund.

Gibson-Graham JK (2006) *A Postcapitalist Politics*. Minneapolis, MN: University of Minnesota Press.

Hofer T (2008a) Socio-economic Dimensions of Tibetan Medicine in the Tibet Autonomous Region, China (Part One). *Asian Medicine* 4: 174–200.

Hofer T (2008b) Socio-economic Dimensions of Tibetan Medicine in the Tibet Autonomous Region, China (Part Two). *Asian Medicine* 4: 492–514.

Hofer T (2018) *Medicine and Memory in Tibet: Amchi Physicians in an Age of Reform*. Seattle: University of Washington Press.

Janes C (2001) Tibetan Medicine at the Crossroads: Radical Modernity and Social Organization of Traditional Medicine in the Tibet Autonomous Region, China. In: Connor L and Samuel G(eds), *Healing Powers and Modernity: Traditional Medicine, Shamanism, and Science in Asian Societies*. Westport, CT: Bergin & Garvey.

Janes C (2002) Buddhism, Science, and Market: The Globalization of Tibetan Medicine. *Anthropology and Medicine* 9(3): 267–289.

Kala C, Dhyani P and Sajwan B (2006) Developing the Medicinal Plants Sector in Northern India: Challenges and Opportunities. *Journal of Ethnobiology and Ethnomedicine* 2: 32.

Kloos S (2016) The Recognition of Sowa Rigpa in India: How Tibetan Medicine Became an Indian Medical System. *Medicine, Anthropology, Theory* 3(2): 19–49.

Kloos S (2017a) The Politics of Preservation and Loss: Tibetan Medical Knowledge in Exile. *East Asian Science, Technology and Society (EASTS)* 11(2): 135–159.

Kloos S (2017b) The Pharmaceutical Assemblage: Rethinking Sowa Rigpa and the Herbal Pharmaceutical Industry in Asia. *Current Anthropology* 58(6): 693–717.

Kloos S (2020) Humanitarianism from Below. Sowa Rigpa, the Traditional Pharmaceutical Industry, and Global Health. *Medical Anthropology* 39(2): 167–181.

Kloos S, Madhavan H, Tidwell T et al. (2020) The Transnational Sowa Rigpa Industry in Asia: New Perspectives on an Emerging Economy. *Social Science & Medicine* 245 (112617).

McKay A and Wangchuk D (2005) Traditional Medicine in Bhutan. *Asian Medicine* 1(1): 204–218.

Muehlebach A (2013) On Precariousness and the Ethical Imagination: The year 2012 in Sociocultural Anthropology. *American Anthropologist* 115(2): 297–311.

Ogden L, Hall B and Tanita K (2013) Animals, Plants, People, and Things: A Review of Multispecies Ethnography. *Environment and Society: Advances in Research* 4: 5–24.

Olsen C and Bhattarai N (2005) A Typology of Economic Agents in the Himalayan Plant Trade. *Mountain Research and Development* 25(1): 37–43.

Petryna A, Lakoff A and Kleinman A (eds) (2006) *Global Pharmaceuticals: Ethics, Markets and Practices*. London: Duke University Press.

Pigg SL (1992) Inventing Social Categories through Place: Social Representations and Development in Nepal. *Comparative Studies in History and Society* 34(3): 491–513.

Pigg SL (1996) The Credible and the Credulous: The Question of 'Villagers' Beliefs' in Nepal. *Cultural Anthropology* 11(2): 160–201.

Pordié L (2008) Tibetan Medicine Today: Neo-traditionalism as an Analytical Lens and a Political Tool. In: Pordié L (ed) *Tibetan Medicine in the Contemporary World: Global Politics of Medical Knowledge and Practice*. Abingdon: Routledge, pp. 3–33.

Pordié L and Gaudillière JP (2014) The Reformulation Regime in Drug Discovery: Revisiting Polyherbals and Property Rights in the Ayurvedic Industry. *East Asian Science, Technology and Society* 8: 57–79.

Pordié L and Kloos S (eds) (2022) *Healing at the Periphery: Ethnographies of Tibetan Medicine in India*. Durham: Duke University Press.

Prost A (2009) *Precious Pills: Medicine and Social Change among Tibetan Refugees in India*. Oxford: Berghahn Books.

Sassen S (2008) Neither Global nor National: Novel Assemblages of Territory, Authority, and Rights. *Ethics & Global Politics* 1(1–2): 61–79.

Saxer M (2013) *Manufacturing Tibetan Medicine: The Creation of an Industry and the Moral Economy of Tibetanness*. Oxford: Berghahn Books.

Schrempf M (2015) Contested Issues of Efficacy and Safety between Transnational Formulation Regimes of Tibetan Medicines in China and Europe. *Asian Medicine: Tradition and Modernity* 10: 273–315.

Stewart K (2012) Precarity's Forms. *Cultural Anthropology* 27(3): 518–525.

Subedi B (2006) *Linking Plant-Based Enterprises and Local Communities to Biodiversity Conservation in Nepal Himalaya*. New Delhi: Adroit.

Subedi M (2018) *State, Society, and Health in Nepal*. New Delhi: Routledge.

Taee J (2017) *The Patient Multiple: An Ethnography of Healthcare and Decision-Making in Bhutan*. New York, NY: Berghahn Books.

Tsing A (2015) *The Mushroom at the End of the World: On the Possibility of Life in Capitalist Ruins*. Princeton, NJ: Princeton University Press.

Van der Geest S (2006) Anthropology and the Pharmaceutical Nexus. *Anthropological Quarterly* 79: 303–214.

Wangchuk P, Pyne S and Keller P (2013) An Assessment of the Bhutanese Traditional Medicine for its Ethnopharmacology, Ethnobotany and Ethnoquality: Textual Understanding and the Current Practices. *Journal of Ethnopharmacology* 148(1): 305–310.

West P (2012) *From Modern Production to Imagined Primitive: The Social World of Coffee in Papua New Guinea*. Durham, NC: Duke University Press.

10 The emergence of the Traditional Mongolian Medicine industry
Communism, continuity, and reassemblage

Stephan Kloos

Traditional Mongolian Medicine (henceforth "TMM")[1] constitutes an important part of Asia's Sowa Rigpa industry today and participates in the large-scale phenomenon of Asian medical industries more generally. Sowa Rigpa is the Tibetan term for "science of healing," and commonly used by scholars to refer to the family of Tibetan, Mongolian, and Himalayan medical traditions based on a singular corpus of classical Tibetan texts and the ethical and epistemological foundation of Tibetan Buddhism. TMM is prevalent in all Asian areas with populations of Mongolian descent or influence, such as Mongolia, parts of China (especially Inner Mongolia), and Russia (Buryatia, Tuva, Kalmykia), and more recently also in the global Mongolian diaspora including, most notably in terms of practitioner numbers, Poland. While in Russia, Sowa Rigpa is called "Tibetan" rather than "Mongolian" medicine and is not properly recognised or industrially developed, TMM is fully integrated into Mongolia's national health system and officially counts as China's third-largest "minority medicine" in terms of economic value. Thus, TMM accounted for 166 million USD or about 25 percent of the total sales value of the transnational Sowa Rigpa pharmaceutical industry in 2017, of which 162 million USD were generated in China and about 4 million USD in Mongolia (Kloos et al. 2020). Even at a superficial glance, then, it is clear that TMM constitutes a significant part of Sowa Rigpa today and that China dominates TMM at least in economic terms. Yet, these observations are neither reflected in the growing scholarly literature on Sowa Rigpa generally, which tends to focus on Tibetan and Himalayan medicine, nor in the scant body of work on Mongolian medicine specifically, which tends to ignore China. This chapter addresses these gaps by tracing the reassemblage of Mongolian medicine during the twentieth century and examining

---

1 Both in Mongolia and in most scholarly literature on the topic, the term "Traditional Mongolian Medicine" is used in English. Although problematic on several levels, it is the product of – and reflects – the historical processes and ethnographic reality described in this chapter. Although, as described below, the term only emerged during the 1950s, for simplicity's sake, it is used here for the Mongolian branch of Sowa Rigpa both before and after the 1950s.

DOI: 10.4324/9781003218074-14

its emergence as an industry in the twenty-first century in both Mongolia and China.

Although TMM's "Mongolian" identity is rarely questioned, it is actually a relatively recent phenomenon. Until at least the middle of the twentieth century, what is now called "Mongolian medicine" (*Mongol anagaakh ukhaan*) was referred to by Mongolians as *"tuvd emneleg"* (Tibetan medicine) or *"lameen emneleg"* (Lama medicine). Indeed, Tibetan medicine constituted Mongolia's sole professional health resource since the seventeenth century, when it was institutionalised there along with the Gelugpa monastic order as part of the Fifth Dalai Lama's expansion of Central Tibetan hegemony. Between 1662 and 1937, over 100 Tibetan medical schools (*manba datsan*) were established in Inner and Outer Mongolia (Ganbayar and Tumurbaatar 2007), and Mongolian doctors wrote over 230 medical texts in the Tibetan language (Bold 2013: 190), some of them becoming part of the wider Tibetan medical canon. Despite adaptations to the Mongolian climatic, ecological, and social context, and the integration of elements of pre- or non-Buddhist medical traditions (Mongolian, Indian, Chinese), Mongolians essentially practiced a variant of Tibetan medicine. How, then, did this regional branch of Tibetan medicine become "Traditional Mongolian Medicine," and how did it subsequently turn into a modern industry? How did an institution that asserted Tibet's hegemonic power over Mongolia transform into a symbol of a separate national identity and finally into an economic resource competing for market shares? In order to trace this remarkable reassemblage, it is necessary to take a wider perspective, expanding the limited historical, geographic, and conceptual scope of existing literature.

According to the scant English-language literature available on this topic, the most remarkable feature of TMM during this timeframe is its discontinuity. Thus, many Western scholars speak of a "revival" of TMM after Mongolia's democratic reforms of 1990, framing communism as a near-death experience (e.g. Gerke 2004; Kletter et al. 2008; Pitschmann et al. 2013), while others go even further, assuming that there was little left to be revived and thus regarding post-communist TMM as a new "invention" (Janes and Hilliard 2008). Counterbalancing such tropes of radical discontinuity and the narrow focus on Mongolia, I suggest that a more productive way of understanding contemporary TMM is to focus on its *continuity* (cf. Scheid 2002). I argue that rather than being completely interrupted or destroyed by a monolithic spectre of communism, TMM – like Buddhism or shamanism (Humphrey 1983; Shimamura 2019) – was actually reassembled in various ways in different locales, which together facilitated its contemporary commercialisation, industrialisation, and gradual alignment with global health (Kloos 2020). Given the undeniable historical ruptures of the twentieth century – the Stalinist purges in Mongolia, the Cultural Revolution in China, and the large-scale introduction of biomedicine being only the most prominent ones – and their profound impact on Asia's medical traditions, then, Sowa Rigpa's outstanding feature is its continuity. Rather than simply a historical achievement, this continuity needs to be understood as an ongoing process that requires constant efforts and adjustments to be secured, whether in the context of communism or neoliberal market reforms.

At the forefront of such contemporary efforts and in marked contrast to foreign scholarship, Mongolian literature on TMM strongly emphasises historical continuity, albeit across much larger timeframes. For example, Mongolian academician Bold Sharav (2013) covers 5000 years of medical history in his book *The History and Development of Traditional Mongolian Medicine*, and renowned Inner Mongolian scholar B. Jigmed traces TMM back to well before the twelfth century CE (Jigmed 1981; Wang and Bao 2017). However, the focus of these historiographies lies on the more distant past, and their scholarly strength and details diminish the closer they approach the present. In short, Mongolian medical historiography only partially fills the gap left by foreign scholarship as far as TMM's development over the last century is concerned. Furthermore, while not sharing the discontinuity bias of English-language literature, it tends to have a strong nationalist bias that equally requires critical scrutiny. Thus, such longue-durée historical narratives suggest both implicitly and explicitly that TMM existed long before Tibetan influence in Mongolia and is therefore originally Mongolian. While foreign influences are generally acknowledged, many Mongolian doctors and scholars systematically highlight TMM's Indian origins (e.g. Ganbayar and Tumurbaatar 2007), thereby reducing Tibet to a mere stopover on the path of medical knowledge from India to Mongolia. Yet despite archaeological findings from the Neolithic, indicating practices like bloodletting, piercing, acupuncture, and trepanation (skull drilling) (Bold 2013: 34–43); pre-Buddhist written sources describing shamanism, herbalism, and various Dhom therapies; as well as a pre-Tibetan influx of Indian medical scriptures, there is no evidence for an *institutionalised, systematic and codified* medical tradition in Mongolia before the introduction of Tibetan medicine.

Without denying the existence of various medical practices among (proto-)Mongolian people, then, TMM as we know it today clearly belongs to the Sowa Rigpa family. As such, this chapter traces its so-far understudied development and transformation from the beginning of the communist era in Mongolia in the 1920s through the democratic reforms and economic liberalisation of the 1990s and into the present day, offering a critical history of the Sowa Rigpa industry in Mongolia and Inner Mongolia. I argue that contemporary TMM and its industry are best understood in terms of a pharmaceutical assemblage (Kloos 2017), shaped by various processes of de- and reterritorialisation, and the coming together of seemingly incompatible elements such as Buddhism, communism, "traditional" medicine, and "modern" science. Using ethnographic data and policy documents collected in Mongolia, the Inner Mongolia Autonomous Region, and Liaoning province between 2014 and 2018, I specifically highlight the important yet ambivalent roles played by the Mongolian and Chinese governments in the emergence of a TMM industry. This chapter is thus structured in three parts. The first outlines the transformation of TMM during communist times, the second traces the policy developments of the 1990s and 2000s that enabled its industrialisation, and the third offers ethnographic insights into the TMM industry today. I conclude with a summary of TMM's trajectory since the early twentieth century, a discussion of the influence of government policies on its development as an industry, and reflections on its configuration as a pharmaceutical assemblage. While necessarily providing only a brief overview of multiple and complex histories, this chapter aims to contribute to a bigger picture of contemporary Sowa Rigpa and its historical development, and lay a solid foundation for further, more specialised research into Mongolian medicine.

Continuity under communism

Mongolia

The establishment of Tibetan medicine in Mongolia coincided with the fall of the Mongol Yuan dynasty in China and the general demise of Mongol power in Asia. In the late seventeenth century, both Outer and Inner Mongolia became part of the Manchu Qing Empire, where they would remain for more than 200 years until its collapse. In 1911, Outer Mongolia claimed independence (Tibet following suit in 1912), while Inner Mongolia, which had been subject to much stronger Chinese influence and control, became part of the newly established Republic of China. While Tibet enjoyed its regained independence relatively undisturbed until 1950, Outer Mongolia became a site of conflict between Mongolian nationalist, Chinese, White Russian, and Bolshevik agendas, until the Mongolian revolution of 1921 ended this tumultuous period with the establishment of an autonomous Mongolian government, closely aligned with the Soviet Union. In the same year, Mongolia's first hospital (the Central Army Hospital) opened, employing one Hungarian and ten lama doctors, and in 1923, the country's first drug store began selling both European and Tibetan medicines (Bold 2013: 218–223). In 1924, after the death of Mongolia's nominal ruler, the *Bogd Khan* Jebtsundamba Khutugtu, the Mongolian People's Republic was established, through which the Soviet Union forcefully installed a communist regime in Mongolia. New biomedical institutions were founded, such as the first more advanced Western-style hospital in 1925 (still also employing lama doctors) and the first biomedical college in 1934, while successive waves of collectivisation, land expropriation and violent political purges placed Tibetan medicine – strongly linked to the Buddhist monastic system – under increasing pressure. In the first major repression in 1933–1934, many lama doctors were arrested, and on 13 March 1937 the Revolutionary Party passed a resolution encouraging the further development of "scientific medicine," as "traditional medicine ... had the potential to become a weapon in the lamas' hands to strengthen religious influence" (quoted in Bold 2013: 223). Shortly thereafter, the 1937–1938 Stalinist purges began. Over 18,000 lamas and thousands of intellectuals, government officials, Buryats, and Kazakhs were executed, and 746 (i.e. almost all) monasteries were destroyed (Sandag and Kendall 1999). Almost as an afterthought, in April 1938, the sale of Tibetan medicine was officially banned (Bold 2013: 223), but by that time, both Tibetan medicine and Buddhism had ceased to exist in Mongolia as institutions.

Yet Tibetan medicine did not completely disappear in Mongolia in 1938. The lama doctors who had received ten-year prison sentences during the 1933–1934 repression not only survived the second, deadlier purge but in some cases were even asked to treat high communist officials from their prison cells. Upon their release in the 1940s, some of them secretly continued their practice and even taught small numbers of students, as did others who had managed to hide in the remote countryside (Banzragch and Gerke 2002). As *Khamba Lama* Damdinsuren Natsagdorj, the founder of the largest private TMM hospital in the country today, told me, "People think that during communism, all of Mongolian medicine was destroyed. But that's not true, only the government thought so. Actually, not even the government ... there were very good old lamas who kept the lineage alive." The names of some of these lamas are listed by Munkh-Amgalan and Tsend-Ayush (2002: 41) and Bold (2013: 224). Indeed, not only did communist officials continue to seek treatment from traditional doctors even after persecuting them but, as old officials and doctors told me, later on they also supplied them with imported *materia medica* to produce medicines that would have been otherwise unavailable. As in Tibet during the Cultural Revolution, it was the perceived clinical efficacy of such medicines – in many cases far superior to the biomedical care available at the time – that prevailed over political ideology.

By the late 1940s and early 1950s, the reputation of TMM was such that Anastasia Filatova, the Russian wife of Mongolian General Secretary Yumjaagiin Tsedenbal, sent a Mongolian *emchi* (practitioner of TMM) to Moscow in order to treat the Russian war hero and previous Chief of Staff of the Soviet Army, Georgy Konstantinovich Zhukov. Marshal Zhukov had commanded the First Soviet-Mongolian Army Group against Japan in 1938–1939, where he not only developed battle maneuvers that he later effectively employed against the Nazis in World War Two but presumably also came in contact with Mongolian lama doctors who had been forced to disrobe and join the army during the purges. While we do not have exact details about this, it appears that Marshal Zhukov remembered the efficacy of TMM when biomedicine failed to improve his condition after a heart attack in 1948 and specifically requested the services of a Mongolian *emchi*. We neither know this *emchi*'s name nor the exact year of his visit to Moscow (mid to late 1950s), but the outcome of his trip suggests that the treatment was successful. Not only did Marshal Zhukov continue to resort to TMM for the rest of his life – albeit through the more easily available Buryat practitioner Lenkhoboev[2] – but news about this also significantly improved its legitimacy, setting in motion developments that would shape TMM in Mongolia until today.

Upon the suggestion of Filatova and with the active support of Tsedenbal, a pharmacology laboratory was founded in 1959 at the Institute of Biology of the Mongolian Academy of Sciences in order to conduct scientific research on the history and pharmacology of TMM (Mongolian Ministry of Health 2012: 33; Bold 2013: 231). In 1973, this laboratory was upgraded to the "Institute for Natural Products Chemistry and Pharmacology" and supplied with high-end instruments from Germany as well as extraordinary staff salaries, with the aim of developing standardised recipes and technological methods (Munkh-Amgalan and Tsend-Ayush 2002: 40) for producing medicines in its "Manufactory of Traditional Medicine" (Pitschmann et al. 2013: 946).[3] In a further upgrade, the Institute for Natural Products was transferred to the Ministry of Health and reorganised as an "Institute of Folk [or People's] Medicine" in 1981. While the Manufactory of Traditional Medicine was the first factory producing multi-compound Mongolian medicines in Mongolia, an unrelated "Herbal Company" had already been established in 1968, cultivating and selling crude Mongolian medicinal herbs to China, North Korea, and domestic Mongolian doctors who secretly manufactured their own medicines. In 1990, that company also began producing Mongolian medicines according to classical recipes and accordingly changed its name to "Traditional Medicine and Herb Company." However, it was the Institute of Natural Products/Folk Medicine and its Manufactory as the only official institution for Mongolian medicine until the 1990 Democratic Revolution that served as the foundation for much of TMM's post-socialist development in Mongolia. In 1996, the institute was expanded into a "Traditional Hospital Health Science Centre." It then became the "Traditional Medical Science, Technology and Production Corporation" (short: "Corporation") in 1998 and was renamed in 2015 as the "Institute of Traditional Medicine and

---

2   See Sablin (2019: 102), who provides a detailed account of Tibetan/Mongolian medicine in the Soviet Union.
3   The account given here is based on original Mongolian government documents and corroborated by information from the website of the Institute of Traditional Medicine and Technology of Mongolia (www.sci-tradmed.mn). I am grateful to D. Gunbilig for his help and recollections regarding this. However, there exist partly conflicting published accounts regarding the history of this institution. According to Bold (2013: 238), research on Mongolian medicine already began in 1950, and a "Traditional Medical Institute" was established only in 1976 (Bold 2013: 231). Munkh-Amgalan and Tsend-Ayush (2002: 41) call the 1959 institution a "Medical Studies Laboratory," while a survey report published by the Mongolian Ministry of Health (2012: 33) calls it "Drug Research Laboratory." The same report mentions that it was expanded as a "Natural Science Institute" in 1973 and an "Academy for Traditional Medicine" in 1980.

Technology." It remains the only government-owned and operated research and production center for TMM today.

The central figure in these developments was academician Tsend Haidav, the director and driving force of the pharmacology laboratory and its successor institutes from 1959 until 1990. A pharmacologist with additional training in phytochemistry, Haidav pioneered modern scientific research on Mongolian medicinal plants and texts, laying the foundations for modern TMM in Mongolia under very difficult political conditions.[4] Between 1960 and 2009, he published over 200 research articles and monographs on "Mongolian folk medicine" or simply "Mongolian medicine" (e.g. Haidav et al. 1962; Haidav and Zakrividoroga 1965; Haidav 1975, 1977), thereby not only providing a scientific basis to what communism had hitherto dismissed as superstitious, feudalist and unscientific but also giving it its contemporary identity as "Mongolian medicine." Despite uneasy and heavily restricted relations between Mongolia and China, this mirrored and was no doubt influenced by developments in Inner Mongolia, where official attempts to modernise and integrate ethnic medicine into the regional health care system began in the late 1950s, culminating in China's official recognition of "Mongolian medicine" as distinct from Tibetan or "lama" medicine in 1962 (Saijirahu 2007).

Haidav was neither a doctor nor a pure scholar but was rather driven by the practical desire to formulate new medicines based on traditional Mongolian *materia medica*, as well as to develop the necessary standards and technologies to mass-produce them. Indeed, during his career, he "discovered" and developed over 100 high-value herbal pharmaceutical compounds, most of them based on TMM (see e.g. Haidav et al. 1985).[5] While this makes him the founding father of Mongolia's modern TMM industry, it also placed him in a controversial position among Mongolia's TMM practitioners. One major criticism was that Haidav never took Mongolian medical knowledge seriously, approaching it not as an authoritative science and epistemology but simply as a resource for scientific-commercial bioprospecting. To some extent, this attitude lives on in his former students, some of whom now hold powerful positions and contribute to contemporary government policies, although it is met with strong resistance from other quarters of the Mongolian TMM community. Even so, Haidav could not have accomplished what he did without the cooperation of old *emchi* (Munkh-Amgalan and Tsend-Ayush

---

[4] For more biographical information on Haidav (in Mongolian), see www.sci-tradmed.mn (About Us, Our Pride-Directors).

[5] These compounds were available in pharmacies already well before 1990, sold under trade names such as Barbadin, Arjiremyn, Dendroniside, Altan Utas ("golden strings"), or Tameta-3. Although based on TMM pharmacopoeia, most of them were not classical TMM formulations but newly developed products.

2002), who had managed to preserve medical texts, instruments, and practical knowledge despite communist persecution.[6] Not surprisingly, however, given Haidav's above-mentioned attitude as well as his failure to acknowledge their contributions in his publications, many of these practitioners remained suspicious of Haidav. As one former communist official told me: "I feel sorry now that whenever I heard about a good *emchi*, I referred him to Haidav. There was always a misunderstanding, because Haidav never took Mongolian medicine seriously, he had a very different worldview. All the doctors went away disappointed after meeting him." Some witnesses even recall that Haidav was in contact with the KGB and denounced doctors who were reluctant to work with him in order to have their old texts confiscated. If discontent with all this could not be openly voiced under communism, it broke out during the first conference on TMM in post-communist Mongolia in 1991. Haidav was verbally attacked by old practitioners who saw themselves and their expertise sidelined even after the democratic reforms and TMM's official rehabilitation. More than a voicing of old grievances, this was a power struggle over who would control the newly legitimate TMM profession and its emerging pharmaceutical industry. Even though the field of TMM has grown larger and more diverse since the early 1990s and is certainly not limited to Haidav's "school," it was Haidav and his students more than the old lama doctors who gave TMM its contemporary form in Mongolia.

Inner Mongolia

Across Mongolia's southern border, Chinese communism similarly reassembled Tibetan medicine in Inner Mongolia and other regions with significant Mongolian populations into a TMM industry, but with important differences. The communist Inner Mongolia Autonomous Region was established in 1947, two years before the People's Republic of China but 23 years after the Mongolian People's Republic. In contrast to Mongolia, TMM in Inner Mongolia remained relatively unaffected by an otherwise tumultuous period between 1911 and 1947, shaped by internal strife, the Japanese invasion, the Chinese civil war, and various Mongolian resistance movements. It was only with the establishment of a communist government in 1947 that the monasteries, which constituted TMM's institutional backbone in the region, were forced to close down. However, although the lama physicians

---

6 In addition to working with old lama physicians who had remained in Mongolia, Haidav also had two monks of partly Tibetan origin repatriated from India. Since they had fled the Mongolian communist government together with Diluwa Khutugtu Jamsrangjab in 1931, this was an extraordinary achievement that testifies to the privileges afforded to Haidav and the importance given to his research on TMM.

had to disrobe and – if young enough – marry, traditional medicine itself was not outlawed, allowing them to continue their medical and pharmaceutical practices privately, and pass on their knowledge to apprentices (often their sons). Official efforts soon began not only to establish a modern biomedical infrastructure but also to reform, modernise, and integrate what was soon called "Mongolian medicine" into the region's health care system. According to Chinese medical historians, the first modern TMM college in China was founded in 1952 in Hohhot (Tao et al. 2017). Then, in 1954, the Inner Mongolia Autonomous Region established a Mongolian-Chinese medicine branch, which expanded into a department in 1956 (IMAR 2015: 27). Such early official initiatives notwithstanding, Inner Mongolian physicians remember the decade between 1947 and 1956/58 as a period of transition, when the old institutional establishment of "lama medicine" had been abolished but not yet replaced by the new institutional infrastructure of "Mongolian medicine."

In many ways, Mongolian medicine's fate in Inner Mongolia was strongly connected to that of Chinese medicine in the rest of mainland China. Initially attacked by the Communist Party, in the mid-1950s Chinese medicine began to be reframed in positive terms as a "legacy of the motherland" and officially recognised as a valid medical system called "Traditional Chinese Medicine" (TCM). A Research Academy for TCM was established in Beijing in December 1955, providing an institutional basis where TCM knowledge was to be standardised into a national curriculum and taught to doctors of Western medicine (Taylor 2005: 84). In Inner Mongolia, this political shift created space for Traditional Mongolian Medicine, or "Mongolian-Chinese Medicine" (often implying a combination of TMM and TCM), to undergo a similar process of recognition, upgrading, and modernisation. In 1957, the first Mongolian-Chinese pharmaceutical company was founded in Hure (the former site of a Tibetan Buddhist monastery, about halfway between Tongliao and Fuxin), with funds provided by high government officials who had been successfully treated by a famous local lama physician. In 1958, TMM began to be officially taught at the Inner Mongolia Medical School in Tongliao (founded in 1956) and the Baotou Medical School, and in 1960 the country's first TMM Research Unit was established in Liaoning (Tao et al. 2017). In these institutions, Tibetan medicine was systematically translated into Mongolian language and script, paving the way for the official recognition of "Mongolian medicine" as a legitimate medical system, distinct from Tibetan or "lama" medicine, on 21 February 1961 (Saijirahu 2007).

The years from 1958 to 1966 thus constituted a more optimistic period of reorganisation and gradual growth. Inner Mongolian biomedical students and doctors were sent to the countryside as village health workers, but also to learn TMM from former lama physicians. The latter, similarly deputed as "barefoot doctors," were also invited to teach in the colleges in the cities. Small district clinics opened in towns, offering rudimentary biomedical care as well as TMM, and hospitals in the bigger cities began to produce and prescribe TMM formulas. TMM physicians also began to publish a corpus of medical case studies, a well-established genre in Chinese medicine (Scheid 2007) but unique in the context of Sowa Rigpa. Although the barefoot doctors' program was expanded after 1965 and became national policy in 1968, the development of TMM was interrupted by the Cultural Revolution (1966–1976). Now it was Inner Mongolia's turn to have its temples and monasteries – which, although closed down, had remained physically intact until then – destroyed, while a large section of the intellectual and cultural elite, including many old TMM physicians, was killed or imprisoned. While research and expansion were impossible, however, even during these difficult times TMM was not completely outlawed, as evidenced by the foundation of the "Mongolian Medicine Company" in 1970 in Fuxin (today: Fuxin Pharmaceuticals Co.), the first official pharmaceutical producer specialised exclusively on TMM in China.

The end of the Cultural Revolution marked the beginning of TMM's modern growth and development phase, which continues in the present day. In contrast to Mongolia, where the impact of communism on TMM was both longer and more severe, the continuity of TMM in Inner Mongolia had never been seriously questioned, even if its reassemblage was similarly radical. Substantial government investment led to the foundation and expansion of TMM institutions, including hospitals, pharmaceutical factories, and colleges. In 1978 alone, for example, research on TMM was officially resumed; the Jelimu Medical College for TMM was founded at the Inner Mongolian National Medical School in Tongliao, later to become the foremost TMM institution in the Inner Mongolian Autonomous Region (IMAR); a TMM hospital was established in Fuxin; and a new production plant was built at the Mongolian Medicine Company in the same city. This gradual resumption of work was coupled with moderate growth from the late 1970s through the mid-1990s, setting the foundation for the emergence of a TMM industry and a much faster pace of development.

The emergence of a TMM industry

In the early 1990s, TMM was well integrated into local and regional public health systems in the Mongolian areas of China, but it was by no means an industry. TMM hospitals and individual practitioners produced their own medicines for direct clinical use, without commercial motives and outside of national pharmaceutical regulations. This began to change in 1992 when China's decision to transition to a "socialist market economy" set in motion TMM's industrialisation. As state subsidies were reduced, TMM hospitals were for the first time confronted with the need to generate income, leading to a gradual expansion and commercialisation of hospital pharmacies into pharmaceutical companies. In 2001, China joined the WTO, which mandated regulatory standards also for the emerging TMM pharmaceutical industry, including the implementation of Good

Manufacturing Practices (GMP) by 2004. Together with the increasing privatisation of hitherto government-owned TMM factories, the introduction of GMP significantly accelerated TMM's industrial development. A major next step was the establishment of a multi-department centralised management structure for the TMM industry, initiated by the IMAR Health Bureau in 2005. As a result, 90 percent of all Inner Mongolian league cities had "Mongolian-Chinese Medicine Bureaus" by 2015 (IMAR 2015). In 2006, the IMAR made the official "Decision to Promote Mongolian-Chinese Medicine Industry Development" that crucially increased financial assistance and salaries, pre-empting similar, subsequent suggestions and policies on the national level (e.g. 17th National Congress 2007, Chinese State Council 2009, 18th National Congress 2012). In another major promotion of the TMM industry in 2013, the IMAR government raised the status and standards of TMM hospitals, banned the reduction of existing TMM facilities, standardised TMM drug processing, included over-the-counter (OTC) TMM drugs into the subsidised category of "basic pharmaceuticals," and lowered the health insurance premium on TMM. If in 2006, 86 TMM hospitals operated in Inner Mongolia (not counting other Mongolian regions of China), by 2015 this number had increased to 122 (IMAR 2015). The 13th Five Year Plan (2016–2020) finally gave equal value to biomedicine and "traditional" medicines including TCM, Tibetan medicine, and TMM, providing yet another boost to the development of these medical industries.

On a much smaller scale and at a slower pace, TMM policy development followed a similar trajectory in post-communist Mongolia. After the peaceful revolution in 1990, Mongolia not only transitioned to democracy and a market economy but, in the words of one TMM practitioner, "suddenly realized that we have a national identity and a traditional medicine." Yet, in contrast to Inner Mongolia, there were no books or experienced teachers, nor any kind of TMM infrastructure. What did exist, still, were oral traditions and a few old texts that a small number of lineage/lama physicians had managed to preserve and, in some cases, pass on to students, as well as Haidav's research centre. While the old physicians and their students began to practice openly and establish clinics in 1990, the main priority was to create official institutions – schools, hospital departments, factories – to build a foundation for modern TMM. Here, Haidav's students and affiliates, already well connected to the Mongolian People's Revolutionary Party (which remained in power until 1996), proved most influential. Haidav was appointed as a government consultant and his research institute became Mongolia's foremost governmental TMM institution, consisting of a drug manufacturing unit, a TMM hospital, and a research center. Also, in 1990, a Traditional Medicine Department was founded at Mongolia's Health Sciences University, with Dr N. Tumurbaatar, a neurologist and acupuncturist with little knowledge of TMM, as its head. The first batch of 24 TMM professionals graduated in

1993, including Dr Tserendagva, the current principal of the International School of Mongolian Medicine, as the oft-renamed Traditional Medicine Department is called since 2016.

TMM's transition in Mongolia into a legitimate part of the country's health care system and later into a small industry is best illustrated by briefly recounting the professional trajectories of four contemporary practitioners. The first account is of Dr Boldsaikhan, head of the Mongolian Association for Traditional Medical Sciences, who represents Haidav's institute and Mongolian state institutions for TMM, but also one of Mongolia's oldest medical lineages. A student at the Health Sciences University of Mongolia in the 1970s, he secretly learned TMM from his father who was a lama physician, and from Otoch Luvsandanzanjantsan (1914–1993), the reincarnation of the founder of Lameen Gegeen monastery and Mongolia's first medical school.[7] Having completed both his official training at university and his unofficial training in TMM, Boldsaikhan joined Haidav's institute in 1980 and in 1990 became head of the research institute on medicinal plants at the Corporation. Later, he also served as the head of the TMM clinic at the Ulaanbaatar Central Hospital Nr. 1, while moving from the Corporation to the System Science Research Center at the Mongolian University for Science and Technology.

Never affiliated to Haidav but also part of the state's medical establishment, Dr Mendsaikhan was the head of the 400-bed Internal Medicine Department of Mongolia's Military Hospital during the communist era. He also secretly studied TMM from old lama doctors since 1984, after he had witnessed them curing diseases that he could not treat with his modern resources. In 1990, he was among the first batch of TMM students to enrol at the Traditional Medicine Department and simultaneously founded Mong-Em, a TMM clinic and drug manufacturer, in an old building of the Military Hospital.[8] "It was difficult to develop Mongolian medicine in the 1990s, because everyone only knew European medicine," he remembers. Still, he persevered, privatised the company in 1996, bought the building with his life savings in 2000, and today runs Mong-Em – comprising a 40-bed hospital, an outpatient clinic, and a TMM factory – together with his wife, daughter, and some 40 staff, while simultaneously serving as director of the State Dermatology Hospital since 2014.

Khamba Lama Natsagdorj, founder and president of Manba Datsan hospital and Otoch Manramba university, recounts that he began to study Buddhism and TMM in 1975 under an old lama named Chatrabal:

---

7   This medical school (*manba datsan*) was established in the 1680s as one of eight colleges of Lameen Gegeen monastery in Bayanzurkh, located in today's Bayankhongor aimag.
8   This 150-year-old Russian building had served as the headquarters of Baron Roman von Ungern-Sternberg during his 5-month stay in Ulaanbaatar (then Urga) in 1921. Due to the building's bad shape and increasingly strict regulations, Mong-Em was forced to demolish this historical building in 2020 and begin construction of a new hospital and factory.

> My teacher did not wear monk's robes, and I of course was no monk then but studied at college. After six years, he gave me permission to treat a few patients and from then on, I practiced medicine secretly. Meanwhile, in 1980 I had ordained as a monk to study at the Mongolian Buddhist University.[9] In 1988, I went to Dharamsala in India to study at the Men-Tsee-Khang. When I came back in 1990, everything had changed. I told my teachers that I wanted to start a Manba Datsan, a TMM school and medical center. They thought it was a good idea, but they were scared. I had no money, so I borrowed money from the government to build Manba Datsan. Such a short time after communism, people had big eyes when they saw me, a monk, going into the government offices to ask for money to build a TMM school! [laughs] But I did it, I founded a small medical center and in 1991, also Otoch Manramba College. All of this was a lot of work.

This was the first private TMM college in Mongolia and has graduated over 500 TMM doctors since then. Today, Manba Datsan operates an 80-bed hospital and a TMM factory, with future plans including new centres in Tuva and Bulgaria, as well as potential joint ventures with Chinese and Taiwanese investors to gain access to these export markets.

If Natsagdorj's brand of TMM is closely aligned with Buddhism, then Dr Baatar emphasises his unbroken medical lineage (*jud*, from Tibetan *rgyud*) of nine generations. A weightlifter and athletic instructor during communism, he suffered an accident in 1980 that left him with chronic health problems. Biomedicine hardly offered any relief, so after six years, he secretly went to an old lama physician, Dorj "Odi" Damdinjav. "He may have been afraid of the communists ...," Dr Baatar remembers. "After checking me, he sent me away with only three doses of medicine. I was disappointed, because I had travelled a long way just to see him, but he told me, 'if this doesn't cure you, I won't be a doctor anymore.' And I was amazed, after only two doses I was completely well again. So I went back to see him again and the same year, I started to learn from him." In 1990, Dr Baatar began to treat patients free of charge and after Dorj's death in 1997, he enrolled in college to get an official medical license. In 2002, he formally established "Otoch Odi" clinic, which soon attracted large numbers of patients, especially those suffering from hepatitis and (liver) cancer, due to Dr Baatar's highly effective lineage recipes. From 2015 onwards, Dr Baatar also founded a medical laboratory, an agricultural company cultivating medicinal plants, a charitable foundation, and a pharmaceutical factory (Oditan) that commercially produces larger quantities of medicines as well as herbal OTC products.

---

9 The Mongolian Buddhist University was established in 1970 at Gandan monastery (Gandantegchinleng Khiid) in Ulaanbaatar, the only major Buddhist monastery in Mongolia that had escaped destruction under communism.

Although brief, these four accounts illustrate some of the diverse strands of contemporary TMM in Mongolia, which complicate simplistic dichotomies such as TMM and biomedicine, Buddhism and communism, old lineages and new institutions. They also share important commonalities. For example, they all reveal a relaxation of restrictions against TMM and Buddhism well before the end of communism, where not only Haidav could openly conduct research on TMM at the Mongolian Academy of Sciences, but also old lama *emchi* could be invited to treat patients at the Military Hospital, and young men could ordain as monks in an official Buddhist University. They all involve personal experiences of TMM's clinical effectiveness, which often constituted a turning point in their personal and professional lives. All of them were also, in different ways, centrally involved in the rehabilitation of TMM, which after more than half a century of communism proved to be a slow and arduous process. While a fundamental understanding and appreciation of TMM may have been lacking among both the general population and officials, the Mongolian government soon began to create a policy and regulation framework for TMM's post-communist development (cf. Mongolian Ministry of Health 2012).

In 1991, the Mongolian Ministry of Health created the position of "Traditional Medicine Specialist," who was charged with drafting the "Main Directions of Development of Traditional Medicine 1991–1995." The second issue of these Main Directions for the period 1996–2000 was drafted and approved five years later, playing a vital role in providing TMM care to the population, especially at the provincial level. Both strategy papers led to the adoption of the "Government Policy on Developing Mongolian Traditional Medicine" in 1999, which provided the first proper legal basis for the development of TMM. This policy included the "Development Agenda 1999–2015," which outlined concrete measures to increase the utilisation of TMM by integrating it into national health services. This was followed in 2001 by a Government Drug Policy that set the regulations for both prescription and OTC herbal medicines. The first official safety requirements for herbal medicines appeared in 2002, subjecting TMM medicines to laboratory tests for bacteria, fungi, and heavy metals. In the same year, the first of three Action Plans to implement the 1999 Policy was approved for the period 2002–2006, while subsequent Plans covered the periods 2006–2010 and 2010–2018. In 2003, an "Encyclopedia for Traditional Medicinal Substances and Prescription Control" was published, with the aim of strengthening quality control regarding 182 substances and 177 traditional formulas. The first General Requirements were instituted for TMM drugs and their manufacture in 2005 (these were updated in 2007 and periodically thereafter), while new State Standards mandated periodic inspections of TMM manufacturers to ensure quality control.

The development of a policy and regulation framework for the industry coincided with that of a professional TMM infrastructure, beginning with the above-mentioned Traditional Medicine Department at the Mongolian

Health Sciences University (1990) and Natsagdorj's TMM College "Otoch Manramba" (1991). After the first domestic conference on TMM in 1991, the First International Symposium on TMM was organised in September 1995 in Ulaanbaatar, bringing together TMM scholars and practitioners not only from Mongolia but also Inner Mongolia, Buryatia, and Tuva. Since then, five more such international conferences have taken place, in Ulaanbaatar (2006, 2016, 2021), in Ulan Ude, Buryatia (2008), and in Hohhot, Inner Mongolia (2012). The fact that four of these six international symposia took place in Ulaanbaatar underscores the Mongolian capital's nodal position in the TMM world. In 1996, the Darkhan City Medical College established a Department for Traditional Medicine to train TMM nurses and in 1999, the Association of TMM Doctors and Researchers was founded in Ulaanbaatar, which over time established branches not only in the city but also across the Mongolian countryside and in Poland. Despite these numerous institutional developments, TMM itself developed only very slowly in Mongolia during the 1990s, having had to start almost from scratch after the end of communism. In the 2000s, industrial development picked up speed, with pharmaceutical production output tripling between 2001 and 2008 (Kloos et al. 2020). TMM's growth also made it a more interesting career option, leading to the foundation of new TMM colleges and college departments. Thus, in 2009 two new departments for TMM opened at the Ach and Etugen private universities; in 2013, the TMM department of Monos Medical University (founded in 2000) split off and became Shine Anagaakh Ukhaan ("New Medicine") College; and in 2014 the private Mongolian National University also established a Department for TMM. With university departments graduating up to 500 TMM professionals a year by 2017, the government introduced a standard TMM curriculum in 2012, about 60 percent of which consists of biomedical subjects.

Between 2010 and 2013, along with the expansion of Mongolia's higher education infrastructure for TMM and a more general economic boom, the TMM pharmaceutical industry underwent rapid growth: in the space of just three years, it more than quadrupled its production volume and value (Kloos et al. 2020). This not only inspired official visions of developing TMM into a profitable export industry but also triggered a new wave of laws and regulations that aimed at least partially at facilitating this development. Thus, in 2014 a new law required all TMM producers to officially register their drugs, a process that was largely completed by 2016. Higher pharmaceutical production standards were also introduced, moving towards full GMP compliance by 2020. In 2017, finally, the first official TMM pharmacopeia, including 80 single herbs and 80 multi-compound formulas, was written by the Corporation and approved by the government.[10] Government initiatives thus combined with considerable

---

10 This pharmacopoeia is based on the Corporation's older manual for TMM doctors, which consists of instructions on which drugs to use for which indications and on recipes provided by Natsagdorj.

individual labour, dedication, and investment to create the necessary policy, regulatory and professional infrastructure for a TMM industry to emerge. Yet despite similar patterns of development in Mongolia and Inner Mongolia, the status quo of TMM north and south of the Gobi differs dramatically.

The TMM industry today

The TMM industry is flourishing in Inner Mongolia and other regions of China with Mongolian populations (notably Liaoning, Jilin, Qinghai, and Xinjiang), generating some 162 million USD in 2017 through pharmaceutical production alone (Kloos et al. 2020). According to official figures (Celimuge et al. 2016), there were 94 TMM inpatient hospitals above township level, 54 licensed pharmaceutical units, and 25 commercial TMM pharmaceutical companies (18 of them in the IMAR) operating in China, not to mention hundreds of private clinics and small pharmaceutical producers. Pharmaceutical companies such as the large Inner Mongolian Mongolian Medicine Co. in Tongliao and the China Mongolian Medicine Factory Center in Hohhot, produce medicines licensed for the regional or national market, according to stringent GMP standards. Licensed pharmaceutical units, on the other hand, are mostly hospital factories that produce exclusively for their own internal hospital use and are required to follow Good Production Practices (GPP), which gives them more freedom to produce medicines according to traditional protocols. Not least for economic reasons, most TMM hospitals operate their own hospital factories, while private practitioners without their own pharmaceutical production rely on more expensive commercial TMM pharmaceuticals. However, there also exist many private practitioners in Inner Mongolia who manufacture and prescribe their own medicines on a small scale according to their own traditional standards, without any government interference.

While many such small manufacturers as well as hospital factories strive to produce the best quality of medicines possible and make efforts to source their raw materials from clean sources in remote Inner Mongolian areas or even Qinghai, commercial factories often use cheap, cultivated herbs and substitute ingredients that are expensive or hard to source. Like substitutes, cultivated herbs are widely considered to have weaker potency and are prone to contamination with pesticides (cf. Wu 2015). Furthermore, large parts of Inner Mongolia are heavily affected by environmental pollution, compromising the quality of both wildcrafted and cultivated herbs. Producers in Mongolia refer to such concerns to highlight the superior quality of their own unpolluted, wildcrafted medicines, but Inner Mongolian practitioners also admit to this problem. One doctor in Tongliao, who ran a private clinic where he sold both Mongolian and Tibetan medicines, told me: "There is a big difference between Tibetan and Mongolian medicines. The quality of Tibetan medicine is very good: if I prescribe 20 days of medicine, the patient usually recovers completely.

Mongolian medicine, on the other hand, is weak - 20 days are not enough." Indeed, it is not uncommon for Inner Mongolian TMM hospitals to prescribe six or more herbal pills as a single dose of medicine to their patients, while in Tibetan medicine and in Outer Mongolian TMM, the standard dose consists of one large or three small pills. A first-hand report from an employee of a large TMM company even described routine counterfeiting practices, where Tibetan medicine is mixed with cheap local herbal powder and repackaged as Mongolian medicine.

Despite this, many Mongolians travel to Inner Mongolia to avail themselves of superior TMM hospital facilities or to take advantage of free university tuition to study TMM.[11] The Inner Mongolia University for Nationalities in Tongliao and the Mongolian Medicine and Sciences University in Hohhot are the two flagship institutions for TMM in China, each graduating about 200 TMM professionals per year, but there are also several colleges and four professional schools offering lower-level TMM degrees. The International Mongolian Hospital of Inner Mongolia in Hohhot is the world's largest TMM hospital – and China's largest minority medicine hospital – with over 1500 beds and some 2000 staff. Built in 1957 as the "Inner Mongolian Chinese and Mongolian Medicine Hospital," it originally offered both TMM and TCM as well as biomedicine, but separated from its TCM branch in 2006 and moved to its present location in 2012. Other outstanding TMM hospitals include the 600-bed Affiliated Hospital of the Inner Mongolia University for Nationalities in Tongliao, founded in 1968, and the 350-bed Liaoning Province Mongolian Medicine Research Hospital in Fuxin, founded in 1980. Although a small city with less than a million inhabitants, Tongliao is considered the main center for TMM in China. It was officially named "Mongolian Medicine City" in 2017, in recognition of its long history of TMM scholarship, its highly regarded TMM school, and its several important TMM hospitals and pharmaceutical companies. Other important centers for TMM are Hohhot, the Inner Mongolian capital and administrative center, as well as Ulanhot, Hulunbuir, Xilinhot, Hure, and Fuxin in Liaoning province.

By comparison, the TMM pharmaceutical industry in Mongolia, valued at roughly 4 million USD in 2017 (Kloos et al. 2020), appears very small. Today, seven official TMM producers – all based in the capital Ulaanbaatar – provide about 15 tons of medicines to some 200 public and private TMM clinics and hospitals[12] and about 200 TMM doctors based abroad (the vast

---

11 According to Tserendagva, the Dean of the International School of Mongolian Medicine at the Mongolian National University of Medical Sciences in Ulaanbaatar, 300–400 Outer Mongolians go to Inner Mongolia every year to study TMM.
12 Official numbers are dated, sometimes refer to even older data, and can be contradictory (Mongolian Ministry of Health 2007, 2012). According to these and informal interview sources, however, there were 175 hospitals and clinics exclusively offering TMM in 2014, compared to 140 in 2012 and 115 in 2007.

majority in Poland). Besides the companies mentioned above – the Institute of Traditional Medicine and Technology ("Corporation"), Manba Datsan, Mong-Em, and Oditan – these include also Ariun Mongol ("Armon"), Dr Khatanbaatar's Liver Disease Center, and a new company run by Dr Ogtonbaatar. In addition, there are up to 50 unofficial manufacturers that produce another estimated 10–15 tons of medicines per year mostly for use in their own clinics, which do not appear in any official statistics but are included in the above-estimated value of 4 million USD. Not included in this number is the relatively large and profitable education sector, with six university TMM departments (all in Ulaanbaatar) and one TMM professional school in Darkhan; hospital and consultation fees; and the rapidly expanding sector of OTC herbal products based on TMM. Some 60–70 percent of medicinal raw materials are imported from China and India, while the remainder – mostly steppe plants – are wildcrafted in the Mongolian countryside by the producers themselves, equipped with official permits.

How can the difference in TMM's industrial development between Mongolia and Inner Mongolia be explained, given the similar patterns of policy development in both places? Why is TMM thriving in China, where Mongolians constitute a disadvantaged minority, while it is struggling in independent Mongolia, the capital of which functions as the centre of the TMM world? Talking to TMM practitioners and producers in both countries, the problem seems easy to sum up: in contrast to China, Mongolia's TMM pharmaceutical industry is scarcely profitable. One simple explanation would be Mongolia's small population and a weak economy, limiting the domestic market for TMM but encouraging a more cosmopolitan, international outlook among practitioners and producers than in Inner Mongolia. Until recently, however, China's Mongolian regions also had small populations and weak economies. Interview data reveals broad agreement on a different explanation, centred on two key factors: Soviet communism and Mongolia's post-communist politics. As Dr Natsagdorj told me, "You have to understand one thing: between 1938 and 1990, there was continuous government propaganda against TMM. Many Mongolians are still under this influence, so there is not much demand for TMM." Dr Ganzorig, a Dharamsala Men-Tsee-Khang trained physician who runs the Naidan Traditional Medicine Center at the Pethub monastery[13] in Ulaanbaatar, similarly explained: "The thing is that the Mongolians' mentality changed under communism. Most people forgot the old concepts of health and illness. So as traditional doctors today, we have to use modern concepts when we talk to our patients, otherwise they won't accept or even understand us." And when I asked Dr Purevjav at Mong-Em in Ulaanbaatar whether TMM was a symbol of Mongolian national pride,

---

13 Pethub Stangey Choskhor Ling monastery was founded in 1999 by the Indian ambassador to Mongolia, the 19th Bakula Rinpoche from Ladakh.

like Tibetan medicine for Tibetans, she replied: "Not really. There was too much Soviet influence for too long. Because of that, even now everything needs to be modern, scientific, proven …"

The market for TMM in Mongolia is thus still very small, even though TMM's popularity has grown considerably since 1990. While the impact of Soviet communist repression is keenly felt by Mongolian TMM practitioners even three decades after its end, they are also well aware of the role of successive post-communist governments. Expressing a widely shared sentiment, Dr Natsagdorj told me: "We have a TMM policy, we have a medicine law that includes TMM, we have a drug law, we have TMM development programs … On paper, it all looks very good, but in reality, there is not much support." Even the Deputy Health Minister Amarsanaa admitted in a 2014 interview: "The government has a good policy and strategy for TMM, but there is no funding, and therefore no implementation … So TMM in Mongolia is only growing naturally, not because of government help." While the Mongolian government is certainly operating with limited means, the absence of funding was also a matter of priority, as one TMM expert told me: "Most politicians have a business background, so they are not very interested in developing TMM." The MoH's Center for Health Development, charged with licensing doctors and overseeing medical education, is a good case in point: when I visited the centre in 2014, only one out of 70 staff was responsible for TMM. Asked whether this reflected the importance given to TMM by the government, the concerned officer laughed and replied, "yes."

Despite the country's impressive TMM policy and regulatory development, then, in the absence of tangible financial and administrative support, the industry has not benefitted from these policies as it has in China. One good example was the government's requirement for all second and third-level hospitals to have a TMM unit/department, the successful implementation of which is documented in official statistics (e.g. Mongolian Ministry of Health 2012: 23). In practice, however, "traditional medical services" offered in such units may be acupuncture, electricity treatment, light, water, oil, and mud therapies, massage, bloodletting, moxibustion, cupping, or physical exercise. The actual coverage of TMM in Mongolia is therefore much lower than such official numbers suggest, stagnating at about 3 percent of all healthcare. Furthermore, this government initiative is undermined by unequal health insurance coverage, where TMM was covered by only up to 117,000 MNT (48 USD) per patient in 2017, as compared to 350,000 MNT (144 USD) for biomedicine. Excess costs have to be paid by public hospitals themselves or, in the case of private hospitals, the patients. Especially in the wake of the 2016 economic crisis, TMM has thus become a financial burden, initiating its slow disappearance from public hospitals and accelerating its shift to the private sector. This, in turn, increasingly moves it out of the reach of poorer and middle-class patients, who formerly constituted its core clientele. Another example of the government counteracting its own TMM development policies was the successful "Family First Aid Kit" distributed by the NGO Vansemberuu. Containing basic TMM formulas along with simple descriptions of their indications and dosage,[14] these kits proved highly popular in rural and nomadic areas. However, the project died when the Mongolian government announced it would take over its funding, causing Nippon Foundation, its original funder, to withdraw, but then never followed up on its promise.

None of this means that the government's management of TMM is the only problem. Another issue, Dr Mendsaikhan from Mong-Em explained, are Mongolian medicinal plants, which in contrast to non-endemic ingredients (which constitute 60–70 percent of Mongolian medicines) cannot simply be bought and imported according to demand: "They are a very limited resource, especially now with climate change and desertification. This is why running a TMM company is not very good business, because we can't expand much." Nor does the comparatively well-developed TMM industry in China mean that all is well there. As mentioned above, environmental pollution, counterfeiting practices, and industrial-scale herb cultivation are all seen to be having negative impacts upon the quality of these medicines.

Even on a more general level, Inner Mongolian doctors and scholars point to mounting difficulties. In his study on the development of the TMM industry, Wu Lan (2015) argues that despite a consistent annual growth rate of 30 percent since 2001, TMM is struggling, having first been replaced by biomedicine and TCM, and more recently outcompeted by Tibetan medicine, which today ranks just behind TCM in popularity in China. One physician in Tongliao district told me:

> Today, TMM doctors have high certificates, there are many new medicines, they are packaged very nicely ... Also, the quantity of TMM produced has increased a lot, our medicines are sold everywhere, and there are more and more TMM doctors and nurses. So it looks like TMM is flourishing. But personally, I don't believe TMM has a good future. The quality of our medicines is going down, it's nothing special anymore. And for TMM to develop well, we need the freedom to follow our own culture and medicine. But the government doesn't give us this freedom, and they don't respect our medical tradition.

A senior doctor from Hure made a similar point:

> Socially, politically and economically, the TMM industry is doing very well here in China, that's true, but this doesn't mean TMM itself is doing

---

14 These kits were partially inspired by the *haichi* household medicine delivery model developed in Japan (see Futaya and Blaikie, this volume).

well. Some rich people make a lot of money with TMM, but TMM is not just for money. Human life is more important, and it's our duty to help people. In my opinion, the biggest problem is that we cannot practice as we want - the government controls us too much, there is no freedom, and government officers don't understand TMM.

Conclusion

Beginning with a brief outline of pre-modern medicine in Mongolia, this chapter has traced the transformation of a regional branch of Tibetan medicine into Traditional Mongolian Medicine and, most recently, the TMM industry. By analysing English, Chinese, and Mongolian textual sources as well as oral histories and interview data of officials, senior practitioners, and Mongolian scholars, it provides a first critical account of the emergence of modern TMM in Mongolia and China. While Western medical anthropological scholarship often focuses on the destructive, disruptive impact of communist rule on Mongolian and Tibetan medicine, the data presented here offers a more nuanced picture. Most obviously, communism was introduced at different times, took different forms, and had different attitudes vis-à-vis "traditional medicine" in Stalinist Mongolia and Maoist China. Furthermore, we have seen that even in Mongolia, where TMM undeniably suffered the brunt of communist destruction, communism proved to be not only a disruptive but also a productive force. Thus, after the brutal deterritorialisation of Tibetan medicine during the Stalinist purges in the 1930s, the communist government began to tentatively reterritorialise it as "Mongolian medicine" two decades later through Haidav, preparing the ground for the emergence of a TMM industry in the post-communist period after 1990. Although in comparatively less violent ways, the same process of de- and reterritorialisation occurred in the Mongolian regions of China, where "lama medicine" was similarly uprooted from its old institutions and reestablished as "Mongolian medicine" in secular, modern, state-controlled facilities, which later played a central role in TMM's industrialisation.

TMM's actual industrialisation began with Mongolia's democratic revolution in 1990 and China's switch to a "socialist market economy" in 1992. It was driven by TMM's increasing integration into the respective states' health care policies, pharmaceutical regulatory frameworks, and administrative structures. While this integration followed similar trajectories in both countries, China's TMM industry today outperforms Mongolia's by a ratio of more than 40 to 1 in terms of economic value. Professionals on both sides of the border explain this discrepancy by referring to the massive destruction and repression under Soviet communism on the one hand and to the absence of effective government support and economic development plans for TMM in Mongolia since the 1990s on the other. Ethnographic data shows, however, that TMM on both sides of the Gobi struggles with the role of the state, as well as shrinking supplies of good quality raw materials, caused not only by the rapid expansion of the industry in the past two decades but also by the effects of climate change, desertification, and environmental pollution. While the TMM industry continues to expand on the domestic and international levels, these issues are likely to grow, as will the profits and stakes involved.

I have argued that the development of TMM during the twentieth century is more productively understood in terms of continuity rather than discontinuity. Recent medical historiography by Mongolian scholars and several decades of government policy interventions, as well as the individual efforts of a large number of practitioners and stakeholders, can all be read as attempts to ensure TMM's continuity. In the contemporary context, continuity thus refers to the selective construction of both a traditional and national past, alongside particular visions of TMM's future as a competitive modern industry. As the brief accounts of different practitioners' professional trajectories illustrate, this transformative process cannot be adequately described or analysed in terms of a clash between tradition and modernity, nor can its result – the TMM industry – be accurately labeled as an instance of "alternative modernity" (e.g. Hsu 2009) or "neo-traditionalism" (Pordié 2008). Rather, it constitutes an assemblage that brings together old and new elements in a new entity, whose past and future continuity still remains to be settled. This particular assemblage, furthermore, is pharmaceutical since, like most Asian medicines today, TMM is largely based on pharmaceuticals and their production, regulation, and distribution (Kloos 2017). In short, the very existence, shape, and development of contemporary TMM is inextricably connected to its pharmaceutical industrialisation, in similar – but perhaps even more direct – ways than TCM (Chee; Campinas, this volume), Kampo medicine (Arai et al.; Futaya and Blaikie, this volume), or Ayurveda (Kudlu; Madhavan and Soman, this volume). We have seen how in both Mongolia and China, medical texts, knowledge, lineages, and what Adams et al. (2011) call a "Sowa Rigpa sensibility" were not only preserved by outstanding lama physicians under most difficult circumstances, but also underwent a radical reassemblage that changed both the contents and the nature of this medical tradition. Based on classical texts and old knowledge as much as modern technology and government regulations, TMM's industrial reassemblage not only acquired a new name and identity, but also a new history and future. What used to be a relatively stable and well-established regional branch of Tibetan medicine thus became a modern industry of Mongolian medicine.

Acknowledgements

Research for this chapter took place in 2014 (Mongolia), 2016 (Mongolia and Inner Mongolia), and 2018 (Inner Mongolia, Mongolia, and Buryatia), interspersed with three shorter trips to meet Mongolian doctors in Poland. The help and hospitality I received in all these places were truly extraordinary, and it would be impossible to name everyone here. Still, I would like to particularly thank academician S. Bold, Dr D. Ganzorig, Dr M. Purevjav,

Khambo Lama D. Natsagdorj, and S. Demberel in Mongolia; a venerable friend who shall remain unnamed in Inner Mongolia; and Oyuuna Rinchinova and Galina Kopeliovich in Russia for their outstanding kindness and support. Thanks also to Harilal Madhavan for his congenial company and collaboration during the first two fieldwork trips. All research and writing for this chapter were funded by the European Research Council (ERC) Starting Grant RATIMED (336932).

Bibliography

Adams V, Schrempf M and Craig S (2011) Introduction: Medicine in Translation between Science and Religion. In: Adams V, Schrempf M and Craig S (eds) *Medicine between Science and Religion. Explorations on Tibetan Grounds*. Oxford & New York: Berghahn Books, pp. 1–28.

Banzragch P and Gerke B (2002) The Tale of a Private Physician Practising Tibetan Medicine in Mongolia. *AyurVijnana* 8: 45–54.

Bold S (2013) *History and Development of Traditional Mongolian Medicine (from Neolithic Age – Early 21st Century)*. Third revised and enlarged edition. Ulaanbaatar: Sodpress Kompanid Khevlv.

Celimuge S, Liu M-j and Tuya S (2016) 蒙医药特色与发展思路 (Characteristics and Development of Mongolian Medicine). 中国中医药图书情报杂志 *(Chinese Journal of Library and Information Science for Traditional Chinese Medicine)* 40(6): 4–9.

Ganbayar Y and Tumurbaatar N (2007) *Ayurveda in Mongolia from Antiquity to 1937. Journal of Sasang Constitutional Medicine* 19(3): 300–307.

Gerke B (2004) Tradition and Modernity in Mongolian Medicine. *The Journal of Alternative and Complementary Medicine* 10(5): 743–749.

Haidav T (1975) *Domo dahinii anagaah uhaanii sudar bichgiin toim (Survey of Sutras on Oriental Medicine)*. Ulaanbaatar.

Haidav T (1977) *Ardiin emnelegt hereglegdej baisan amitnii garaltai em (Drugs of Animal Origin used in Mongolian Folk Medicine)* Vol. 1. Ulaanbaatar.

Haidav T, Altaichimeg B and Varlamova TC (1985) лекарственные растения в монгольской медицине *(Medicinal Plants in Mongolian Medicine)*, 2nd edition. Ulan-Bator: Gosizlatel'stvo.

Haidav T, Tsognemeh J and Badam B (1962) *Mongol omii emiin zarim urgamal (The Medicinal Plants of the Mongolian People's Republic)*. Ulaanbaatar.

Haidav T and Zakrividoroga SP (1965) *Kratkaya Istoriya Mongolskoi Meditsini (Brief History of Mongolian Medicine)*. Ulaanbaatar.

Hsu E (2009) Chinese Propriety Medicines: An "Alternative Modernity?" The Case of the Anti-Malarial Substance Artemisinin in East Africa. *Medical Anthropology* 28(2): 111–140.

Humphrey C (1983) *Karl Marx Collective: Economy, Society and Religion in a Siberian Collective Farm*. Cambridge: Cambridge University Press.

IMAR (Inner Mongolia Autonomous Region Health and Family Planning Commission of the Mongolian-Chinese Medicine Management Bureau) (2015) 内蒙古自治区蒙医药中医药事业发展成就 *(1947–2015) [Accomplishment of the Mongolian Medicine Industry of the Inner Mongolia Autonomous Region (1947–2015)]*. Hohhot, China: IMAR Health and Family Planning Commission.

Janes C and Hilliard C (2008) Inventing Tradition: Tibetan Medicine in the Post-Socialist Contexts of China and Mongolia. In: Pordié L (ed) *Tibetan Medicine in the Contemporary World: Global Politics of Medical Knowledge and Practice*. London & New York, NY: Routledge, pp. 35–61.

Jigmed B (1981) Survey of Mongolian Medicine: The Three Stages of Development from Ancient to Modern. *Journal of Chinese Medical History* 4.

Kletter C, Glasl S, Thalhammer T et al. (2008) Traditional Mongolian Medicine – A Potential for Drug Discovery. *Scientia Pharmaceutica* 76(1): 49–63.

Kloos S (2017) The Pharmaceutical Assemblage: Rethinking Sowa Rigpa and the Herbal Pharmaceutical Industry in Asia. *Current Anthropology* 58(6): 693–717.

Kloos S (2020) Humanitarianism from Below. Sowa Rigpa, the Traditional Pharmaceutical Industry, and Global Health. *Medical Anthropology* 39(2): 167–181.

Kloos S, Madhavan H, Tidwell T, et al. (2020) The Transnational Sowa Rigpa Industry in Asia: New Perspectives on an Emerging Economy. *Social Science and Medicine* 245: 112617.

Mongolian Ministry of Health (2007) *Report of Market Research on Mongolian Traditional Medicinal Drugs*. Ulaanbaatar: WHO.

Mongolian Ministry of Health (2012) Assessment of National Traditional Medicine Policy and Strategy in the Context of WHO "Regional Strategy for Traditional Medicine in the Western Pacific (2011–2020)": Survey Report. Ulaanbaatar: Mongolian Ministry of Health.

Munkh-Amgalan Y and Tsend-Ayush G (2002) Academician Tsend Haidav – Innovator of Traditional Mongolian Medicine. *AyurVijnana* 8: 40–44.

Pitschmann A, Purevsuren S, Obmann A, et al. (2013) Traditional Mongolian Medicine: History and status quo. *Phytochemistry Reviews* 12(4): 943–959.

Pordié L (2008) Tibetan Medicine Today: Neo-Traditionalism as an Analytical Lens and a Political Tool. In: Pordié L (ed) *Tibetan Medicine in the Contemporary World. Global Politics of Medical Knowledge and Practice*. London & New York, NY: Routledge, pp. 3–32.

Sablin I (2019) Tibetan Medicine and Buddhism in the Soviet Union: Research, Repression, and Revival, 1922–1991. In: Hokkanen M and Kananoja K (eds) *Healers and Empires in Global History: Healing as Hybrid and Contested Knowledge*. London: Palgrave Macmillan, pp. 81–114.

Saijirahu (2007) 论 20 世纪内蒙古传统蒙医学的发展 (On the Development of Traditional Mongolian Medicine in the 20th Century Inner Mongolia). *Chinese Journal of Medical History* 37(2): 88–93.

Sandag S and Kendall H (1999) *Poisoned Arrows: The Stalin-Choibalsan Mongolian Massacres, 1921–1941*. Boulder, CO: Westview Press.

Scheid V (2002) *Chinese Medicine in Contemporary China*. Durham & London: Duke University Press.

Scheid V (2007) *Currents of Tradition in Chinese Medicine, 1626–2006*. Seattle, WA: Eastland Press.

Shimamura I (2019) Magicalized Socialism: An Anthropological Study on the Magical Practices of a Secularized Reincarnated Lama in Socialist Mongolia. *Asiatische Studien – Études Asiatiques* 73(4): 799–829.

Tao S, Li X and Wang H (2017) 辽宁省蒙医药现状及发展思路 (Status quo and Direction of Mongolian Medicine in Liaoning Province). 中国民族医药杂志 *(Chinese Journal of Nationality Medicine and Pharmacy)* 2017(9): 64–66.

Taylor K (2005) *Chinese Medicine in Early Communist China, 1945–63*. Oxon & New York, NY: Routledge.

Wang X and Bao L (2017) 巴·吉格木德教授论蒙医药历史的分期方法 (Prof. B. Jigmed's Conception on the Division of Stages of History of Mongolian Medicine). 中华医史杂志 *(Chinese Journal of Medical History)* 47(2): 103–106.

Wu L (2015) 蒙医药产业发展研究 (The Development of the Mongolian Medicine Industry). 中国民族医药杂志 *(Chinese Journal of Nationality Medicine and Pharmacy)* 2015(12): 59–62.

Conclusion
Assembling Asian pharmaceuticals

Calum Blaikie

What can we learn about Asian medicines through a sustained scholarly focus on their historical trajectories and current configuration *as industries*? What can observations generated through such research tell us about regional and global patterns of pharmaceutical development, production, regulation, and flow, or indeed about contemporary Asia more broadly? Constituting one of the first collective enquiries into Asian medical industries, this volume invites reflection upon these questions and a host of others besides. Exploring a broad range of contexts from a variety of disciplinary perspectives, these case studies offer numerous insights into the specific regions and medical traditions upon which they focus. At the same time, they present us with a range of commonalities that not only facilitate comparative analysis but also show these industries to be much more than an assortment of localised, unconnected, and inward-looking "traditional medicine" production sectors. What the chapters collectively reveal instead is a distinct phenomenon that is gathering momentum and carrying increasing significance at various scales, yet has not been adequately defined or investigated to date.

Each medical tradition discussed in this volume clearly has its own unique history, identity, and lived reality. A vast literature attests to the importance of medical texts in establishing the epistemological and theoretical foundations of these traditions, as well as to the way medical lineages, institutions, and fields of practice have both sustained and transformed them over time, in relation to wider social and medical change.[1] All of these factors have shaped medicine production and circulation in highly specific ways, resulting in a diverse array of socioeconomic, institutional, industrial, and pharmaceutical forms. When placed within a comparative framework, however, the medical industries of China, India, Japan, Mongolia, and Nepal also appear as parts of something much

---

1 For example, see: Leslie (1976), Zimmermann (1987), Leslie and Young (1992), Scheid (2002, 2007), Taylor (2005), Unschuld (2010 [1985]), Berger (2013), Lei (2014), Gyatso (2015), and Salguero (2017).

DOI: 10.4324/9781003218074-15

larger, with many shared or similar characteristics, dynamics, and problematics. Although each industry is deeply embedded in its local context, we propose approaching them as one object of study, albeit a dynamic, unstable object with emergent properties and fuzzy, shifting, and contested boundaries. Asian medical industries do not sit easily within any one field or framework. They defy simple narratives and transcend familiar analytical categories. Reducing them to their individual parts and studying each part in isolation can only take us so far.

This reflective final chapter seeks to identify some of the main cross-cutting themes that run through the book and thus further ground these industries in a single field of inquiry. It traces connections not only between the industries of Chinese Medicine, Ayurveda, Kampo, and Sowa Rigpa but also across seemingly disparate domains such as the collection of medicinal plants in remote areas and vast GMP-compliant factories, cottage industry pharmacists and global governance regimes, well-known classical formulas and lab-based reformulation practices, localised pharmaceutical development efforts and globally oriented nation branding exercises. The discussion focuses on three important domains that emerge from the case studies: the role of the state, regulation and reformulation, and the supply of raw materials. Many emergent characteristics of Asian medical industries are located within and across these domains, and these are drawn out further with reference to several current analytical concepts, notably sociotechnical imaginaries (Jasanoff and Kim 2015), reformulation regimes (Pordié and Gaudillière 2014b, c), and frontier assemblages (Cons and Eilenberg 2019). These ruminations then enable fruitful reflection back on to the questions posed in Stephan Kloos' introductory chapter: To what extent are these industries global in scope, transnational in the constitution, and capitalist in orientation? What similarities and differences are evident in the way industrial actors formulate, produce and market drugs? What symbolic, economic, and social values are ascribed to Asian medical industries and medicines by different actors?

As noted in the introduction, the field of Asian medical industries is vast and in constant flux, so the current volume can only take small steps towards mapping and exploring this new territory. Similarly, this concluding chapter can only briefly pick up on some of the main themes highlighted in the chapters, offer some preliminary and partial answers to the questions posed above, and draw attention to potential avenues for further research. These reflections are aided by a specific, comparative analytical framework, the "pharmaceutical assemblage" (Kloos 2017), which underpins the volume as a whole. This approach emphasises dynamism, contingency, and emergent temporality over fixed structures, teleologies, and stable categories. Pharmaceutical assemblages connect material and non-material elements across local, national, and transnational fields, bringing heterogeneous components into more or less stable configurations, whose convergence and articulation provide the main focus of enquiry. From such a perspective, the multitude of knowledge forms, practices, processes, materials and flows that constitute Asian medical industries today can be studied in and of themselves *and also* as parts of a larger phenomenon, one that has gained sufficient critical mass to exert distinct social, economic, political and medical forces of its own.

States and pharmaceuticals

The chapters in this volume attest to the crucial roles played by national governments in both the historical formation and contemporary dynamics of Asian medical industries. Political forces were key to the emergence of each of these industries, contributing greatly to their initial shape and orientation under various colonial, postcolonial, imperial, and post-imperial conditions, as well as differing Cold War and post-Cold War positions (Chen 2010). State governments also play vital roles in the contemporary operation of these industries. They are participants in global regulatory regimes, as well as being responsible for the design, implementation, and enforcement of policies concerning the industrial activities taking place within their national borders. States also manage public healthcare and health insurance systems, shape the general business and investment environment, intervene in the ways markets are structured and operate, and oversee the management of natural resources. The chapters describe various patterns of state involvement at different junctures, which appear along continuums of repression and tolerance, indifference and active support, top-down intervention and more laissez-faire modes of governance. All show state governments as key actors that interact with and influence medical industries in numerous ways.

Recent scholarship argues that "the state" can no longer be approached as a singular, easily defined entity with clear boundaries, agendas, and modes of operation (Fuller and Benei 2001; Chatterjee 2004; Das and Poole 2004; Corbridge et al. 2005). States are arguably better thought of as clusters of individuals, institutions, procedures, tactics, knowledge, policies, and technologies, broadly oriented towards the task of governance. Governmentality operates through the production and control of knowledge/power, the propagation of discourses, and the deployment of resources and technologies, both within state bureaucracies and through external institutions broadly aligned with their aims. My analytical focus is thus on the way various state elements articulate with components of Asian pharmaceutical assemblages, co-producing aspects of one another under varying conditions of accord and antagonism. This analysis is further focused through the notion of sociotechnical imaginaries, which refers to "collectively held, institutionally stabilized, and publicly performed visions of desirable futures, animated by shared understandings of forms of social life and social order attainable through, and supportive of, advances in science and technology" (Jasanoff and Kim 2015: 4). Such an approach highlights the role that national-level aspirations and visions of the future play in shaping state agendas, strategies and policies regarding "traditional" pharmaceutical industries, as well as the negotiations and tensions that surround their positioning within broader medical, scientific, and technological fields.

Several contributions to this volume show how particular historical junctures, political contexts, ideological frameworks, and socioeconomic conditions contributed to the emergence of particular kinds of the pharmaceutical industry. National governments not only established the legal status of medical traditions and the degree of support they received, but also shaped the initial form and scale of their medicine production activities. The chapter by Stephan Kloos illustrates this particularly clearly by contrasting the impacts of the longer and more repressive Soviet-influenced political regime on Mongolian medicine's development in Outer Mongolia with the shorter and (relatively) less destructive effects seen in Inner Mongolia, which was under Chinese control. Kloos demonstrates the significance of these early phases to the continuity of currents of medical knowledge, the structure of medical institutions, and the patterning of state patronage for industrial development, as well as the public demand for the medicines being produced. Differences in the initial conditions of industrial emergence partially explain the faster growth and larger scale of the traditional medicine industry in Inner Mongolia compared to the slower start and lower growth rates seen in Outer Mongolia. This chapter also shows how recent differences in degrees of state support, as well as in factors such as population size, market access, and the availability of raw materials, played key roles in the later development and contemporary trajectories of these industries.

Although under much less repressive circumstances, the chapters by Ichiro Arai, Julia Yongue, and Kiichiro Tsutani, and Tomoko Futaya and Calum Blaikie reveal how the negative stance of the early Meiji-era Japanese government towards traditional forms of medicine had crucial yet contrasting effects on the way the Kampo and *haichi* industries developed. The newly centralised Japanese state forced major transformations in the way these nascent industries were structured, as well as how they sourced, formulated, produced, and marketed their medicines. This was achieved through waves of increasingly stringent regulation, the dissolution of the medicinal merchant's guilds, the delegitimisation of practitioners, and changes to tax laws. These aggressive policies severely damaged the producers of Kampo medicines, who did not begin to recover until the mid-twentieth century. The *haichi* manufacturers of Toyama did not suffer as badly and the patent medicine market continued to grow, although firms were forced to radically reorganise their formulation and production practices.

The contributors argue that these initially disruptive top-down interventions also led to productive and galvanising effects, such as the formalisation of manufacturing companies, standardisation of formulas, introduction of new technologies, and development of innovative pharmaceutical techniques.

These forced modernisation processes later proved instrumental in the government's shift to a more supportive policy stance during the mid-twentieth century, which in turn ushered in a new period of intensive institutional expansion, research, innovation, and public health integration. In Toyama, prefectural state bodies worked collaboratively with manufacturers and academics to help the industry adapt to new regulatory regimes, acting as a counterweight to the stricter policies emanating from the centre. Powerful lobbies within the central government intervened during the reforms of the 1970s to protect the Kampo industry against its harshest detractors, while state-led regulators took a relatively lenient approach to the re-evaluation of Kampo drugs, which facilitated their subsequent coverage under the national health insurance scheme. Thus, an initial phase of state suppression can be seen, albeit retrospectively, as crucial to the process of industrial reorganisation and pharmaceutical transformation that eventually enabled the incorporation of Kampo drugs into Japan's single system of healthcare and *haichi* medicines to retain a foothold in the national market.

Liz Chee's study of "new" drug development in Chinese medicine shows how a particular state-industry configuration allowed a specific reformulation regime to emerge, which remains central to the industry in the present day. The Maoist state's takeover of formerly private, Republican-era laboratories and manufacturing facilities enabled it to strictly control research, development, and manufacturing agendas, which focused on combining elements of Chinese medicine and biomedicine in order to achieve pharmaceutical self-sufficiency. This core aim effectively continued into the Deng era and subsequent periods of economic reform, while the laboratories and factories involved re-oriented themselves towards the pursuit of profit as government support waned. The Chinese state shifted to the role of relatively lax regulator and industrial enabler, oriented towards facilitating industrial and market growth while providing a sizable proportion of medicines for public healthcare without the need for large imports. In stark contrast to Japan, the state dedicated very little effort or resources to matters of quality control, centralised drug registration, or efficacy testing until the end of the twentieth century. This reflects China's strongly growth-driven priorities, as well as the much longer period in which medicines of traditional origin were widely accepted by both state bodies and the general public as major components of national healthcare provision.

Manuel Campinas' chapter illustrates another dimension of Chinese state engagement with the herbal medicine industry. By officially bringing the nation's many ethnic minority medical traditions under the umbrella of Chinese medicine in 2016, the central government gained greater influence and control over them while simultaneously furthering its political agenda of limiting discontent towards the state in minority areas. State policies presented the development of minority pharmaceutical industries as the main field in which minorities could "catch up" with the mainstream Chinese medicines industry, which was itself seen to be lagging behind global pharmaceutical trends. As Campinas shows, catching up proved highly problematic for groups that had failed to gain a foothold in national markets during the late twentieth century period of easy proprietary drug registration. Despite the efforts of researchers, academics, entrepreneurs, and local practitioners to launch a Qiang medicines industry, the absence of nationally marketable proprietary medicines and the obstacles facing attempts to gain new licenses severely hampered progress. Instead, the main thrust of development was directed towards raw materials, both through the controversial ethnic labelling of medicinal plant species and cultivars, and through large-scale cultivation initiatives intended to supply existing manufacturers at the national level. Thus, while ostensibly promoting an ethnically inclusive model of pharmaceutical and rural development, the Chinese state furthered its agenda of finding agricultural solutions to the twin crises of rising industrial demand and declining wild stocks, while Qiang doctors saw their ethnic and medical identities increasingly manipulated by outsiders, primarily for marketing purposes and political ends.

The chapters by Harilal Madhavan and Sajitha Soman, and Chitprabha Kudlu, illustrate two different ways by which elements of the Indian state have attempted to intervene in the contemporary Ayurvedic industry and turn it to governmental advantage at national and global scales. In each case, governmental agendas came up against a powerful and growing industry that developed largely beyond the state's purview. Both chapters underscore the state's indifference to the Ayurvedic industry during the early post-colonial period, which enabled large firms to consolidate, expand and capture significant market shares in relative independence from governmental regulation or intervention.[2] In Madhavan and Soman's case, the state's main interests were (1) improving product quality, safety, and innovation, particularly for smaller firms; (2) supplying major public health schemes; and (3) increasing Ayurveda's share of the global market. Kudlu discusses the Modi government's agenda of expanding its geopolitical soft power and competing with China in the global herbal medicines market while seeking to revive cultural nationalist symbolism based on Hindu identity claims through the medium of Ayurveda.

Both chapters show how the Indian government's aim of global market expansion was thwarted by Ayurvedic manufacturers' ongoing reliance on the national market as their main source of revenue. Combined with the regulatory and marketing hurdles facing efforts to expand Ayurveda's overseas markets, this severely limited export-oriented investment.[3] Madhavan and Soman also argue that by misunderstanding the structure of the existing industry in Kerala and the respective needs of its various sectors, a state-inspired industrial clustering initiative failed to make significant progress

---

2 See also: Bode (2008), Banerjee (2009), and Berger (2013).
3 See Kudlu and Nichter (2019).

towards its stated goals. Kudlu further shows how the nationalist state failed to resolve major discrepancies between its envisioning of Ayurveda as a singular, uniform, and scientifically validated medical system, which was crucial to its imagined global future, and the multiple versions of Ayurveda that were actually being practiced on the ground. These disjunctures mean that even as government representatives, industry spokespeople, and the mainstream media increasingly internalise and amplify the discourse of pharmaceutical standardisation, the major manufacturers continue to resist state-driven efforts in this direction.

The chapter by Calum Blaikie and Sienna Craig considers how the *absence* of state recognition, support, and regulation affects Sowa Rigpa pharmacy in Nepal. For a cottage industry struggling to survive and navigate a locally appropriate development path in a precarious state, the lack of government intervention has many constraining and destabilising effects. However, it also grants *amchi* pharmacists a large degree of freedom over the mode and orientation of medicine production, which many realise would likely be curtailed under more formalised arrangements. Thus, governmental indifference feeds a sense of precarity and vulnerability while leaving space for small-scale manufacture to flourish, continuing to produce what many consider high-quality medicines, often within lineage-based streams of knowledge and practice. These medicines are prescribed at low cost in small clinics, according to ethical precepts that are widely contrasted with the profit-oriented motivations associated with industrial mass production and over-the-counter (OTC) distribution (see also Craig et al. 2020). This example highlights the ambivalence that many practitioners and manufacturers of Asian medicines feel towards state intervention in their activities, which resonates across several of the cases discussed in this volume. Because Sowa Rigpa practice spans several contiguous nation-states and those involved in this cottage industry hail not only from Nepal but also from Tibetan areas of China, India, and Bhutan, the chapter also shows how pharmaceutical assemblages can be at once transnational and deeply embedded within specific national spaces.

Taken together, these contributions attest to the hugely important role that the agendas and policies of various state institutions have played in the emergence and consolidation of Asian medical industries and continue to play in the present day, as well as to the way sociotechnical visions (and apparitions) have driven or modified these relations. We have seen instances where state repression has crushed medical traditions to the brink of annihilation, only for them to later re-emerge and flourish into sizeable industries making major economic, medical, and social contributions. In other cases, unsupportive state agendas and policy postures have had enduring effects on the form, scale, and orientation of these industries, even long after these policies have been superseded. Several contributors also point to areas in which state powers meet their limits and where industries have sufficient independence to resist direct attempts to intervene in their operations or to co-opt their material or symbolic potential for other agendas.

In each case, the increasing significance of Asian medical industries to their wider polities, societies, and economies is abundantly clear, as is the positioning of states as crucial components of pharmaceutical assemblages that exert powerful, but not always inexorable, effects on many other constituent elements. There is also ample evidence here to support current theoretical revisionings of "the state" which highlight its complexity, multiplicity, permeability, and plasticity, such as when central and regional state bodies take different stances towards pharmaceutical development, when policy positions take sudden or unexpected turns, or when state and industry discourses and roles overlap to the point of becoming virtually indistinguishable. Even though most of the governmental interventions discussed in this volume focused primarily on their national contexts, we have also seen how global market aspirations and nation branding efforts can exert significant influence on state discourses and policies relating to medical industries, with various outcomes and degrees of success. Thus, patterns of convergence and disjuncture between local, national, and global frames shape both sociotechnical imaginaries and concrete policies at the nation-state level, but the consequences these have for Asian medical industries are not always predictable, intended, or easy to disentangle from the other factors at play.

Regimes of regulation and reformulation

Two central themes running through many of the chapters concern the regulatory policies and laws with which Asian medical industries engage, and the reformulation regimes within which medicines are adapted, invented, popularised, and marketed. These fields merit careful consideration in their own right and have indeed become the focus of significant academic attention over recent years.[4] This work has shown how the governance, reformulation, and circulation of Asian medicines are closely intertwined, influencing one another in important ways as pharmaceutical assemblages take shape across Asia. These convergences are particularly visible in laboratory-based reformulation practices, in the articulation between global and national regulatory policies, notably concerning Good Manufacturing Practices (GMP), and in the application of new technologies for production and quality control. It is these clusters of external interventions, internalised responses, and subsequent feedback effects that I wish to draw out for closer consideration here.

As Arai, Yongue, and Tsutani describe in detail, the global pharmaceutical regulatory regime embraced GMP from the late 1960s onwards and

---

4 See the works edited by Pordié and Gaudillière (2014a), Pordié and Hardon (2015), and Coderey and Pordié (2020), as well as Banerjee (2014), Pordié and Gaudillière (2014c), Kuo (2015, 2009), and Schrempf (2015).

is now moving towards "GxPs," which incorporate Good Post-Marketing Surveillance Practices (GPMSP), dealing with issues of safety and iatrogenesis, and Good Clinical Practices (GCP), which focus on efficacy. These GxPs are supranational, biomedically defined, normative and technoscientific, and can themselves be seen as assemblages of vast scale and complexity (Quet et al. 2018). Global regulations are increasingly powerful forces shaping the development, production, and circulation of all kinds of medicines, contributing to general trends of pharmaceuticalisation, pharmacovigilance, and surveillance within the realm of "Global Health" (Petryna et al. 2006; Biehl and Petryna 2013; Gaudillière 2014). Within this pattern of global regulatory and market convergence, the implications of GxPs for Asian medical industries are multiplying, particularly for those with large existing export markets and those wishing to expand further into these markets. It is also notable that questions of safety, quality, and bioscientific validity are of mounting importance for the general public in many Asian nations, which reflects the region's emergence as a leading force of economic, scientific, and technological advance, as well as a general pattern of convergence with global norms in this field (Kuo 2009, 2015; Ong and Chen 2010; Banerjee 2014; Ma 2020).

Although pharmaceutical regulations developed at the global level by organisations such as the WHO and WTO aim towards deterritorialised homogeneity, they are adapted and reterritorialised as each national government inscribes them into policies, laws, and guidelines (Coderey 2020; Saxer 2013). Thus, in articulation with these "global forms" (Collier and Ong 2005), nation states develop their own regulatory frameworks, pharmaceutical laws, and pharmacopoeial standards over long periods of time, resulting in a variety of systems and modes of enforcement. Several chapters discuss the challenges that emerged when GMP and other regulatory mechanisms were introduced into industries unused to external oversight, stringent rules and complex, unfamiliar technical and administrative procedures (Arai et al.; Chee; Futaya and Blaikie; Kudlu, this volume).

The standardisation of raw materials and formulas represents a major thrust area in Asian states' efforts to "develop" traditional medical industries and promote them in national and global markets (Saxer 2013; WHO 2013, 2018; Kuo 2015; Kumari and Kotecha 2016; Wang et al. 2016). This volume shows how governments placed varying degrees and forms of pressure on industries to standardise formulas and products, often as precursors to the introduction of GMP or in its early stages. Some interesting contrasts emerge between India, China, and Japan in terms of the periodicity and veracity of their regulatory interventions, as well as their subsequent effects on industrial development and market positioning.

In Japan, state pressure to standardise formulas began to mount in the early twentieth century, well before the advent of GMP, with a series of laws and directives that levied harsh financial penalties for non-compliance.

Despite initial reluctance, companies gradually standardised their formulations and this became the norm for the Kampo and patent medicine industries from then on. Although forced upon manufacturers from above, such early and effective standardisation processes contributed to making the later adoption of GMP a far less onerous task than it was in other Asian countries. It is notable that Japan's drive to tightly regulate these industries, standardise their formulas and later adopt GxPs emerged from a largely inward-looking sociotechnical orientation, focused primarily on the national market and public healthcare system, with little evidence of global market aspirations. With this initial impetus in the background, Arai et al. argue that, with certain provisos, Japan's current regulatory framework treats Kampo medicines identically to biomedicines, subjecting them to the same pharmacovigilance and new drug approval systems. This remains a unique achievement and is worthy of much more academic and applied interest than it has so far received, not least because it further blurs the boundaries that formerly separated herbal medicines from biomedicines in Japan. It is also notable that all large Kampo manufacturers design and manage their own in-house quality control systems, particularly for testing the quality and contaminant levels of raw materials, which extend beyond GMP requirements. Arai et al. recognise that such self-imposed "quasi standards" have contributed to the largely collaborative and consensus-based regulatory regime that pertains in contemporary Japan.

In stark contrast to Japan, standardisation and other forms of regulation were not major state priorities in either India or China, so regulatory systems remained weak and fragmentary until the end of the twentieth century (Chee, and Kudlu, this volume; Kudlu and Nichter 2019). It was China's pursuit of WTO accession and the associated drive to secure its leading role as an exporter of both raw materials and finished "traditional" medicines within global regulatory norms, which inspired its push towards higher levels of standardisation and quality control during the early 2000s. This rapid drive to implement GMP and other regulatory measures did not only affect the Chinese medicine industry but also had enormous implications for the many ethnic minority traditions operating within the PRC (Campinas), proving particularly disruptive and transformative for producers of Tibetan medicines (Adams et al. 2001; Craig 2011, 2012; Saxer 2013).

According to Kudlu, the Government of India was even slower to react to global trends and begin implementing regulatory reforms. When they finally emerged, these efforts were explicitly framed in terms of expanding Ayurveda's global market share so as to compete with China, as well as more recently being linked to nation branding and Hindu nationalism. Kudlu deftly illustrates how the Indian government's subsequent efforts to standardise Ayurveda and implement GMP were entangled in deeply contradictory dynamics both internal to Ayurveda and existing between its main industrial players and the state. As these contradictions continue to play out, they reveal "a gulf between policy discourses of standardisation and regulation on the one hand, and a ground reality of entrenched pluralism on the other, which not only shapes the contemporary Ayurveda industry in India but also highlights some of the complexities of nation branding and transnational nationalisms in Asian medical industries more generally."

Blaikie and Craig consider the implications of the *absence* of regulation for Sowa Rigpa medicine production in Nepal. Despite the lack of external regulatory frameworks, *amchi* pharmacists are increasingly aware of regulatory effects upon Sowa Rigpa and Ayurvedic industries elsewhere. They begin to imagine and discuss amongst themselves the impacts that GMP *could* have on their activities. Some change their packaging materials, adapt their formulas or adopt new production processes in light of what they read or hear from colleagues and friends in other countries. They discursively link tighter regulations with the pressure to scale up production volumes, as well as the need to charge higher prices to their patients in order to cover the extra expenses that regulation would likely incur. Here we glimpse how regulation, scale, market dynamics, and profitability are linked in sociotechnical and ethical imaginaries, despite the absence of regulation as a feature in contemporary terrains of production. We also see how notions of medicine quality and efficacy that remain embedded in small-scale, highly personalised modes of production reverse the polarity of global regulatory discourses. Rather than looking at modern Sowa Rigpa factories with envy or as further evidence of their own underdevelopment, Nepal-based *amchi*-pharmacists frequently question the impacts of mechanised mass-production, sterilisation, and other GMP-related procedures on the properties and effectiveness of industrially produced herbal medicines, while also raising ethical questions over the way they are distributed.

Several contributions to this volume also consider aspects of reformulation, building upon the excellent empirical and theoretical foundations laid by Laurent Pordié and Jean-Paul Gaudillière (2014a, b, c). It is in this field that Asian medical industries have pushed furthest into new experimental realms, transcending the boundaries that were formerly seen to circumscribe "traditional medicine" and separate it from biomedicine. Through processes such as reverse engineering, the "mining" of classical texts and the recombination of familiar components, interdisciplinary teams from traditional medical and bioscience backgrounds work both separately and together in laboratories, research institutes, and factories to adapt existing medicines and develop new drugs, while in so doing, arguably develop their own "alternative modernities" (Chatterjee 1986; Gaonkar 2001; Hsu 2009; Pordié and Gaudillière 2014b).

The chapter by Liz Chee shows how a specific reformulation regime developed in China from the 1950s onwards, beginning in earnest with Mao's dictum "to combine Chinese and western medicine" but later moving in directions that could not have been predicted from this starting point. She shows how two distinct approaches to achieving this "combination" ran simultaneously in Chinese laboratories throughout the latter half of the twentieth century and continue into the present day. The first aims to "re-network" well-known Chinese herbs into new medicines, minus the corpus of theory and practice surrounding their use. This model corresponds closely to "pharmaceuticalisation" in Madhulika Banerjee's (2009) sense of the term. Another approach was to "scientise" (or inscribe science onto) Chinese medicine and thus prove its efficacy according to biomedically recognised criteria, even as it was being presented and practiced as an explicit alternative to biomedicine.[5] These parallel tracks continue to run through contested terrain, resulting in a complex of partially overlapping and partially contradictory reformulation regimes.

Drug discovery in the company on which Chee focuses, Guangzhou Huahai, proceeds largely through reverse engineering. The company targets a biomedically recognised condition or set of symptoms that are undertreated by existing Chinese medicines or do not respond well to biomedical treatment, before matching these to well-documented Chinese medicine syndromes. Interdisciplinary teams locate known prescriptions for these syndromes and add or reduce components to make a novel combination. They then decide how to extract the necessary components, combine them together and finalise them as a "new medicine" before standardising and testing it. Other methods include simplifying classical recipes or seeking active ingredients from single plants via extraction. There are many similarities here with the ways the large companies develop new medicines from existing textual and applied sources of knowledge within Indian "techno-Ayurveda" (Pordié 2014; 2015; Pordié and Gaudillière 2014b, c). Chee further shows how tensions remain between proponents of the different approaches, with the single extract method popular among those with "hard science" backgrounds and the new multi-compound drug route favoured by those with Chinese medicine training. These tensions reflect the dynamism, contingency, and controversy inherent to processes of pharmaceutical innovation, which in this case have arguably resulted in the simultaneous construction of several coexisting alternative modernities. Some commentators may view such reformulation practices as further evidence of the "death of Chinese medicine" as an independent system of knowledge and action (Unschuld 2010 [1985]: xi). Others see internal debate and divergence as signs of a vibrant, living tradition (Scheid 2007), while recognising the hugely complex dynamics at play (Scheid 2014).

The chapters by Arai et al., and Futaya and Blaikie, chart the emergence of reformulation practices in Japan's Kampo and *haichi* medicines industries. *Haichi* household medicine production effectively took the form of a

---

5 See also Lei (2014) and Scheid (2014).

patent medicine industry early in its history and many manufacturers experimented with new drug development from the eighteenth century onwards, including combining raw materials of Eastern and Western origin. The Meiji government's clear preference for biomedicine offered tacit support for such hybrid forms, while the manufacturers apparently saw no inherent contradiction in these experimental combinations, so long as customers found them efficacious and therefore kept consuming them. Even though it emerged under strict regulatory oversight and distinct modernising pressures, this suggests a relatively pragmatic and opportunistic mode of reformulation, which developed without the involvement of multidisciplinary teams working under laboratory conditions. Such a regime was certainly facilitated by the fact that the *haichi* industry does not claim origins in a single medical tradition, and therefore lacks the inertia that comes with textually inscribed classical formulas and a body of practitioners upon whom the development, acceptance, and prescription of new pharmaceutical forms depend. Further research is called for in order to better understand the trajectory, inner workings, and wider implications of this mode of reformulation, particularly because combinations of Eastern and Western medicinal resources raise all sorts of potentially productive questions but have not yet been closely studied in the social science literature.[6]

The innovations Arai et al. chart in the Kampo industry emerged largely in response to regulatory interventions and technological developments. The adoption of rapid spray-drying and extraction techniques for herbal materials offers a particularly intriguing example of how reformulation practices entangle materials, technologies, regulations, and economics. This technology-led innovation altered the production process and material form of the vast majority of Kampo medicines from the 1960s onwards. In response to regulatory changes during the 1980s, laboratory techniques were developed to establish the levels of active ingredients in dried extracts and compare them with benchmarks taken from "traditional" decoction forms of the same named formulas. Initial results showed that neither the quantity nor the quality of selected chemical markers in dried extracts were equivalent to standard decoctions, suggesting that this widely adopted industrial process actually resulted in far less potent medicines. Binding standards were subsequently introduced but allow for dried extracts to be considerably less potent than decoctions. This discrepancy highlights the tensions and trade-offs involved in the Kampo industry's attempts to mass-produce drugs that meet the same quality criteria as biomedicines and compete with them in the same markets. This chapter also shows how

---

6 Hybrid medicines combining herbal and chemical components became popular in Vietnam during the late colonial period (Monnais 2019). Similar combination practices exist in contemporary Cambodia (Pordié 2021), but further studies are needed to delve deeper into the origins, materials, logics and impacts of such formulations.

the Kampo industry's positioning in regulatory and public health spheres currently serves to limit innovation and reformulation, especially when compared to the highly experimental and innovative regimes that pertain in India and China. Kampo firms see the barriers to new drug registration as being too high and have little interest in developing new overseas markets, so appear content to continue producing well-known formulations that are either covered by national health insurance or sell well in the domestic OTC market.

Regimes of regulation and reformulation emerge from this volume as fields in which a heterogeneous array of actors engage in continuous processes of translation between material, technical, economic, and social realms at various scales (see Callon 1986; Latour 1991; Brown 2002; Jasanoff 2004; Jasanoff and Kim 2015). We have seen how industry actors creatively work around problems, overcome contradictions and exploit new opportunities under varying degrees of accommodation on behalf of their counterparts in national governments and agencies. Asian medical industries provide numerous excellent examples of these translation processes in action, while also reflecting larger struggles over identity, modernity, nation building, development, and progress that are playing out as their societies undergo far-reaching change. Pharmaceutical regulation appears simultaneously as a field of top-down governance and control and as a horizontal plane on which various agendas converge to enable industrial growth and public health promotion. Similarly, the way that processes of industrialisation, pharmaceuticalisation, and globalisation combine to form particular reformulation regimes result in different articulations between scientific modes, medical epistemologies, technologies, regulations, and markets, involving various innovation pathways and new categories for classifying formulations and product types (Coderey and Pordié 2020; Chee, this volume, 2020; Lei 2014; Pordié and Gaudillière 2014a, b, c; Schrempf 2015).

It is noteworthy that the reformulation practices developed by Asian medical industries are shaping not only the field of therapeutics but also medical epistemology, etiology, and nosology. These industries can thus be seen as major forces driving the transformation of medical thought, knowledge, and practice more broadly. These transformations occur through myriad practices of hybridisation involving adapted "traditional" notions of syndromes and humours, biologically defined signs and biomedically defined symptoms, regulatory systems, material restrictions, and market logics. New medicines thus emerge along with new understandings of what diseases or disorders are, how they develop and how they can be addressed. Zooming into any Asian pharmaceutical product reveals a composite of old and new elements, both material and non-material. The dialectics of alternative modernity involved in such phenomena constantly challenge and redefine the boundaries between tradition and modernity, society, medicine and technology, the universal and the particular, rendering them ever less analytically useful as exclusive, standalone categories. The conceptual framework of the pharmaceutical assemblage helps to make these emergent processes visible and to trace out the connections between individual cases across various contexts and scales.

Raw materials in motion

Asian medical industries depend existentially upon medicinal plants and other raw materials of natural origin.[7] Although seemingly self-evident, this observation opens onto a whole raft of issues that are becoming increasingly critical for a wide range of actors, as several contributors to this volume underscore. To understand how these issues manifest themselves and to appreciate their role in shaping Asian medicines, we need to keep in mind how medicinal plants exist simultaneously as biological entities, symbols of cultural heritage and objects of laboratory research, wild-crafted items and agricultural products,[8] locally valued objects and globally traded commodities, ingredients in classical textual formulas and components in reformulated drugs, as well as being the focus of governance regimes at various levels. Medicinal plants also set herbal strands of pharmaceutical production apart from the biomedical sector in important ways, resisting the processes of convergence and hybridisation at play in domains such as drug discovery, reformulation, and productive technology, while directly participating in other fields of transformation.

Asian medicinal plants are in many ways quintessential global commodities. Many species have been traded for centuries or even millennia[9] and are today products with massive and growing global flows.[10] Their collection, cultivation, and trade have been subject to continuous change over long periods, but as several chapters in this volume note, recent decades have seen a sharp increase in the scale and force of transformation. Indeed, the remarkable growth of Asian medical industries has created an ever-increasing demand for hundreds of medicinal plant species, many of which remain wild-crafted, cultivated on a small scale, or restricted to specific locations and ecological niches. This has inevitably led to mounting

---

7 Although many Asian medicines include minerals, metals, or animal products, medicinal plants are by far the most widely utilised and provide the main focus of discussion in this volume.
8 Modes of medicinal plant stewardship and cultivation vary widely, but "wildness" and "domesticity" are more accurately seen as points along a continuum than as clearly distinct categories (Craig and Glover 2011; Springer 2015, 2016, 2019).
9 On the more than 3000-year history of global trade in nutmeg and cloves, see Andaya (1993) and Ellen (2003).
10 Recent estimates suggest that the global trade in medicinal and aromatic plants has an annual value between 3.6 billion USD (Vasisht et al. 2016) and 6.2 billion USD (Tripathi et al. 2017). This trade is growing at 2.4 percent per annum in terms of volume, but 9.2 percent in terms of value, showing how prices are rising significantly faster than the quantity traded (Vasisht et al. 2016).

pressure on stocks and thus to widespread shortages, price instability, and increasingly competitive sourcing activities (Thomas et al. 2005; Larsen and Olsen 2007). Over a similar period, discourses of biodiversity conservation and resource management have gained considerable prominence, combining with the interests of state and market actors to produce new modes of governance and control that extend from the global level through to national, local, and micro scales. Medicinal plants and those involved in their stewardship, cultivation, collection, and trade are coming into ever closer articulation with pharmaceutical manufacturers and with institutions, policies, laws concerned with resource management, conservation, trade, and regulation, within a broader global pattern of growing neoliberal hegemony. These developments hold enormous implications for Asian medical industries and for our understanding of pharmaceutical assemblages, several of which I draw out for further consideration here.

Despite an extensive literature concerning the medicinal plants of Asia, remarkably little published work positions itself to tackle the dynamic ways that industrial demands, regulatory regimes, political economies, and plant flows shape one another. Similarly, recent work has shed welcome light on the circulation and regulation of Asian pharmaceutical products (Pordié 2021; Pordié and Hardon 2015; Coderey and Pordié 2020), and the intellectual property dimensions of bioprospecting and drug discovery (Dutfield 2014; Gaudillière 2014; Dutfield et al. 2020; Madhavan and Gaudillière 2020), but largely overlooks the relationship between physical flows of raw material and medical industries. The chapters by Campinas, Dejouhanet and Sreelakshmy, and van der Valk make important critical contributions towards a clearer understanding of these dynamics. Several other chapters note the importance of control over the raw materials trade to the initial emergence of Asian medical industries, or consider how trade dynamics and medicine production shape one another in the present day. Blaikie and Craig, Campinas, and van der Valk also examine the positioning of medicinal plants within contemporary forms of governance, as well as the roles they play in emerging patterns of capitalist extraction and accumulation. These are all excellent starting points from which to explore relations between spatial, temporal, material, economic, political, and regulatory dimensions of Asian medical industries.

Such exploration is facilitated by Dejouhanet and Sreelakshmy's observation that raw material supply systems themselves can be understood as complex assemblages, which interact with and depend upon pharmaceutical constellations while remaining distinct from them. With this in mind, we can focus on fields where raw material and pharmaceutical assemblages intersect and mutually constitute one another, as well as locate areas where their components and dynamics differ. A further analytical step in this direction is offered by recent scholarship revolving around the concept of "frontier assemblages" (Cons and Eilenberg 2019). This work highlights the convergence of two phenomena in Asia over recent decades: the transformation of remote, mountainous, forested and agrarian spaces into sites for export-oriented extraction, and the transformation of these same spaces into sites for new forms of production. By approaching these as conjoined projects, the notion of frontier assemblages helps us to "move away from an exclusive focus on extraction and understand resource frontiers also as sites of creative, if often ruinous, production" (ibid.: 2). Zones of experimentation, innovation, and hybridity have emerged in frontier spaces across many parts of Asia in recent times, in which formerly stable boundaries are pushed at, existing limits, laws and models questioned, and relations transformed (ibid.: 7). The frontier assemblage approach is attuned to the powerful impetus of capitalist expansion in these processes of transformation, yet resists their reduction to mere functions of accumulation, urging caution so as not to conflate processes with complex origins and multiple causal elements with an overdetermined, exaggerated notion of neoliberalism (ibid.: 10).

There is much here that resonates with several themes running through the current volume, providing conceptual space in which to unite them in search of further insights. Medicinal raw material extraction is reaching further and deeper into every corner of Asia, at the same time as medical industries are establishing themselves, often in remote, marginal, or "underdeveloped" regions, where they transform raw materials originating across Asia's resource frontiers into products destined largely for distant markets. These new combinations of extraction and production are taking place within a field of experimentation and creative hybridity, not only in terms of the medicines themselves but also through new articulations of material, social, cultural, economic, and political resources that enable their production and circulation. Furthermore, while we can comfortably connect the accelerating medicinal plant flows, scaled-up production processes, and larger distribution networks associated with the consolidation of Asian medical industries to forms of profit-seeking and capitalist accumulation, it would be reductionist to propose these as the only forces driving such processes.

Several chapters, notably those focusing on Japan, show how vital the transnational trade in medicinal plants was to the historical development of medical industries in particular locations, as well as its continued importance for contemporary production. Arai et al. note the importance of herbs imported to Japan from China in the sixth century to the early development of Kampo. Along with Futaya and Blaikie, they also show how the later development of major Japanese plant trading hubs played crucial roles in the foundation of traditional - and later biomedical - pharmaceutical industries in specific locations, providing fertile ground for their subsequent interaction. Arai et al. also underscore the mounting difficulties Kampo manufacturers face in securing reliable supplies of high-quality raw materials in the present day. As 80 percent of the raw materials used in Kampo production are imported from China and demand for these resources is growing there also due to the expansion of the Chinese medicine industry, many large Japanese companies are developing their own closed supply chains by working directly with growers in China and beyond. Recent decades have also seen concerted efforts on behalf of various Japanese ministries and industry actors to reduce import dependence and simultaneously improve quality and GMP traceability by subsidising agricultural production of medicinal herbs inside Japan. These contributions illustrate how trade flows shaped the early development of Japan's herbal industries, as well as the growing importance of medicinal plants in wider economic, regulatory and geopolitical dynamics, including the expansion of resource frontiers across China and Southeast Asia.

Manuel Campinas' chapter explores several ways that medicinal plants are being manipulated in efforts to simultaneously establish a Qiang medicines industry and feed the broader Chinese medicine sector's growing demands. He first focuses on contested issues surrounding the ethnic labelling of medicinal plants and cultivars. Largely conducted by non-Qiang academics and entrepreneurs, such activities used "place of origin, assumed 'historical use' and Qiang-led cultivation in order to materialise Qiang ethnicity in a medicinal product, specifically for marketing purposes." Intensive cultivation efforts focusing on locally growing species with large national market demands resulted in new cultivars that defy the morphological parameters of the national pharmacopoeia. Disconnects subsequently multiplied between the scientists and entrepreneurs, who insist their cultivars have comparable potency to their wild counterparts, local people and Qiang doctors who continue to favour wild plants with familiar morphological forms and potencies, and the large firms producing medicines for national and global markets, who are happy to accept cheaper materials so long as they conform to their own minimum standards and increase their profit margins. Thus medicinal plants become objects of multiple fields of contestation as they are renamed, assigned ethnicities, selectively bred, collected from the wild, brought under cultivation and marketed, within a broader pattern of articulation from biological entity to industrial input.

The second important contribution of this chapter is the way it outlines the formation of a frontier assemblage par excellence. Here the broad political and economic objectives of China's transnational "Belt and Road" initiative combined with both regional economic stimulus programs and local conservation and development plans to result in the intensive agricultural production of medicinal plants. The aim of these coordinated policies is to supply huge quantities of raw materials to medical industries located within Sichuan, thus explicitly merging remote area extraction with production, as well as to feed factories elsewhere in the country and beyond. Campinas raises complex questions of quality control relating to the unregulated use of agricultural inputs and the voluntary nature of agricultural regulations. He shows how the disparagement of local herb collectors accompanies the championing of highly questionable "win-win" conservation and development scenarios, as well as how an ostensibly inclusive mode of development sidesteps local interests and needs, offering limited tangible benefits for the Qiang or their medical tradition. Thus, a vast state-industry-market assemblage co-opts a localised ethnic minority medicine while extending its resource frontiers to enable intensification of both regular and "salvage" (Tsing 2015) forms of capitalist accumulation.

A different strand of critical analysis emerges from the chapters focusing on South Asia. This questions the growing influence of quantitative, microeconomic readings of medicinal plant flows in shaping policies, laws, regulations, and academic discourses. Such reductionist approaches are epitomised in commodity-chain analyses and market surveys in which demand, supply, price, volume, quality, trade channels, and future access are key (and often the only) criteria. The trade is widely assumed to be vertically integrated and linear, with decision-making based on principles of rational profit maximisation. For many larger pharmaceutical manufacturers, such approaches have become the basis for supply chain management while they also inform the bulk of policymaking and regulatory intervention within state institutions. The chapters by Blaikie and Craig, Dejouhanet and Sreelakshmy, Madhavan and Soman, and van der Valk all illustrate, in different ways, how inadequate these models are to explaining how plants actually flow and how their values are indexed, and thus how inappropriate they are as the basis for state and industry-led efforts to control or modify plant circulations.

Dejouhanet and Sreelakshmy show how Keralan medicinal plant supply networks are responsive to a "changing combination of factors as diverse as: local history, caste and class hierarchy, geographical and social proximity, industrial dynamics, market demands, national or state policies on conservation or socioeconomic development, and interstate relations." They meticulously document multi-dimensional and multi-scalar plant flows, which are embedded in complex social networks and involve a wide range of relationship forms. The opaqueness of the actual dynamics at play when viewed from a linear, vertical, and single-channel perspective contributed to the failure of several government schemes to secure reliable industrial supply or improve the livelihoods of those engaged in collection and trade. Madhavan and Soman provide another example in support of this argument. They show how the CARe Keralam project underestimated the Ayurvedic industry's "dependence on long-established, trust-based raw material sourcing mechanisms," leading to miscalculated interventions and the inability of the scheme to meet its main objectives. Controlling and stabilising medicinal plant supplies is shown to be a crucial precursor to the government's aims of simultaneously raising production volume, efficiency, and quality, improving drug supplies for the 'mainstreaming' of Ayurveda into public health, and increasing export volumes. The scheme's failure highlights the many contradictions between these aims, especially in an era of substantial corporate consolidation in the sector, as well as a fundamental misreading of the dynamics at play in networks of material supply.

The chapter by Jan van der Valk highlights the inherent contradiction between continuous, profit-driven pharmaceutical industry growth and the sustainable management of largely wild-crafted plants, as well as tracing out emerging connections between scientific knowledge production, neoliberal policies, and regulatory systems. It argues that national-scale, technoscientific discourses of plant management and conservation in India[11] are not only based on inaccurate assumptions but are also implicated in inequitable and ineffective policies, with contradictory and often harmful outcomes. In this sense, his argument echoes and amplifies those expressed in the chapters concerning Kerala and Sichuan. Taking this line of critique further, van der Valk argues that current Indian regulatory interventions mainly serve to transfer control of resources, rights, profits, and legitimacy from heterogeneous, diverse, and small-scale actors to powerful bureaucracies and corporations. Heavily bureaucratic, largely ineffective in terms of its stated aims and itself riddled with corruption, this system forces plant collectors and traders to operate in legal grey zones or indeed in breach of the law, while facilitating "accumulation by dispossession" and "accumulation by conservation" for those in positions of power, including large pharmaceutical firms.

This chapter offers an incisive critical framework through which articulations between pharmaceutical, raw material, and regulatory assemblages can be traced, both through macro-scale developments in the spheres of policy and ground level readings from the perspective of those involved in small-scale plant trade. Such a framing takes us to the very heart of the paradox facing Asian medical industries. Their continued growth depends on ever-larger supplies of precarious natural resources, the provision of which involves large numbers of people struggling to adapt to governance regimes that often work against their interests, while furthering those of local elites and contributing to global patterns of accumulation that, in turn, further threaten the resource base and those most dependent upon it. This formulation resonates with other contributions to this book and with a good deal of recent literature across several academic fields, providing a valuable counterpoint to the (exhausted, but still widespread) narrative that continuous industrial expansion, ecological sustainability, and inclusive socioeconomic development are not only commensurable but readily achievable through macro-scale policy, regulatory, and institutional interventions.

While such critical approaches are vital for accurate understandings of contemporary dynamics, caution is required lest we lapse into reductive readings of complex, historically contingent and multi-causal phenomena. For example, neoliberalism is a highly malleable concept that has been defined and deployed in several ways over the last two centuries (Brisbois et al. 2021; Collier 2012; Ferguson 2010; Harvey 2007; Ong 2006; Ortner

---

11 See Gaudillière (2014a) for further details.

2011). It has become too unwieldy and contested a term to use without lengthy qualification, so while its application in relation to natural resource management and biodiversity conservation appears increasingly necessary, it is also fraught with problems (Büscher et al. 2012). If all medicinal plant related activities, policies, and interventions that engage with capitalist markets are dismissed out of hand as being inherently neoliberal, the term further loses analytical specificity and serves more to obfuscate than reveal contemporary political-economic-ecological dynamics. Critical perspectives are crucial to distinguish between different approaches, aims, and implications within this field; to call out those that exacerbate precarity and normalise exploitation while supporting those working towards more equitable and resilient interventions. While remaining attuned to the powerful and arguably ruinous role that emerging forms of capitalist accumulation play in animating Asian medical industries and in shaping the raw material assemblages they depend upon, it is necessary to clearly specify our technical terms and consider both their contested theoretical underpinnings and the complex ground realities they ostensibly index.

Blaikie and Craig touch on these issues while tracing similar processes to those described for India unfolding in Nepal. They take the viewpoint of *amchi* pharmacists working in cottage industries, who are also dependent on complex and precarious networks of plant trade. As conservation and management discourses gain traction and regulations tighten, informal networks animated by personal ties are weakening and being replaced by middlemen and commercial traders better able to navigate bureaucratic obstacles. Top-down regulatory and management systems criminalise local collectors and informal traders at the periphery, favouring large industrial players located mostly outside Nepal and thus enabling the generation of profits through "salvage accumulation" (Tsing 2015). We glimpse here both direct and indirect relationships between large factories producing Asian herbal medicines and the small-scale manufacturers who remain crucial healthcare providers across much of the continent. Large firms based in India and China can bribe their way around regulations in order to collect massive volumes while also outbidding smaller operators for the plants available in the marketplace, forcing up prices and reducing availability for ordinary buyers. These combined trends are pushing cottage industry manufacturers to scale up and become more profit-oriented, despite the reluctance of many to do so. The authors also note the resilience of personal networks and moral economic principles in animating plant flows, despite the increasingly capitalist formations within which medicine production and circulation are subsumed. This is epitomised in the lone trader upon whom large numbers of commercial Sowa Rigpa pharmacists in India and Nepal depend for access to crucial plants. He sells to them at deliberately low prices and nurtures long-standing relationships rather than using his customers' dependence as leverage to maximise short-term gains. Echoing aspects of the Keralan and North Indian networks discussed above, this case also points to the limits of reductive microeconomic models for understanding plant flows, as well as to the failure of mainstream conservation and development discourses and interventions to result in effective, let alone equitable or locally appropriate, management policies.

It is worth briefly noting here that many reformulation practices reflect the declining availability and protected status of certain raw materials (Pordié 2014), while at the same time, GMP-linked requirements of "traceability" (Dejouhanet and Sreelakshmy, this volume; Lubbe and Verpoorte 2011; WHO 2018) are bringing notions of origin, "terroir" and territoriality into a picture that was, until recently, one of relatively undifferentiated and seemingly limitless raw material stocks and flows. Similarly, mounting concerns over pollution and contamination levels in medicinal plant materials (Arai et al., this volume; Dwivedi and Dey 2002; Govindaraghavan 2008; van der Valk, this volume) are both adding new questions over the safety of herbal medicines and pushing resource frontiers outwards in the search for "pure" sources of supply. It appears that Asian medicine producers will be increasingly forced to confront questions of raw material substitution, traceability, and contamination over the years to come, which will, in turn, impact upon collection and cultivation practices as well as reshaping formularies, regulatory regimes, and market dynamics.

To sum up, the raw material domain of Asian medical industries emerges from this volume as a constantly shifting configuration of heterogeneous components, including (but not limited to): plants as biological entities and the ecologies that sustain them; the people involved in all stages of their collection, cultivation, and trade; the governance and regulatory systems concerning them at various scales; patterns of local and industrial demand; and the various material, economic, symbolic and analytical uses to which they are put. Whether we think of these as assemblages, multi-species entanglements (Ogden et al. 2013), or actor-networks (Law and Hassard 1999; Latour 2005), it is clear that multiple, contingent elements are always involved in the transit of raw materials from their places of origin to the pharmacies and factories that depend upon them for their continued existence. Isolating one or a set of these variables as the basis for regulation and management always involves political and economic decision-making, and how these decisions are framed on high and implemented on the ground holds huge implications for the plants, collectors, growers, traders, practitioners, and industries concerned, as well as for those observing them from the outside.

Assembling tentative conclusions

In light of the above discussion, as well as the case studies and broader literature that informed it, this final section proposes some tentative conclusions concerning the configuration, orientation, and dynamics of Asian medical industries. Given the diversity and complexity of the factors at play, these reflections serve only to draw together some common threads in search of larger patterns, highlight areas of tension, and draw attention to issues that demand further research.

Firstly, focusing on Asian medicines as industries reveals remarkable similarities in terms of the characteristics, dynamics, and problematics involved. Although the cases discussed both here and elsewhere[12] concern specific medical traditions, historical trajectories, socioeconomic-political circumstances, and cultural configurations, which make each case unique, there are numerous parallels that merit brief reiteration here. All of these industries depend on raw materials of natural origin and as they expand in scale, are exerting mounting pressure on these resources. This is resulting in heightened internal and transnational competition over these materials, the expanding and deepening of resource frontiers, as well as a range of more or less contentious governance systems and regulatory interventions. All these industries are engaged to some degree in reshaping medicines at the level of their constitution through various innovation practices and reformulation regimes, as well as in terms of their production processes and final form through new technologies and packaging. All are in articulation with emergent forms of pharmaceutical governance at various scales, including global and national regulatory regimes, epitomised in GMP and other "good practices." These emerging modes of reformulation, production, and regulation all bring Asian medicines into closer interaction with discourses, practices, and standards derived from biomedicine and bioscience, forging new modes of adaptation, integration, and hybridity, which are expressed in material, social and discursive registers. We have also seen how industries across Asia are extending their reach within the domestic sphere, both through public health systems and private sales and in some cases, are pushing (or aspiring to push) further into global markets. Furthermore, in many cases, tensions are evident as proponents of different understandings of medical tradition and different approaches to pharmaceutical development coexist or compete in overlapping terrains of production. While remaining sensitive to their many unique features, it thus appears valid to approach these industries as one field of enquiry and to study them using a common analytical framework.

The editors of this volume propose assemblage thinking as a fruitful way to approach the complexity, fluidity, creativity, and emergent properties of the phenomena described within it. This approach keeps analysis open to the wide range of material and non-material components involved in the production, regulation, and circulation of Asian medicines. By placing the convergence and articulation of these heterogeneous components at the centre of enquiry, we can resist assumptions of structural solidity or simple causality. This allows us to glimpse moments of pharmaceutical,

---

12 See: Bode (2008), Banerjee (2009), Lei (2014), Pordié and Gaudillière (2014a), Pordié and Hardon (2015), and Coderey and Pordié (2020).

governance, and raw material assemblages in flux, as well as the way they interact with and coproduce one another. Each contribution to the volume traces aspects of these interactions and alignments, helping to place each case both in its specific context and in relation to the others. Although theorists such as Deleuze and Guattari (1987) and DeLanda (2006, 2016) have advanced a sophisticated "view of reality in which assemblages are everywhere, multiplying in every direction" (DeLanda 2016: 7), we apply the framework in a deliberately loose, descriptive manner rather than as a unified theory of everything. Without wishing to be drawn into complex philosophical reflections and theoretical debates, we focus on particular constellations and on interactions within and between them while striving also to do justice to the experiences of the people and organisations involved. With this in mind, it is vital that researchers across several academic disciplines continue to conduct fine-grained, topically focused, and spatially delimited studies into particular aspects of Asian medical industries. Such research is necessary and important in its own right while also potentially providing accurate data and insights to enable further analytical work from an assemblage perspective.

My second tentative conclusion supports Stephan Kloos' assertion in the introduction of the need to move beyond "Asian medical systems" as the basic framework for understanding non-biomedical forms of healing across the continent. This volume offers ample evidence of Asian medicines as dynamic, vibrant, and messy fields, suggesting that assumptions of stasis, boundedness, coherence, and inward orientation no longer hold. Indeed, it is arguably time to go further and question the extent to which Asian medical traditions were ever stable, coherent, bounded, or distinct. Recent work in anthropology and history supports a robust challenge to this view, suggesting a multiplicity of partially overlapping traditions characterised by continuous debate, rupture, and reconfiguration (Sivaramakrishnan 2005; Attewell 2007; Scheid 2007; Pati and Harrison 2008; Hardiman and Mukharji 2012; Kumar and Basu 2013; Mukharji 2016). This is not to deny the extent to which many forms of Asian medicine remain deeply embedded within specific medical epistemologies, cultures and histories, ethnic and religious identities, or ethical frameworks. However, such fields of continuity must now be placed in a theoretical framework that can also handle the pace and implications of far-reaching processes of interconnection, transformation, adaptation, and innovation, or the emergence of an ongoing series of hybrid forms, which are especially pronounced in the pharmaceutical realm. We thus need to be open to applying similar methodological tools and theoretical approaches to "traditional medicine" as we do to biomedicine or other fields where science, technology, society, and culture intertwine. Asian medicines, increasingly formed around and represented by their industries, demand approaches that are contemporary, critical, and comparative, not static, romanticised, or relativistic. For example, the urgent need for more engaged, critical scholarship linking issues of resource extraction, governance, and medicine production stands out strongly in several chapters. Further research into patterns of state and private investment, ownership, and corporate consolidation in Asian pharmaceutical companies, as well as studies of profit flows and development strategies, also appears timely. Such studies will be severely hampered if tied to notions of bounded, independent, and homogenous medical systems. Similarly, our collective understanding of innovation and reformulation practices cannot progress far if research retains assumptions of clear dividing lines between medical traditions, bioscience, and other knowledge forms, the universal and the particular, the global and the local, rather than seeing how these fields increasingly interpenetrate and coproduce one another.

My third point tempers and grounds the second. Although this volume attests to industrialisation, pharmaceuticalisation, reformulation, and market expansion as clear trends that are either well-established or gathering momentum across Asia, it does not suggest that they are consistent, uniform, inexorable or totalising processes. As Blaikie and Craig demonstrate for Nepal, Campinas shows for Sichuan and the chapters regarding Kerala allude to, small pharmacies remain important producers of medicine in many areas, just as individual – and often officially unrecognised – practitioners remain crucial healthcare providers for large numbers of Asian people.[13] Far from invalidating the arguments presented in this book, such observations highlight the importance of careful and ongoing evaluation of the evolving relationships between Asian medical industries and the many diverse, non-industrialised, and locally valued forms of production and medical practice that coexist with them (Adams, Schrempf and Craig 2011; Craig 2012; Blaikie 2013; Blaikie et al. 2015). Finding ways to describe and analyse these often conflicting elements together presents many challenges but is surely necessary in order to accurately understand contemporary Asian medicines and reflect upon the changing role of drug production within them.

While continuing to trace out the evolving forms of Asian medical industries, future research must take into account the divisions, debates, and growing power differentials that have often accompanied their emergence. For example, the large pharmaceutical corporations we have read about in China, India, and Japan generate sizable profits for owners or shareholders by behaving in many similar ways to biomedical firms or companies in other sectors. They are resolutely profit motivated and growth oriented, seeking competitive advantage through technological advance and innovation, mergers or the incorporation of smaller firms, and extensive marketing campaigns. This orientation reflects what Blaikie and Craig call "big pharma with traditional characteristics." Although by no means ubiquitous,

---

13 See also: Craig (2008, 2012), Blaikie (2011, 2013, 2015, 2018), Hardiman and Mukharji (2012), Sujatha and Abraham (2012), Hofer (2018), Kloos et al. (2020), and Pordié and Kloos (2022).

we can detect a general trend among such firms towards the targeting of middle-class, wealthy, and overseas consumers, which without doubt contributes to pushing industrially produced herbal medicines increasingly out of the reach of the rural and urban poor. Furthermore, several chapters in this volume show how the increasing capture of raw material flows by large firms is raising prices and making access difficult for smaller producers and individual healers, increasing their precarity while jeopardising access to drugs for those sections of the population already facing limited therapeutic options. At the same time, larger scales of production that increasingly focus on reformulated and OTC medicines are eliciting strong critical responses from some smaller-scale producers and practitioners, for whom classical formulas, low-tech production, and healer-mediated, individually tailored treatment regimens epitomise their vision of medical tradition. These debates frequently take on ethical, social, and economic, as well as medical, technical, and epistemological dimensions, all of which must be taken seriously as scholarship concerning these issues progresses.

My fourth point of conclusion highlights the way new drug forms (particularly OTC) contribute to the global trend of pharmaceuticalisation, with significant implications not only for pharmacy but also for medical epistemology and practice, popular understandings of disease, and treatment modality. Until recent decades, Chinese medicine, Ayurveda, Sowa Rigpa, and Kampo treatments were founded in personal interactions between patients and practitioners. Diagnosis proceeded according to textually inscribed theories and embodied techniques, based on very different models of the body, disease, and remedy to those of biomedicine. Treatments were, ideally, tailored to individual cases (according to bodily constitution, phase of disease, etc.) and might include simple or compound drugs but also behavioural advice and external treatments, as well as rituals and mantras in some cases. Although these kinds of clinical interactions still take place in many locations, the shift towards the mass-production of reformulated and OTC drugs in Asian medical industries reflects a very different model. Here, symptomatic categories based on biomedical concepts lead to the self-prescription of standardised drugs that correspond to these categories. Thus, reformulation in Asian medicines contributes directly to pharmaceuticalisation by de-emphasising the role of practitioners in medical treatment and further raising drugs above all other forms of remedy (Kudlu 2016). This "transfer of power from the doctor to the medicine" (Pordié 2014: 71), in turn, plays a major role in the replacement of canonical and medical tradition-based understandings of health, disease, and treatment with biomedically derived symptomatic indices, as well as the bypassing of practitioners and the rejection of individually tailored therapeutic responses in favour of largely self-administered "one-size-fits-all" products. Future studies of reformulation, new drug delivery forms, and marketing strategies must take careful account of these transformative interrelations between pharmaceutical practice, medical epistemology, disease representation, self-care practice, and sociomedical organisation.

The fifth reflection concerns the centrality of domestic markets to the growth, consolidation, and orientation of Asian medical industries. While this volume confirms these industries as increasingly global in scope, it also shows domestic markets as key to patterns of pharmaceutical development across Asia. Despite the continued growth of the Complementary and Alternative Medicine (CAM) market in the global north (Tovey et al. 2004) and the aspirations (particularly in China and India) to reach further into them, it is primarily national concerns that drive these industries forward and dictate their production and marketing activities. As Kudlu illustrates so elegantly in her chapter, discrepancies between imagined futures of global market expansion and the realities of Ayurvedic companies' domestic focus continue to reverberate, feeding back to create tensions both in regulatory spheres and between Ayurveda's diverse constitution on the ground and the idealised image of it as projected by the nationalist state. These arguments further nuance her earlier work (Kudlu and Nichter 2019), which shows just how challenging, expensive, and risky it is for Asian firms to try to gain access to North American and European markets, making such attempts unrealistic for all but the largest and most confident firms. More research is called for to untangle claimed global market aspirations from concrete efforts to increase overseas sales at the national and firm levels, to establish the medicine forms and volumes that are actually circulating transnationally, and to critically evaluate the role of regulatory regimes in the global north in shaping transnational flows of Asian medicines (Schwabl 2009, 2015; Wang 2020). It also appears important for future studies to continue assessing the ways in which global aspirations shape national regulatory policies within Asia, as well as how they affect reformulation practices and the reclassification of medicines as supplements, nutraceuticals, or food products in order to enter otherwise restricted markets both at home and abroad (Chee, this volume, 2020; Kuo 2009, 2015; Coderey and Pordié 2020; Ma 2020).

The centrality of the domestic sphere also reflects the integration of Asian medicines into national public healthcare systems. Chee's chapter shows how Chinese medicine's longstanding role in public healthcare provision has significantly shaped its industry. Arai et al. demonstrate how such factors crystallised more recently in Japan, with Kampo medicines being widely prescribed by doctors under national insurance coverage from the 1960s onwards, contributing enormously to the industry's subsequent growth and transformation. Integration patterns have thus exerted significant effects on the industry in both these countries, particularly in relation to regulatory regimes, productive technologies, economies of scale, and the dynamics of reformulation. Further research is needed to clarify these relations, especially as it appears that public healthcare demands shape industrial pharmaceutical production in quite different ways to private market concerns. While the former tends towards mass production of classical and other well-known formulas at low cost, the latter encourages far greater degrees of innovation and reformulation, as well as a clear focus on branded OTC products. The 2005 launch of the National Health Mission heralded the beginning of large-scale public supply of traditional medicines in India (Madhavan and Soman, this volume; Priya and Shweta 2010; Blaikie 2019). The effects these new state-managed demands have upon the Ayurveda, Unani, Siddha, and Sowa Rigpa industries also offer fruitful avenues for future research, including questions of corporate consolidation and the role of state-industry "syndicates" (Hardiman 2009) in an era of expanding public-private partnership.

The final set of conclusions reflect upon instability and tension, both as particularly salient characteristics of Asian medical industries to date and as useful concepts through which to think about their contemporary dynamics and possible futures. Much of this book addresses these industries' struggles to adapt to constantly changing conditions, tracing their passage through periods of decline and growth, fracture and reconstitution. Although the "industrial revolution" of recent decades has brought considerable economic growth, sociopolitical legitimation, and institutional consolidation in many cases, it has also involved a great deal of flux and tension. Industry actors continue to navigate shifting relationships with state governments, healthcare systems, and regulatory regimes, to push into new markets or reposition themselves in existing ones, and to experiment with hybrid research paradigms, new technologies, and modes of reformulation. Although these transformative processes have different starting points and varying trajectories, they are ongoing in every case and are in many ways central to the identity, operations, and dynamics of these industries. This leads me to conclude that Asian medical industries have not cohered into stable apparatuses with firmly established structures and properties, or predictable modes of action and interaction.

Asian medical traditions have changed and adapted throughout their histories, as a large body of literature attests. What, then, does this book show that is new or different about this most recent phase of transformation? What does it tell us about the position and role of pharmaceutical industries within this changing context, or about how we might better conceptualise the observed phenomena? To begin with, each chapter focuses in one way or another upon *interconnections between clusters of heterogeneous components*. They show how industry actors at different levels interact with medicinal plants and their suppliers, with state bureaucracies, laws, policies, and regulations, with concepts of traditional and biomedical origin, with old and new technologies, with sociotechnical and ethical imaginaries, and with forces associated with globalisation and capitalism. Despite the many particularities of each case, when looked at together they all suggest a significant multiplication and deepening of interconnections, as well as an accelerating rate at which they are formed and modified, which correspond with this recent period of industrial emergence and consolidation. Assemblage thinking helps to see these as open-ended processes of emergence, or ongoing states of becoming. New articulations are continually being forged between components while others weaken, hierarchies are reordered through phases of stratification, and pharmaceutical assemblages recompose themselves through relations of contingency. Instead of being assumed to be clearly defined entities that are "influenced" or "shaped by" external forces, contemporary Asian medical industries can rather be understood to be *constituted of*, and *existing through*, these myriad articulations of material and expressive components. Pharmaceutical assemblages exhibit varying patterns of internal coherence and tension; they overlap and interact with numerous other constellations; and continually recompose themselves through processes of de- and re-territorialisation. Taken as an analytical framework rather than an explanatory theory, this approach enables us to account for complexity, variability, and dynamism, and to appreciate both continuity and change while resisting the lure of grand narratives, simple causality, or teleology.

Identifying Asian medical industries as a larger phenomenon with many shared characteristics, dynamics, and problematics does not deny diversity, the specificity of individual cases, or the validity of other analytical approaches to these matters. It also does not suggest that we should only focus on the "big picture," as the tightly focused contributions to this book amply demonstrate. However, it does suggest that this larger shared context cannot be ignored in future studies of Asian medicine, which will surely need to position themselves within it, or in relation to it. This offers fresh approaches to studying local particularities, different questions to ask of them, and new ways of understanding and contextualising them in relation to one another, as well as to broader patterns of change. Alongside other recent literature widely cited within it, this book highlights several fields of tension whose resolution (or not) over the years to come will contribute in crucial ways to the further composition of Asia's herb-based pharmaceutical industries, as well as providing important foci for further research. For example, tensions surrounding raw materials, sustainability, growth, and equity; debates over science, epistemology, and hybridity; or the relationship between corporate consolidation and smaller scales of production all demand detailed and critically informed study. Such research will only gain analytical acuity and comparative scope by being placed within the larger framework identified here.

By establishing viable industries, developing larger markets, and carving out roles for themselves in public healthcare systems Asian medicines have gained far greater status, legitimacy, and influence than seemed possible a few decades ago. Asian medical industries have become integral parts of societies that have themselves been through rapid and profound change. They thus offer a lens through which these wider transformations can be viewed and made sense of, while also suggesting fresh avenues of approach to processes of knowledge production, capitalist expansion, globalisation, governance, resource management, and pharmaceuticalisation at various scales.

Acknowledgements

The author is grateful for the support received from the *Reassembling Tibetan Medicine* project (ERC 336932) during the early phases of writing this chapter, and to the *Integrating Traditional Medicine* project (Austrian Science Fund / FWF P34010-G) during the latter stages.

Bibliography

Adams V, Schrempf M and Craig SR (eds) (2011) *Medicine between Science and Religion: Explorations on Tibetan Grounds.* Oxford: Berghahn Books.

Adams V, Miller S, Craig SR, et al. (2005) The Challenge of Cross-Cultural Clinical Trials Research: Case Report from the Tibetan Autonomous Region, People's Republic of China. *Medical Anthropology Quarterly* 19(3): 267–289.

Andaya L (1993) *The World of Maluku: Eastern Indonesia in the Early Modern Period.* Honolulu, HI: University of Hawaii Press.

Attewell G (2007) *Refiguring Unani Tibb: Plural Healing in Late Colonial India.* New Delhi: Orient Longman.

Banerjee M (2009) *Power, Knowledge, Medicine: Ayurvedic Pharmaceuticals at Home and in the World.* Hyderabad: Orient Blackswan.

Banerjee M (2014) Contemporary Conversations between Ayurveda and Biomedicine – from Reformulating Drugs to Refashioning Parameters. *Asian Medicine* 9(1–2): 141–170.

Berger R (2013) *Ayurveda Made Modern: Political Histories of Indigenous Medicine in North India, 1900–1955.* Basingstoke: Palgrave Macmillan.

Biehl J and Petryna A (eds) (2013) *When People Come First: Critical Studies in Global Health.* Princeton, NJ: Princeton University Press.

Blaikie C (2011) Critically Endangered? Medicinal Plant Cultivation and the Reconfiguration of Sowa Rigpa in Ladakh. *Asian Medicine* 5: 243–272.

Blaikie C (2013) Currents of Tradition in Sowa Rigpa Pharmacy. *East Asian Science, Technology and Society* 7: 425–451.

Blaikie C (2015) Wish-fulfilling Jewel Pills: Tibetan Medicines from Exclusivity to Ubiquity. *Anthropology & Medicine* 22(1): 7–22.

Blaikie C (2018) Absence, Abundance and Excess: Substances and Sowa Rigpa in Ladakh since the 1960s. In: Deb Roy R and Attewell G (eds) *Locating the Medical: Explorations in South Asian History.* New Delhi: Oxford University Press, 169–199.

Blaikie C (2019) Mainstreaming Marginality: Traditional Medicine and Primary Healthcare in Himalayan India. *Asian Medicine* 14: 145–172.

Blaikie C, Craig S, Hofer T et al. (2015) Co-Producing Efficacious Medicines: Collaborative Ethnography with Tibetan Medicine Practitioners in Kathmandu, Nepal. *Current Anthropology* 56(2): 178–204.

Bode, M (2008) *Taking Traditional Knowledge to the Market: The Modern Image of the Ayurvedic and Unani Industry.* Hyderabad: Orient Blackswan.

Brisbois B, Feagan M, Stime B et al. (2021) Mining, Colonial Legacies, and Neoliberalism: A Political Ecology of Health Knowledge. *New Solutions* 31(1): 48–64.

Brown S (2002) Michel Serres: Science, Translation and the Logic of the Parasite. *Theory, Culture & Society* 19(3): 1–27.

Büscher B, Sullivan S, Neves K et al. (2012) Towards a Synthesized Critique of Neoliberal Biodiversity Conservation. *Capitalism Nature Socialism* 23(2): 4–30.

Callon M (1986) Some Elements of a Sociology of Translation: The Domestication of the Scallops and the Fishermen of St. Brieuc Bay. In: Law J (ed) *Power, Action and Belief: A New Sociology of Knowledge?* London: Routledge & Kegan Paul.

Chatterjee P (1986) *The Nation and Its Fragments: Colonial and Postcolonial Histories.* Washington: University of Washington Press.

Chatterjee P (2004) *The Politics of the Governed: Reflections on Popular Politics in Most of the World.* New York, NY: Columbia University Press.

Chee LPY (2020) Health Products at the Boundary between Food and Pharmaceuticals: The Case of Fish Liver Oil. In Coderey C and Pordié L (eds) *Circulation and Governance of Asian Medicine*. London: Routledge, pp. 103–117.

Chen K-H (2010) *Asia as Method: Toward Deimperialization.* London: Duke University Press.

Coderey C (2020) Governing Medical Traditions in Myanmar. In Coderey C and Pordié L (eds) *Circulation and Governance of Asian Medicine*. London: Routledge, pp. 63–82.

Coderey C and Pordié L (eds) (2020) *Circulation and Governance of Asian Medicine*. London: Routledge.

Collier S (2012) Neoliberalism as Big Leviathan. *Social Anthropology* 20(2): 186–195.

Collier S and Ong A (eds) (2005) *Global Assemblages: Technology, Politics and Ethics as Anthropological Problems.* Oxford: Blackwell.

Cons J and Eilenberg M (eds) (2019) *Frontier Assemblages: The Emergent Politics of Resource Frontiers in Asia.* Chichester: Wiley.

Corbridge S, Willams G, Srivastava M, et al. (2005) *Seeing the State: Governance and Governmentality in India.* Cambridge: Cambridge University Press.

Craig SR (2008) Place and Professionalization: Navigating *Amchi* Identity in Nepal. In Pordié L (ed), *Tibetan Medicine in the Contemporary World.* Abingdon, VA: Routledge, pp. 62–90.

Craig SR (2011) 'Good' Manufacturing by Whose Standards? Remaking Concepts of Quality, Safety, and Value in the Production of Tibetan Medicines. *Anthropological Quarterly* 84(2): 331–378.

Craig SR (2012) *Healing Elements: Efficacy and the Social Ecologies of Tibetan Medicine.* Berkeley, CA: University of California Press.

Craig SR and Adams V (2008) Global Pharma in the Land of Snows: Tibetan Medicines, SARS, and Identity Politics across Nations. *Asian Medicine* 4: 1–28.

Craig SR and Bista G (2005) Himalayan Healers in Transition: Professionalization, Identity and Conservation among Practitioners of *gso ba rig pa* in Nepal. In Thomas Y, Karki M, Gurung K and Parajuli D (eds), *Himalayan Medicinal and Aromatic Plants: Balancing Use and Conservation.* Kathmandu: Government of Nepal Ministry of Forests and Soil Conservation.

Craig SR, Gerke B and Sheldon V (2020) Sowa Rigpa Humanitarianism: Local Logics of Care within a Global Politics of Compassion. *Medical Anthropology Quarterly* 34(2): 174–191.

Craig SR and Glover D (2011) Conservation, Cultivation, and Commodification of Medicinal Plants in the Greater Himalayan-Tibetan Plateau. *Asian Medicine* 5: 219–242.

Das V and Poole D (eds) (2004) *Anthropology in the Margins of the State*. Santa Fe, NM: School of American Research Press.

DeLanda M (2016) *Assemblage Theory*. Edinburgh: Edinburgh University Press.

DeLanda M (2006) *A New Philosophy of Society: Assemblage Theory and Social Complexity*. New York, NY: Continuum Books.

Deleuze G and Guattari F (1987) *A Thousand Plateaus*. Minneapolis, MN: University of Minnesota Press.

Dutfield G (2014) Traditional Knowledge, Intellectual Property and Pharmaceutical Innovation: What's Left to Discuss? In David M and Halbert D(eds) *The Sage Handbook of Intellectual Property*. London: Sage.

Dutfield G, Wynberg R, Laird S, et al. 2020. Benefit Sharing and Traditional Knowledge: Unsolved Dilemmas for Implementation. *The Challenge of Attribution and Origin: Traditional Knowledge and Access and Benefit Sharing*. Voices for BioJustice: Policy Brief.

Dwivedi S and Dey S (2002) Medicinal Herbs: A Potential Source of Toxic Metal Exposure for Man and Animals in India. *Archives of Environmental Health* 57(3): 229–231.

Ellen R (2003) *On the Edge of the Banda Zone: Past and Present in the Social Organisation of a Moluccan Trading Network*. Honolulu, HI: University of Hawaii Press.

Ferguson J (2010) The Uses of Neoliberalism. *Antipode* 41(S1): 166–184.

Fuller CJ and Benei V (eds) (2001) *The Everyday State and Society in Modern India*. London: Hurst.

Gaonkar DP (ed) (2001) *Alternative Modernities*. Durham: Duke University Press.

Gaudillière J-P (2014) Herbalised Ayurveda? Reformulation, Plant Management and the 'Pharmaceuticalisation' of Indian Traditional Medicine. *Asian Medicine* 9(1–2): 171–205.

Govindaraghavan S (2008) Quality Assurance of Herbal Raw Materials in Supply Chain: Challenges and Opportunities. *Journal of Dietary Supplements* 5(2): 176–212.

Gyatso J (2015) *Being Human in a Buddhist World: An Intellectual History of Medicine in Early Modern Tibet*. New York, NY: Columbia University Press.

Hardiman D (2009) Indian Medical Indigeneity: From Nationalist Assertion to Global Market. *Social History* 34(3): 263–283.

Hardiman D and Mukharji PB (eds) (2012) *Medical Marginality in South Asia: Situating Subaltern Therapeutics*. London: Routledge.

Harvey D (2007) *A Brief History of Neoliberalism*. Oxford: Oxford University Press.

Hofer T (2018) *Medicine and Memory in Tibet: Amchi Physicians in an Age of Reform*. Seattle: University of Washington Press.

Hsu E (2009) Chinese Propriety Medicines: An "Alternative Modernity?" The Case of the Anti-Malarial Substance Artemisinin in East Africa. *Medical Anthropology* 28(2): 111–140.

Jasanoff S (ed) (2004) *States of Knowledge: The Co-Production of Science and Social Order*. London: Routledge.

Jasanoff S and Kim S-H (eds) (2015) *Dreamscapes of Modernity: Sociotechnical Imaginaries and the Fabrication of Power*. London: Chicago University Press.

Kadetz P (2015) Problematizing the 'Global' in Global Health: An Assessment of the Global Discourse of Safety. *Fudan Journal of the Humanities and Social Sciences* 9: 25–40.

Kadetz P (2016) Safety Net: The Construction of Biomedical Safety in the Global 'Traditional Medicine' Discourse. *Asian Medicine* 10(1): 1–31.

Kloos S (2017) The Pharmaceutical Assemblage: Rethinking Sowa Rigpa and the Herbal Pharmaceutical Industry in Asia. *Current Anthropology* 58(6): 693–717.

Kloos S, Madhavan H, Tidwell T, Blaikie C and Cuomu M (2020) The Transnational Sowa Rigpa Industry in Asia: New Perspectives on an Emerging Economy. *Social Science & Medicine* 245 (112617).

Kudlu C (2016) Keeping the Doctor in the Loop: Ayurvedic Pharmaceuticals in Kerala. *Anthropology & Medicine* 23(3): 275–294.

Kudlu C and Nichter M (2019) Indian Imaginaries of Chinese Success in the global Herbal Medicine Market: A Critical Assessment. *Asian Medicine* 14: 104–144.

Kumar D and Basu RS (eds) (2013) *Medical Encounters in British India*. New Delhi: Oxford University Press.

Kumari R and Kotecha M (2016) A Review on the Standardization of Herbal Medicines. *International Journal of Pharmaceutical Sciences and Research* 7(2): 97–106.

Kuo W-H (2009) The Voice on the Bridge: Taiwan's Regulatory Engagement in Global Pharmaceuticals. *East Asian Science, Technology, and Society* 3(1): 51–72.

Kuo W-H (2015) Promoting Chinese Herbal Drugs through Regulatory Globalisation: The Case of the Consortium for Globalization of Chinese Medicine. *Asian Medicine* 10(2): 316–339.

Lama YC, Ghimire S and Aumeeruddy-Thomas Y (2001) *Medicinal Plants of Dolpo: Amchi's Knowledge and Conservation*. Kathmandu: WWF Nepal Program Publication Series.

Larsen HO and Olsen CS (2007) Unsustainable Collection and Unfair Trade? Uncovering and Assessing Assumptions Regarding Central Himalayan Medicinal Plant Conservation. *Biodiversity Conservation* 16: 1679–1697.

Latour B (1991) Technology Is Society Made Durable. In: Law J(ed) *A Sociology of Monsters: Essays on Power, Technology and Domination*. London: Routledge.

Latour B (2005) *Reassembling the Social: An Introduction to Actor-Network-Theory*. Oxford: Oxford University Press.

Law J and Hassard J (eds) (1999) *Actor Network Theory and After*. Oxford: Blackwell.

Law W and Salick J (2005) Human-Induced Dwarfing of Himalayan Snow Lotus, *Saussurea laniceps* (Asteraceae). *PNAS* 102(29): 10218–10220.

Lei SH-L (2014) *Neither Donkey nor Horse: Medicine in the Struggle over China's Modernity*. Chicago: University of Chicago Press.

Leslie C (ed) (1976) *Asian Medical Systems: A Comparative Study*. Berkeley, CA: University of California Press.

Leslie C and Young A (eds) (1992) *Paths to Asian Medical Knowledge*. Berkeley, CA: University of California Press.

Lubbe A and Verpoorte R (2011) Cultivation of Medicinal and Aromatic Plants for Specialty Industrial Materials. *Industrial Crops and Products* 34(1): 785–801.

Ma E (2020) Science as a Global Governance and Circulation Tool? The *Baekshuoh* Disaster in South Korea. In: Coderey C and Pordié L(eds) *Circulation and Governance of Asian Medicine*. London: Routledge, pp. 48–62.

Madhavan H and Gaudillière J-P (2020) Reformulation and Appropriation of Traditional Knowledge in Industrial Ayurveda: The Trajectory of Jeevani. *East Asian Science, Technology and Society* 14(1): 1–19.

Monnais L (2019) *The Colonial Life of Pharmaceuticals: Medicines and Modernity in Vietnam*. Cambridge: Cambridge University Press.

Mukharji PB (2016) *Doctoring Traditions: Ayurveda, Small Technologies, and Braided Sciences*. London: University of Chicago Press.

Ogden L, Hall B and Tanita K (2013) Animals, Plants, People, and Things: A Review of Multispecies Ethnography. *Environment and Society: Advances in Research* 4: 5–24.

Ong A (2006) *Neoliberalism as Exception: Mutations in Citizenship and Sovereignty*. Durham: Duke University Press.

Ong A and Chen NN (eds) (2010) *Asian Biotech: Ethics and Communities of Fate*. Durham: Duke University Press.

Ortner S (2011) On Neoliberalism. *Anthropology of This Century* 1. http://aotcpress.com/articles/neoliberalism/

Pati B and Harrison M (eds) (2008) *The Social History of Health and Medicine in Colonial India*. London: Routledge.

Patwardhan B and Mashelkar R (2009) Traditional Medicine Inspired Approaches to Drug Discovery: Can Ayurveda Show the Way Forward? *Drug Discovery Today* 14(15–16): 804–811.

Petryna A, Lakoff A and Kleinman A (2006) *Global Pharmaceuticals: Ethics, Markets, Practices*. London: Duke University Press.

Pordié L (2014) Pervious Drugs: Making the Pharmaceutical Object in Techno-Ayurveda. *Asian Medicine* 9(1–2): 49–76.

Pordié L (2015) Hangover Free! The Social and Material Trajectories of PartySmart. *Anthropology & Medicine* 22(1): 34–48.

Pordié L (2021) Unstable Pharmaceutical Values: The Grey Political Economy of Drug Circulation in Cambodia. *BioSocieties* 16: 342–362.

Pordié L and Gaudillière J-P (2014a) The Herbal Pharmaceutical Industry in India. *Asian Medicine* 9(1–2): 1–305.

Pordié L and Gaudillière J-P (2014b) Introduction: Industrial Ayurveda - Drug Discovery, Reformulation and the Market. *Asian Medicine* 9(1–2): 1–11.

Pordié L and Gaudillière J-P (2014c) The Reformulation Regime in Drug Discovery: Revisiting Polyherbals and Property Rights in the Ayurvedic Industry. *East Asian Science, Technology and Society* 8(1): 57–79.

Pordié L and Hardon A (2015) Special Issue - Drugs' Stories and Itineraries: On the Making of Asian Industrial Medicines. *Anthropology & Medicine* 22(1).

Pordié L and Kloos S (eds) (2022) *Healing at the Periphery: Ethnographies of Tibetan Medicine in India*. Durham: Duke University Press.

Priya R and Shweta AS (2010) *Status and Role of AYUSH and Local Health Traditions under the National Rural Health Mission*. New Delhi: National Health Systems Resource Centre.

Quet M, Pordié L, Bochaton A, et al. (2018) Regulation Multiple: Pharmaceutical Trajectories and Modes of Control in the ASEAN. *Science, Technology and Society* 23(3): 485–503.

Salguero CP (ed) (2017) *Buddhism and Medicine: An Anthology of Premodern Sources*. New York, NY: Columbia University Press.

Saxer M (2013) *Manufacturing Tibetan Medicine: The Creation of an Industry and the Moral Economy of Tibetanness*. Oxford: Berghahn Books.

Scheid V (2002) *Chinese Medicine in Contemporary China*. London: Duke University Press.

Scheid V (2007) *Currents of Tradition in Chinese Medicine 1626–2006*. Seattle: Eastland Press.

Scheid V (2014) Convergent Lines of Descent: Symptoms, Patterns, Constellations, and the Emergent Interface of Systems Biology and Chinese Medicine. *East Asian Science, Technology and Society* 8(1): 107–139.

Schrempf M (2015) Contested Issues of Efficacy and Safety between Transnational Formulation Regimes of Tibetan Medicines in China and Europe. *Asian Medicine* 10(1–2): 273–315.

Schwabl H (2009) It Is Modern to be Traditional: Tradition and Tibetan Medicine in the European Context. *Asian Medicine* 5(2): 373–384.

Schwabl H (2015) Wie kann die Verfügbarkeit von pflanzlichen Arzneimitteln in der Europäischen Union verbessert werden? *Schweizerische Zeitschrift fur GanzheitsMedizin* 27: 370–372.

Shankar D, Unnikrishnan P and Venkatasubramanian P (2007) Need to Develop Inter-Cultural Standards for Quality, Safety and Efficacy of Traditional Indian Systems of Medicine. *Current Science* 92(11): 1499–1505.

Sivaramakrishnan K (2005) *Old Potions, New Bottles: Recasting Indigenous Medicine in Colonial Punjab, 1850–1945*. New Delhi: Orient Longman.

Springer L (2015) Collectors, Producers, and Circulators of Tibetan and Chinese Medicines in Sichuan Province. *Asian Medicine* 10(1): 177–220.

Springer L (2016) Safeguarding Chinese Materia Medica: One Family as a Case of Transmitting Trans-Regional Pharma-Craft and Scholarly Science in Contemporary China. *AAS Working Papers in Social Anthropology* 30: 1–18.

Springer L (2019) Taibai Materia Medica: Unofficial 'Herb Physicians' in North Western China. *EchoGéo* 47 [Online].

Subedi B (2006) *Linking Plant-Based Enterprises and Local Communities to Biodiversity Conservation in Nepal Himalayas*. New Delhi: Adroit Publishers.

Sujatha V and Abraham L (eds) (2012) *Medical Pluralism in Contemporary India*. Hyderabad: Orient Blackswan.

Taylor K (2005) *Chinese Medicine in Early Communist China, 1945–63: A Medicine of Revolution*, London: Routledge.

Thomas Y, Karki M, Gurung K et al. (eds) (2005) *Himalayan Medicinal and Aromatic Plants: Balancing Use and Conservation*. Kathmandu: Government of Nepal Ministry of Forests and Soil Conservation.

Tovey P, Easthope G and Adams J (eds) (2004) *The Mainstreaming of Complementary and Alternative Medicine: Studies in Social Context*. Abingdon, VA: Routledge.

Tripathi H, Suresh R, Kumar S, et al. (2017) International Trade in Medicinal and Aromatic Plants. *Journal of Medicinal and Aromatic Plant Sciences* 39(1): 1–17.

Tsing A (2015) *The Mushroom at the End of the World: On the Possibility of Life in Capitalist Ruins*. Princeton, NJ: Princeton University Press.

Unschuld P (2010 [1985]). *Medicine in China: A History of Ideas*. Berkeley, CA: University of California Press.

Vasisht K, Sharma N and Karan M (2016) Current Perspectives on the International Trade of Medicinal Plants: An Update. *Current Pharmaceutical Design* 22(27): 4288–4336.

Wang S (2020) Circumventing Regulation and Professional Legitimization: The Circulation of Chinese Medicine between China and France. In: Coderey C and Pordié L(eds) *Circulation and Governance of Asian Medicine*. London: Routledge, 139–157.

Wang J, Guo Y and Li GL (2016) Current Status of Standardization of Traditional Chinese Medicine in China. *Evidence-Based Complementary and Alternative Medicine*. DOI: 10.1155/2016/9123103

World Health Organisation (2013) *Traditional Medicine Strategy 2014–2023*. Geneva: WHO.

World Health Organization (2018) Annex 2: Guidelines on Good Manufacturing Practices for the Manufacture of Herbal Medicines. *Expert Committee on Specifications for Pharmaceutical Preparations 52*. Geneva: WHO.

Zimmermann F (1987) *The Jungle and the Aroma of Meats: An Ecological Theme in Hindu Medicine*. Berkeley, CA: University of California Press.

Index

Note: Page references in *italics* indicate figures, **bold** indicates tables and "n" indicates footnotes.

Aba Tibetan and Qiang Autonomous Prefecture 55
Academy of Chinese Medical Sciences 47
Access and Benefit Sharing 157
Acetanilide 120
acupuncture 2, 5, 12, 33, 282, 298
Adams, V. 3n4, 8, 100, 230, 301
adivasi 236n15; collectors 200, 203, 205–207, 211, 218, 236; rights to forest lands and resources 218; workers 201
agents in Ayurvedic plant trade 209–210
Alter, J. 140
alternative modernity 52, 131, 143, 276, 301, 318; *see also* modernity
amchi (Sowa Rigpa practitioners) 230–231, 231n8, 254–255, 311, 315, 325; engaged in clinic+pharmacy model 254–255, 273; entrepreneurial 262; and industrialisation regimes 271, 315; and pharmaceutical development 257; physician-pharmacists 254, 275, 311, 315, 325; professional 258; rural 256, 258–259, 262, 270; urban 256, 259, 270
Amygdalin 101n34
Annual Statistical Report on Production in Toyama Prefectural Pharmaceutical Industry 121, 123
Anoop Pharma 182
"anthropology of pharmaceuticals" 12
artemisia annua 1n3
artemisinin 32–33, 35, 37, 48
Arya Vaidya Pharmacy 159, 174
Ashtangahridayam 174n6

Ashtangahridaya Samhita 6
Ashtavaidya culture 174n6
Asian Industrial Medicines (Pordié and Hardon) 9
Asian medical industries: as assemblages 14–17, 306, 312, 328, 331–333; characteristics of 10–15, 331–333; contemporary transnational identities of 140; *see also* specific types
Asian Medical Systems (Leslie) 4–5, 9, 227, 328–329
assemblages *see* pharmaceutical assemblages
Association of Southeast Asian Nations (ASEAN) 129
authenticity: Ashtavaidyas 174; Ayurveda's, in the West 146; and medical industries 14; of medicinal materials 75; morphology of 61–62; pharmaceutical assemblages 15
Ayurdhara Pharmaceuticals 198, 200, 201, 201n9, 205, 210–211, 211n9
Ayurveda 1n2, 2–3, 6, 10, 17–18, 131; and biomedicine 161; branding India 139–163; canonical 142; cultural-nationalist symbolism 144–146; global economic value 152; globalisation 141, 149, 155, 157, 162; modernisation and professionalisation 7; as pharmaceutical industry 7; reformulation regime in 132n9; spiritual-holistic 149; state channel for NTFPs used in *200*; and state patronage 144–145; traditional 14

342 *Index*

Ayurvedic companies 159, 174, 197–199, 208, 208n16, 211, 213, 215–217, 220, 331; direct suppliers 209; public 200–202; *see also* Ayurvedic industry
Ayurvedic Drug Manufacturers Association of India (ADMA) 177
Ayurvedic Formulary 157
Ayurvedic industry 18–19, 34, 47, 143, 150, 161, 172n3, 310, 315, 323; approaching complexity 194–196; channels and networks 206–213; cultural-nationalist symbolism 144–146; discourse *vs.* market realities 155–158; expansion 197; implications for 139–163; national uniformity 152–155; pressures of scientific modernity 148–152; private 205; producing Brand India through Brand Ayurveda 146–148; raw material supply for 194–220; regulating 161; rural collectors in 216; small-scale 154; spatial connections, enlarging 213–217; and state bureaucracy 158–162; state *vs.* private sector supply 199–205; turnover, in India 172n3; unequal competition 199–205; watershed moment 197–198; *see also* Ayurvedic companies
Ayurvedic Manufacturers Association of India 173
Ayurvedic Medicine Manufacturers Organisation of India 211n18
Ayurvedic plants: agents as brokers of the industry 209–210; companies' direct suppliers 209; complexity of networks 211–213; middlemen 206–209; multi-layered flows of 206–213; supply in Central Kerala 198–199; supply organisation 211–213; villagers as suppliers 211; wholesalers 210–211
Ayurvedic Vicks® 3
AYUSH (Ayurveda, Yoga and Naturopathy, Unani, Siddha, Sowa Rigpa, and Homeopathy) 145, 147, 150, 171–172; clusters 175; Department Task Force 160; exports 158, 173; mainstreaming in public healthcare 171–172, 188; products 156; proprietary medicines 157; *see also* Brand India; India

baekshuoh disaster 98n29
Banerjee, M. 7, 156, 157, 316

Basic Policy for New Drug Approval 98–99
Bhattarai, N. 208, 209n17
Bian, H. 217
biocapital 4
biomedicine 1, 3–5, 14, 39, 41, 47–48, 85, 85n8, 86–88, 99, 101, 104, 132, 152, 154, 257, 281, 284, 290, 292–293, 296, 298–299, 309, 314–317, 327–328, 330; anti-cancer 101; Ayurveda's combative attitude towards 161; Chinese 84; firms 85n11, 102; forceful introduction of 8; GMP standards 94; and GxP 82, 84; histories of biomedicine in China 17; industrialisation of 82; Japanese pharmacopoeia standards 94; and Kampo medicine 81–82; manufacturers' associations 92; market for 84; modern 7, 83; NHI coverage for 103; regulation of 82; as sole legitimate form of healthcare 10; state patronage for 144; synthetic 12; Western 84
bioprospecting 3, 32, 35–36, 47, 139, 286, 320
bioscience 43, 315, 327, 329; -based laboratory protocols 34; -based regulation of "traditional" medicines 34; and Chinese medicines 33–34, 47; -influenced regulatory regime 44; research protocols of 33
Birla Kerala Vaidyasala (BKV) 174–175
Black, M. 74n8
Bode, M. 7, 310n2, 327n12
Bourdieu, P. 202
Brand Ayurveda 141, 143; Brand India promotion through 146–148; promoting 147
Brand India: and AYUSH 150; campaigns 150; overview 145; promotion through Brand Ayurveda 18, 141, 146–148; and yoga 141
broad-leaved *qianghuo* 59; *see also qianghuo*
Brockington, D. 70
Bubandt, N. 234
Buddhism 6, 281, 292–293
Büscher, B. 228n1, 246n22

canon-based classical medicines 143
capital: financial 258; social 176, 202, 218; start-up 181; working 181

Index 343

capitalism 228, 246, 257, 332; late 227; millennial 230, 235; neoliberal 233–235; non-cultural 11; pharmaceutical 4; predatory 246; supply chain 230
Caraka Samhita 6
CARe Keralam 169–191; Ayurveda industry cluster project 177–179; cluster development scheme 179–181; conflicting structures 182–188; constraints of industry at various nodes **178**; initial costs of **177**; "Kerala brand" 177–179; markets and clusters 171–177; policy framework 171–177; profitable nutraceuticals and surviving pharmaceuticals 182–188
Central Health Ministry (India) *see* AYUSH
Central Kerala, Ayurvedic plant supply in 198–199
Central Medical Council of India 151
changshan 32
channels of Ayurvedic plant supply: liberalisation of 203–205; and networks 206–213; state-structured 200–202; towards the end of state regulation of 203–205
Charak 159
Chaudhary, J. 159–160
Chen Weiwu 45n16
Chicken Blood Therapy 37
China: Good Agricultural Practices (GAP) 72–73; "new drugs" in 35–37; Soviet protocols were adopted in 36; transition to a market economy 5; "Western Development Plan" 68; WTO entry 5
China Food and Drug Administration (CFDA) 37–39, 42, 44–45
China Medical Association of Minorities (CMAM) 51
Chinese medicine/medicinals 3, 31–50, 51–80; authentic 17; classical 5; defined 31n1; as food 45–46; medicinals and research protocols 37–40; modern 33; raw materials used in 54; "re-networking" Chinese drugs into 36, 52, 316; state-driven 163; *see also* Traditional Chinese Medicine
Chinese Medicine Law of 2016 51
Chinese Pharmacopoeia 54n2, 60–62, 70n6
Chinese proprietary medicines 6, 55, 57, 61; *see also* Chinese medicine

Circulation and Governance of Asian Medicines (Coderey and Pordié) 9
classical decoction method 89, 92n22, 92–93, 316
classical formulas 131, 261, 263, 268, 306, 317, 330; in Ayurvedic and Sowa Rigpa industries, 131, 132n9, 261; in Kerala, 190; and SMEs, 184, 191; in traditional pharmaceutical industries, 131
classical prescriptions 39
Clinical Trials Draft Bill 2008 (India) 156
clusters/clustering 18; Ayurveda, in India **176**; CARe Keralam 171–181; defined 43, 170; development scheme 179–181; dimensions of 172; industrial, and *Haichi* household medicines 110–133; markets and 171–177; pharmaceutical manufacturers 110, 122; potential 188–188; promotions in developing countries 170; and SMEs 175, 186; Toyama prefecture 124
Coartem® 3
Cohen, L. 149
Coimbatore Arya Vaidya Pharmacy (AVP) 174–175, 182, 198
Cold War 33, 307
Comaroff, J. 11, 230, 235, 246n22
communism: and Buddhism 293; Chinese and Tibetan medicine 287; Soviet 297, 300; and Traditional Mongolian medicine (TMM) industry 283–289, 293, 300
Complementary and Alternative Medicine (CAM) 231n9, 331
conceptual bilingualism 151
Confederation of Ayurvedic Renaissance – Keralam Limited *see* CARe Keralam
conservation: neoliberal 228, 228n1, 229n4, 232, 235, 246n22, 247, 324–325; Tibetan conceptions of 231n8
Conservation, Cultivation, and Commodification of Medicinal Plants in the Greater Himalayan-Tibetan Plateau (Craig and Glover) 231
copy-cat products 38
corruption: anthropologists on 234; and Brand India 150; and capitalism 233–235; institutionalised 245; in medicinal plant trade 232, 233–235
COVID-19 57

344 *Index*

Cultivating the Wilds (Craig) 230
cultural: heritage 13, 218, 319; identity 13, 18, 139, 144, 162; nationalism 144, 146–147, 310; symbolism 139, 141; *see also* nationalism
Cultural Revolution 31, 37, 281, 284, 289
cupping 12, 298

Dabur 159
daiokanzoto 100
decoctions 85, 85n7, 89, 92–93, 92n22, 317
DeLanda, M. 328
Deleuze, G. 328
Deng Xiaoping 33, 35, 37, 309
Dharkye, T. 272–273
discourses 16, 162–163; cultural 270; of cultural nationalism 162; of economic nationalism 152; of Indian medicine globalisation 140; *vs.* market realities 155–158; modernist 16; neoliberal 227; neoliberal conservation 195n4, 229n4, 232, 245–246; Nepali development 270; of pharmaceutical standardisation 311; of predatory capitalism 247; religious 15; of scientific modernity 162; of scientisation 162; surrounding Ayurveda 141, 143, 147, 149–150, 152, 153, 155; systemic corruption 234; technoscientific 228, 324
"Divine Farmer's Materia Medica Classic" 57
Dorjee, K. 266
double-blinded randomised controlled trials (DB-RCTs) 99–100
drug re-evaluations: incorporating features of Kampo medicines into 98–103; results of 100–101
Duffy, R. 70
duoyuan yiti 55

East Asian Medicine in Urban Japan (Lock) 83
EFTA (European Free Trade Association) 93n24
"Encyclopedia for Traditional Medicinal Substances and Prescription Control" 293
"e-tender" system 214–215
ethnicity 32, 54–55, 58, 63, 66; of artemisinin 32; of cultivated *qiang beimu* 54; Qiang 63–64, 322; of *qianghuo* 58
ethno-preneurialism 67
Eunjeong Ma 98n29
European Union 58n3, 101–102; as major drug market 102
evidence-based medicine (EBM) 87n15, 99n30

fake *qianghuo* 59–67
Falconer, H. 240
Federation of Pharmaceutical Manufacturers Association of Japan (FPMAJ) 92
Fifth Dalai Lama 8, 281
Filatova, A. 284
Fletcher, R. 228
food, Chinese medicine as 45–46
Foshan Dezhong Pharmaceuticals Co. Ltd 41
Foshan Feng Liao Xing Pharmaceuticals Co. Ltd. 41n10
Franz, M. 208n15, 219
Fritillaria Cirrhosae 68
Fritillaria unibracteata var. *wabuensis* 54, 60–62
frontier assemblages 20, 321, 322
fufang 36–37
Fu Fengyong 36

Gandhi, Mahatma 144
Gaudillière, J-P. 7, 33–34, 229, 315
Ge Hong 31
Gibson-Graham, J. K. 257
Global Ayurveda 148, 150–151
globalisation: and Ayurveda 141, 149, 155, 157, 162; branding India 139–163; regulatory 10–11, 34, 161
GMP (Good Manufacturing Practices) 12, 72–73, 312–315; and Ayurveda 155–158, 186; Food and Drug Administration (USFDA) introduction of 91; and *haichi* medicines industry 121–122; and Indian medicine industry regulation 145; and Japanese pharmaceutical manufacturers 91; and Kampo medicine extract standards 92–94; regulations in the 1990s and 2000s 94–95; standards 45–46; and TMM 290; and Toyama Prefectural Pharmaceutical Research Institute 122

Index 345

God Monkey Medicine Industry 265, 267
Good Agricultural Practices (GAP) 72–73, 156
Good Manufacturing Practices (GMP) 12, 45, 46n18, 47, 61, 72–73, 81–109, 121–122, 145, 155–158, 160, 185–186, 271, 290, 294, 312–315; *see also* GMP (Good Manufacturing Practices)
Good Vigilance Practices (GVP) 98
Goraya, G. S. 238n17
Graan, A. 146
Guang De 57
Guangzhou Huahai Pharmaceuticals Co. Ltd 33, 40–45, 47
Guattari, F. 328
Gupta, A. 233
gvubgea 60
Gyushi (Four Tantras) 8

haichi household medicines 110–136: development of Toyama 111–115; and industrial clustering 110–133; and intersectoral collaboration 110–133; and Meiji period 115–118; reinvention of 18; *see also* Toyama pharmaceutical industry
Haidav, Tsend 286–287, 291, 293
Hangontan 112, 114–115, 131
Hangontan Agency 115
Han method medicine 81
Happy Intestine Granules 43
health supplements 2, 38–39, 141, 142, 157, 159, 180, 182, 183, 184, 231n9, 331; *see also* supplements
Healthy Medicine Holdings Ltd, Hong Kong SAR 45–46
Helsinki Declaration 102n35
The Herbal Pharmaceutical Industry in India (Pordié and Gaudillière) 7
Himalayan Amchi Association (HAA) 256, 260, 274
Himalayan Buddhist medicine 7
Hindustan Unilever Ltd 174
hindutwa 147
Hiroshi, K. 86
Hisao, Y. 83
The History and Development of Traditional Mongolian Medicine (Bold) 282
Home Medicine Association of Japan 85n11

Homeopathy 144n3, 145n4, 171
Hsu, E. 32, 152
Huangdi Bashiyi Nanjing (Yellow Emperor's Canon of Eighty-One Difficult Issues) 5
Huangdi Neijing (Yellow Emperor's Inner Canon) 5
Hundred Flowers Movement 36
hybridity 31n1, 33, 39, 111, 118, 131, 132, 317, 317n6, 318, 328, 332
hybrid medicines 39, 111, 118, 131–132, 317, 317n6
hybrid networks 202–203; itineraries of NTFPs through *204*

ICH (International Conference in Harmonisation of Technical Requirements for the Registration of Pharmaceuticals for Human Use) 102
India 3, 6–8, 18–19; approved Ayurveda clusters in **176**; and biomedicine 144; branding 139–163; corruption in 232, 233–235; Incredible India campaign 145; medicine policies 162–163; *see also* CARe Keralam; Kerala
India Brand Equity Foundation 145
Indian Drugs and Cosmetics Act (DCA) 1940 143n2
Indian ethnomedicine 148; *see also* Ayurveda
Indian National Guidelines on Access to Biological Resources and Associated Knowledge and Benefits Sharing Regulations 217
An Indian Path to Biocapital (Gaudillière) 227
industrial clustering *see* clusters/clustering
Ingram, V. 245
Inner Mongolia Autonomous Region 287–289
Institute for Natural Products Chemistry and Pharmacology 285
Institute of Natural Medicine of Toyama University 129
Institute of Traditional Medicine and Technology, Mongolia 285
intellectual property rights (IPR) 7, 8, 11, 16, 139, 148, 178, 254, 320
International Development Research Centre 244
Islam, N. 7

346 *Index*

Janes, C. 8
Japan: economic takeoff 88; good practices and health policy making in 81–105; High Growth Period 88; as major drug market 102; as member of Pharmaceutical Inspection Co-operation Scheme (PIC/S) 93; pharmacovigilance system 97; prescription and OTC Kampo medicines sales in 90; regulatory regime for Kampo medicines manufacturing 91–92; trade disputes with US 102n36
Japanese Medical Association (JMA) 89
Japan External Trade Organisation (JETRO) 124
Japan International Cooperation Agency 129
Japan Kampo Medicines Manufacturers Association (JKMA) 82n5, 84–85, 85n8, 92–94, 99
Japan Pharmacopeia (JP) 82n3, 91
Japan Self-Medication Industry Association 85n11
Japan Society for Oriental Medicine (JSOM) 87, 87n15, 88–89, 104
Jia Qian 38
Jigmed, B. 282
John, S. P. 181
Jyokan, M. 112

Kampo boom 83, 95–96
Kampo medicines: affordability of 104; application of GxP to 82n4; *baiyaku* 87; and biomedical drug laws and regulations 3; classical decoctions, use of 89; development 84–91; drug re-evaluations 98–103; effects of GxP on manufacturing of 91–95; extract standards in 1980s 92–94; future of 103–105; as humanised goods 89; ICH GCP 102, 104; industrialisation of 82; integration of biomedicine and 81; Japan's regulatory regime for manufacturing of 91–92; "Kampo boom" 83, 95–96; "the myth of Kampo medicine safety" 97–98; and national medical examination system 86; "new" GCP and impact on 101–103; new manufacturing technologies 88; and NHI coverage 84–85, 103; OTC 84–85, *90*, 103; post-marketing practices 95–98; practitioners 86; prescription 81n1, 84, *90*, 93, 95–97, 103–104, 331; production value of 126; regulation of 82; results of drug re-evaluations 100–101; revival of 87–89; roots of 81; scientisation of 87; standards for physician training in 88; transliteration of 82n3
Kanegafuchi Spinning Company 85n10
kanpō seizai (Kampo formulation) 88
Karimpuzha, R. 186
Kaur, R. 147, 150
Kefauver Harris Amendments 99
Keisetsu, O. 89
Kerala: approaching complexity 194–196; Ayurvedic plant supply in 198–199; captured official channel 202–203; from channels to networks 206–213; hybrid networks 202–203; Kerala brand Ayurveda 147, 154, 174; liberalisation of the channel 203–205; multi-layered flows of Ayurvedic plants 206–213; public Ayurvedic companies 200–202; state regulation, end of 203–205; state-structured channel 200–202; watershed moment 197–198; *see also* India
Kerala Ayurveda Health Centres Ordinance 2007 156
Kerala Ayurveda Ltd (KAL) 174
Kerala Forest Research Institute 199n8
Kerala Industrial Infrastructure Development Corporation (KINFRA) 177, 190
Kerala State Industrial Development Corporation (KSIDC) 177
Kerala Vaidyasala 174
Khalikova, V. 145
Kitamaebune 113
Kokando Company 118, 127–128
Korean Hanbang 2, 6
Kottakal AVS 177, 182, 183, 185, 198, 201, 205, 210
Kumar, G. P. 240n20
Kuniyal, C. P. 240
Kunphen Medical Centre: and borders 264–270; and quality control 264–270; state recognition 264–270
Kuo, Wen-Hua 34, 312n4
Kuracie 85, 100
kusushi 95n25
Kyōritu Toyama Pharmaceutical School 119

Laetrile 101n34
Lazzarini, S. 213n20
Ledeneva, A. 234
Lei, S. 32
Leslie, C. 4–5, 9, 139, 227
Lock, M. 83–84, 89n18
Luvsandanzanjantsan, O. 291
Lyu Guiyuan 43

manbyōyaku 116
Manchu Qing Empire 283
Mao Zedong 33, 35–37
market-oriented, sector-specific talks (MOSS) 102n36
markets: articulating Qiang medicines for growing 65–67; CARe Keralam 171–177; and clusters 171–177; cultivation in service of 51–76; paternalism in service of 51–76; *qiang beimu* 62–64; spiritualized 162
Masatoshi, Lord Maeda 112
Matsui Gen'emon (Mastuiya) 112, 114
Mattathur Labour Cooperative Society in Thrissur 185n9
Meconopsis spp. 232n11
medical parallelism 151
medical systems 4–10, 14–15, 131, 142, 328–329; Asian (Leslie) 4–5, 9, 227, 328–329; Ayurveda as cohesive 155; biomedicine-based 83; Indian 144, 147–148, 171; Japan's 103–104; Meiji period 95; state-approved 56
medicinal plants/herbs 52, 57–61, 94, 125, 145, 148, 153, 170, 180–181, 184–185, 188, 190, 209n17, 215–219, 319–323, 332; and AYUSH 171–173; as biocultural objects 196; collection 195, 206, 208, 306; conservation 229n3; cultivation 196, 208n16, 210, 235, 239, 240n18, 242, 244, 262–263, 292, 319; and government interventions 245–246; high-altitude 258; Himalayan 229; in Ladakh 240n20; Mongolian 285–286, 299; as open-access resource 195; plant trade 153, 199n7, 227–228, 229n3, 229n4, 230, 246, 263, 275, 325; regulatory landscape in India 245–246; research 171; in Sichuan 69–72; spoiling of 210; supply networks of 219; trans-Himalayan 240n20; in Uttarakhand 203n10; *see also* Tibetan medicinal plants

Medicinal Plants Research in Asia (vol. 1) 217n23
The Medicinal Plants Sector in India (Holley and Cherla) 244
medicines *see specific types*
Meiji Restoration 83; *haichi* household medicines expansion following 115–118; *haichi* medicine regulation and transformation following 115–118
Men-Tsee-Khang 231–232, 241, 247, 260
Miao medicine industry 2, 53
middlemen: Ayurvedic plants 206–209; and collection activity 206–209
"The Million Taxes" 45n17
"minor forest products" (MFPs) 229n5
modernity: alternative 52, 131, 143, 276, 301, 318; scientific 148–152
Modi, N. 150, 240
Mongolia 8, 280–304; communism 283–287; communist era in 282; establishment of Tibetan medicine in 283; *haichi* medicine companies of Toyama 129; *haichi* mode of drug delivery 133; Inner 287–289, 290, 294–296, 308; Sowa Rigpa industries in 13, 19
Mongolian Academy of Sciences 285
Mongolian Buddhist University 292, 292n9
Mongolian-Chinese Medicine Bureaus 290
Mongolian Medicine *see* Traditional Mongolian Medicine
Mongolian Medicine Company 289
Mongol Yuan dynasty 283
mongrel medicine 5
moovila (Pseudarthia viscida) 201
moral economy 207n14, 231, 254, 257, 268, 270, 273
"moral economy of the peasant" 207n14
morphology of authenticity 61–62
multi-layered flows of Ayurvedic plants 206–213
Muraleedharan, P.K. 203n10

Nagarjuna Group 174, 182
nagpo guchor pills 273, 273n6
Naigai Yakuhin Company 128
Nanjing Pharmaceutical Institute 40
National Accreditation Board for Hospitals, India 156
National AYUSH Mission 158

National Health Insurance (NHI) 81, 84–85, 87–90, 87n13, 95–96, 101, 103–104
National Health Mission (NHM), India 172, 332
national identity 139–141, 146, 151, 162, 281
National Medical Products Administration (NMPA) 67
National Medicinal Plants Board (NMPB, New Delhi) 148, 229
nationalism 13, 141; cultural 144, 146–147, 162; economic 152; ethno- 56; Hindu 314; transnational 140, 143, 315
national trade surveys 246
national uniformity 152–155
nation branding 7, 13, 18, 33, 139–141, 143, 146–147, 162–163, 312, 314–315
Natsagdorj, D. 284, 291, 292, 294, 294n10, 297–298
Nehru, J. L. 144
neoliberal capitalism and occult economies 233–235
neoliberal conservation 228, 228n1, 229n4, 232, 235, 246n22, 247
neoliberalism 228n1, 246n22, 321, 324
"neo-traditionalism" 261, 301
Nepal 253–279: big pharma with traditional characteristics in 263, 329; clinic+pharmacy mode in 258, 267; lineage-apprenticeship model in 260; making Tibetan medicine in 253–277; wild plant collection and marketing in 195, 262–264
netchains 213n20
networks: complexity of 211–213; supply organisation, mapping 211–213; wholesalers as nodal position in 210–211
new drugs: discovery of 42–45; in Mao's China 35–37; in traditional Chinese Medicine 31–48
Nippon Foundation 299
Nizhakathakadi Kashaayam 180
"non-timber forest products" (NTFPs) 197, 199–202, *200*, *204*, 204–205, 229n5, 229n6, 229n7, 245
Norbu, K. 264
Northern India: losing track of Tibetan medicinal plants 227–247; Tibetan medicinal plant trade in 227–247; *see also* India
Novartis 3

occult economies 233–235
Olsen, C. S. 195, 208, 209n17
One Belt One Road initiative 51, 51n1, 74, 322
Oriental medicine 86
orila (Desmodium gangeticum) 201
OTC Kampo medicines 85
Oushadham 211
Oushadhi 198, 200–201, 205, 210; mapping changes in supply of 214–215
Oushadhi – The Pharmaceutical Corporation (I.M.) Kerala Ltd *see* Oushadhi
over-the-counter (OTC) medicines 2, 84–85, 87, *90*, 93, 95, 98, 103, 123, 127–129, 173, 190–191, 290, 292, 293, 311, 330

PADMA (Swiss pharmaceutical company) 231–232, 235–237, 241, 247
Palakkad gap 198, 198n6
Pana-wan 127, 127n6
Pantaloons Retail (India) Ltd 174
Patent Medicine Affairs Law of 1914 119
patent medicines 36, 39, 47, 83, 87, 115–122, 133, 308, 314, 317
Patent Medicine Sales Tax Law 119
paternalism: Qiang medical industry 67–72; in the service of market 51–76
Pauls, T. 208n15, 219
Pedon, T. 266
Peluso, N. L. 74n8
PepsiCo India 174
Pethub Stangey Choskhor Ling monastery 297n13
Pharmaceutical Affairs Law (PAL) 91, 93, 98, 127–129, 133
pharmaceutical assemblages 15–17, 34, 53, 171, 196, 218, 227, 247, 254, 282–283, 306–307, 311–312, 319–320, 333; defined 15; partially overlapping 14, 52; of Sowa Rigpa 9, 256–257, 262, 264, 267, 269–270, 275–276; transnational and capitalist 3
Pharmaceutical Inspection Co-operation Scheme (PIC/S):

inspections 94; Japan as member of 93
pharmaceutical nexus 3–4, 254
Pharmaceutical Quality Control Workshop 122
pharmaceuticalisation 3, 7, 12, 15, 33, 75, 132, 313, 316, 330; of Ayurveda, 7, 141, 169; of Chinese medicine, 6, 163; of traditional medicines, 36
pharmaceuticals: profitable nutraceuticals and surviving 182–188; states and 307–312; *see also specific industries*
Phenacetin 120
Plan for the Protection and Development of Chinese Medicinal Materials (2015–2020) 68, 73
policy framework: and CARe Keralam 188; markets and clusters 171–177
Pordié, Laurent 7, 33–34, 315
post-marketing practices and Kampo medicines industry 95–98
Pratchett, T. 233n12
prescription Kampo medicines 81n1, 84, 90, 93, 103–104, 331; institutional factors 95–97; rise in 95–97
Procter & Gamble 3
profitable nutraceuticals and surviving pharmaceuticals 182–188
"Project of Scientizing Chinese Medicine" 144
proprietary medicines: and Ayurveda industry 183; categories of 157; Chinese 6, 14, 51–52, 55, 57, 61–63, 65–66; drug licensing conditions for 157; herbal 74; Indian 132n9; Qiang 63; registered 52, 54, 310; standardisation 143

qiang beimu: competing in Sichuan and beyond 64–65; marketing of 62–64; morphology of authenticity 61–62; new ethnic possibilities 60–65
qianghuo: collecting 58–59; described 54; fake 59–67; and Qiang medicine 54–59; real 59–67
Qiang medical industry 53–54, 57, 63–67, 69, 75; GAP and workings of standardisation 72–73; industrial disconnect 73–76; medicinal materials 56–59; and paternalism 67–72; Qiang medicine doctors 53;

qianghuo 58–59; raw materials 67–72; and sustainability 67–72
Quality Council of India 156
Quality Migrant Admission Scheme 45

rampō (Dutch medicine) 86
raw materials: in motion 319–326; pharmaceuticals 319–326; Qiang medical industry 67–72; supply for Ayurvedic industry 194–220
reformulation 2, 7, 9, 12, 13, 19, 33, 34, 47, 52, 63, 130, 132, 183, 190, 228, 236n14, 246, 306, 309, 312–319
regimes of regulation and reformulation 312–319
regulation(s), 312–319; AYUSH, on Ayurveda, 157–160; biomedical, 3, 18; Chinese medicinals and research protocols 37–40; for clinical trials in Japan, 102; GMP, 94–95, 312–319; of medicinal plants, 145; Tokugawa *haichi* medicines, 115–118; of traditional medicines, 34; US FDA, on Chinese medicines, 39–40, 45
regulatory globalization 10, 34, 161
Reliance Retail 174
Review of the Status of Saussurea Costus 240
Roche 3
Routledge Handbook of Medical Anthropology (Manderson) 4n5

salvage accumulation 275, 323, 325
Sanchez, A. 233–234
Sasidharan, N. 203n10
Saxer, M. 8, 156, 245, 263
scientific modernity 148–152; *see also* modernity
Scott, J. C. 207n14
Seethalakshmi, K. K. 203n10
Sensai, N. 86
shamanism 281–282
Shang Hanlun (Treatise on Cold Damage Disorders and Miscellaneous Illnesses) 5
Shankar, A. 203n10
Sharav, B. 282
shosaikoto 97–98, 100, 103
shoseiryuto 97n28, 100–101
Sichuan: authentic medicine certification service 58n3; competing in 64–65; earthquake

350 Index

in 71; environmental sustainability initiatives in 68; herbal pieces (*yinpian*) 55; human-medicinal relations in 54–56
Sichuan College of Chinese Medicine 59
Sichuan Province Chinese Medicine Industry Development Plan 2018–2025 58n3, 64n5, 69
Sida cordifolia 236, 236n14
Siddha 1n2, 2, 145n4, 147, 171, 332
Sitaram Ayurveda Pharmacy 198, 210
Sivadasan, T. 154–155
Sixth National Ethnic Medicine Inheritance and Innovation Development Forum 51
small and medium enterprises (SME) 169–170, 172–173, 175, 179–180, 183–188, 191
SMON scandal 89, 98
SNA Oushadhasala 182, 198, 210
social capital 176, 202, 218
Song dynasty 5
sourcery: neoliberal capitalism and occult economies 233–235; Tibetan medicinal plants 233–235
Sourcery (Pratchett) 233n12
South India: Ayurvedic industry managers in 194; Ayurvedic pharmaceutical production in 169–191; *see also* India
Southwest China: ethnicity in 51–76; medical industry in 51–76; *see also* China
Sowa Rigpa 2–3, 7–14, 17–19, 131, 160, 220, 227, 232, 247, 254–276
Sowa Rigpa International College (SRIC) 256
Sowa Rigpa sensibility 270, 301
standard decoctions 92–93, 92n22, 317
standardisation 9–10, 117, 141–143, 149–150, 152, 154–155, 160, 162, 169, 186, 314–315; advocating 150; company-enforced 72; corporate-led 230; discourse on Ayurvedic globalisation 157, 161; of formulas 119–130, 308, 313; Good Agricultural Practices and workings of 72–73; of raw materials 313; state-led 230
start-up capital 181
State Food and Drug Administration (SFDA, China) 37, 67

state: bureaucracy 158–162; liberalisation 203–205; and pharmaceuticals 307–312; *vs.* private sector supply 199–205; regulation 10, 293, 312–315; role of 300–301, 307–312; state-structured channel 200–202
Stewart, K. 255, 257, 269
stock-keepers 202–203, 207n13, 243n21
"A Strategy to Modernize and Develop Chinese Drugs" report 38
Structural Impediments Initiative (SII) 102n36
supplements (dietary, food, health, herbal) 2, 38–39, 141, 142, 157, 159, 180, 182, 183, 184, 231n9, 331
Supplementary Regulations on the Registration and Management of Chinese Medicine 38
suppliers 211; Ayurvedic companies' direct 209; supply organization 211–213; villagers as 59, 207, 211, 262–263
Sushruta Samhita 6
sustainability and Qiang medical industry 67–72
Svoboda, R. 145
synthetic biomedicine 12

Taikyo Phamaceutical Company 128
Takeda 83n6, 85n8, 88
Takemi Tarō 89–90
Tamiflu® 3
Tanabe 83n6
Tibet 7–8, 253, 260, 263–265, 282, 284
Tibetan Buddhism 8, 280
Tibetan medicinal plants 227–247; corruption 233–235; cultivator and trader from Lahaul 240–244; dark art of sourcing 244–247; exporter in Gurgaon 235–240; failed liberalization 244–247; and governance 244–247; neoliberal capitalism and occult economies 233–235; sourcery 233–235; *see also* Ayurvedic plants
Tibetan medicine 7–8, 253n1, 281, 283–284, 287–288; contested discourses of scaling-up production 270–274; Kunphen Medical Centre 264–270; in Nepal 253–277; quality 295–296; quest for recognition of in Nepal 270–274; terrains of production of 257–264; *see also* Sowa Rigpa

Tokyo and Osaka Crude Drugs Associations 85n11
Toyama City Hygiene Division 120
Toyama Clan Products Agency 115
Toyama Megumi Pharmaceutical Company Limited 128
Toyama Pharmaceutical Federation 124
Toyama pharmaceutical industry 110–133; expansion following Meiji restoration 115–118; *haichi* medicines 111–115, 118–122; medicine manufacturing and sales system 127–129; origins of *haichi* medicines 111–115; regulation following Meiji restoration 115–118; transformation following Meiji restoration 115–118; in twenty-first century 122–127; *see also haichi* household medicines
Toyama Prefectural Drug Testing Laboratory 122
Toyama Prefectural Institute 127
Toyama Prefectural Patent Medicine Dealer Association 122
Toyama Prefectural Pharmaceutical Affairs Laboratory 121
Toyama Prefectural Pharmaceutical Research Institute 122, 124–125
Toyama Prefectural Vocational School for the Pharmaceutical Industry 119
Toyama Prefecture Committee for the Revitalization of the Pharmaceutical Industry 125
Toyama Shakuyaku 125
Toyama University 87–88, 87n16, 129
trade liberalization 246n22
Traditional Chinese Medicine: Chinese medicinals and research protocols 37–40; Chinese medicine as food 45–46; discovering new drugs in 31–48; Guangzhou Huahai Pharmaceuticals Co. Ltd 40–42; Healthy Medicine Holdings Ltd 45–46; inside laboratory of Guangzhou Huahai 42–45; "new drug" discovery 42–45; "new drugs" in Mao's China 35–37; *see also* Chinese medicine
Traditional Knowledge digital database (TKDL) 148
traditional medicine 9, 274, 282, 284, 288, 290, 305, 308, 314–315, 328, 332; affordable 159; bioscience-based regulation of 34; China promoting 140–141; development of 75; global attitudes towards 139; global market potential of 145; in Maoist China 300; pharmaceuticalisation of 36; popular image of 130; raw material supply for 196, 199; RCTs on 103; resurgence of scholarship on 87; safety and efficacy of 100; in Stalinist Mongolia 300; trading routes 83; unscientific 148
Traditional Mongolian Medicine (TMM): and Buddhism 292–293; and communism 283–289; emergence of 289–295; government's management of 299; Inner Mongolia Autonomous Region 287–289; Mongolian literature on 282; physicians 289; post-communist 281; recent developments 295–300; revival of 281
Trinley, J. 265
Tsedenbal, Y. 284
Tsenam, T. 265
Tsering, N. 266, 267
Tsing, A. 11, 73, 206n12, 255
Tsumura & Co. 85
Tsumura Jūsha II 89
Tumurbaatar, N. 290
Tu Yao (or Tu You You) 31–32, 35

Umemura, M. 83, 101, 126
Unani 1n2, 2, 7, 145n4, 147, 171, 332
UNESCO (United Nations Educational, Scientific and Cultural Organisation) 13
United States: clinical trial practices in 101–102; Kefauver Harris Amendments 99; as major drug market 102; trade disputes between Japan and 102n36
unscientific traditional medicines 148
US Food and Drug Administration (FDA) 38–39, 45, 101n34

Vaidyaratnam Oushadalayam Pvt. Ltd. 185, 198, 210, 217n22
Vana Samrakshana Samithi (VSS) 204
van der Geest, S. 35
Vangal, R. 174
Varghese, J. 182
Ved, D. K. 238n17
Vedic Period 6
villagers as suppliers 59, 207, 211, 262–263

wabu beimu 54–55, 60–64, 73
Wahlberg, A. 147
Wakanyaku 81, 86, 110, 110n1, 116, 118, 120, 125–126, 132
Washington Post 256n2
Western biomedicine 84; *see also* biomedicine
Western laboratory protocols 36
Western medical ideas and practices 116
wholesalers: Ayurvedic plants 210–211; as nodal position in networks 210–211
women: harassment of 207; as targets of witchcraft accusations and witch hunts 234n13; and *Wakanyaku* 120
working capital 181
World Ayurveda Congress (WAC) 148–149
World Bank 244
World Health Organisation (WHO) 91, 100, 121, 228, 313; Ayurveda recognized by 151; Good Agricultural and Collection Practices (GACP) 72; guidelines on GACP 74; on herbal medicines 81n2, 160; Traditional Medicine Strategy 74, 142n1
World War II 87n14, 97, 116, 120, 128, 284
WTO 5, 289, 313–314
Wujastyk, D. 6
Wuji Baifeng Wan 46
Wynberg, R. 245

Xu Guojun 41
Xu Luoshan 41

Yang Xionghui 41n10
Yash Birla Group 174
Yasuo, O. 89
Yellow Letter Warning 98
Ye Zhuguang 38–39
You Yun 47, 47n19

Zhan, M. 151
zhongyao 39, 41
Zhou Hou Fang (Ge Hong) 31
Zhukov, G. K. 284–285
Zuiken, K. 113

Printed in the United States
by Baker & Taylor Publisher Services